PROMOTING STROKE RECOVERY

PROMOTING STROKE RECOVERY

A Research-Based Approach for Nurses

KATHRYN SCHOFIELD BRONSTEIN, RN, PhD, CS

Neurosurgery Clinical Specialist, Division of Surgical Nursing
University of Chicago Hospitals, Chicago, Illinois

JUDITH M. POPOVICH, RN, MS, CRRN

Doctoral Candidate, Rush University, College of Nursing;
Former Assistant Unit Leader, Neuroscience Unit Department of Medical Nursing
Rush-Presbyterian-St. Luke's Medical Center, Chicago, Illinois

CHRISTINA STEWART-AMIDEI, RN, MSN, CNRN, CCRN

Clinical Consultant; Neuroscience Clinical Nurse Specialist
Loyola University Medical Center, Maywood, Illinois

With **85** *illustrations*

Illustrations by **Lydia M. Johns**

Mosby Year Book

St. Louis Baltimore Boston Chicago London Philadelphia Sydney Toronto

Mosby Year Book

Dedicated to Publishing Excellence

Editor: William Grayson Brottmiller
Developmental Editor: Winifred Sullivan
Project Manager: Mark Spann
Production Editor: Daniel J. Johnson
Book and Cover Design: Gail Morey Hudson

A Mosby imprint of Mosby–Year Book, Inc.

Printed in the United States of America

Mosby–Year Book, Inc.
11830 Westline Industrial Drive
St. Louis, Missouri 63146

Library of Congress Cataloging-in-Publication Data

Bronstein, Kathryn Schofield.
Promoting stroke recovery: a research-based approach for nurses/ Kathryn Schofield Bronstein, Judith M. Popovich, Christina Stewart -Amidei: illustrations by Lydia Johns.
p. cm.
Includes bibliographical references.
Includes index.
ISBN 0-8016-6229-X
1. Cerebrovascular disease—Nursing. I. Popovich, Judith M. II. Stewart-Amidei, Christina. III. Title.
[DNLM: 1. Cerebrovascular Disorders—nursing. WY 152.5.B869p]
RC388.5.B75 1991
616.8′1—dc20
DNLM/DLC
for Library of Congress 90-6641
CIP

GW/D/D 9 8 7 6 5 4 3 2 1

Contributor

Karen J. Ferguson, RN, MS, CRRN, CNRN, CGNP
Clinical Nurse Specialist, Stroke Service
Department of Neurological Sciences
Rush-Presbyterian-St. Luke's Medical Center
Chicago, Illinois

TO
STROKE VICTIMS AND THEIR FAMILIES
whose struggles during recovery inspired the writing of this book,
AND TO NURSES
who promote and strive for excellence by applying research to their practice

Foreword

More than two million people in the United States today are living with neurologic impairment secondary to stroke. This number is indeed dramatic. It is even more compelling when one closely studies the **personal** disruption created by such a catastrophic event as stroke.

This book is a landmark effort to share the practical knowledge of caring for individuals who have had a stroke. Kathryn Schofield Bronstein, Judith M. Popovich, and Christina Stewart-Amidei have an abundance of clinical and theoretical experience in neuroscience nursing. It is most appropriate for them to share the expert knowledge they have gained in a publication such as this. Through sharing their expert nursing knowledge, they remind all caregivers, educators, and researchers what is important in the human struggle of stroke.

First, the authors have provided a comprehensive work that includes detailed description of stroke as a disease **process,** as well as stroke as an illness **experience.** This perspective is unique to nursing, and I applaud the authors for their contribution of this perspective to the growing body of scientific literature on stroke.

Second, nurses are empowered by the knowledge that living with stroke goes far beyond living with physical impairment. As the authors suggest, living with stroke is marked by the often slow return to a meaningful life, marked by activities and concerns that matter to the person. The authors address issues that are paramount to living with stroke. Alterations in mobility, sensation, communication, and sexual activity enormously disrupt one's life. In their discussion of these issues, the authors emphasize the importance of individual assessment and planning. This discussion is essential for health care providers. All too often, individuals are admitted to acute care settings and are known only in terms of the current admission. However, for people who have had a stroke, life before the stroke stands as a point of reference for recovery. If health care providers are to assist and mobilize people to recover, they must have accurate and detailed historical knowledge of the daily concerns, values, and habits of the people they are caring for.

Third, this book addresses the importance of early discharge planning, home assessment, and community reintegration. Although the neurological manifestations of stroke occur very suddenly, often without warning, home and community reintegration frequently occur over many years. In my own experience of caring for stroke survivors, I too have found that most individuals are encouraged by a view toward **long-term progress,** rather than a finite view of improvement, such as reaching "the end of recovery."

Living with stroke is the story of adapting to a new, often foreign, body and struggling to regain a sense of personal and social reintegration. **Promoting Stroke Recovery: A Research-Based Approach for Nurses** takes into account the many dimensions of this reintegration, and empowers all health care providers to accurately and humanely care for the person who has had a stroke.

Nancy D. Doolittle, RN, PhD

Preface

Over the past three decades there has been a tremendous increase in research and general knowledge regarding stroke mechanisms and treatment. This research-based book is an exploration of the research literature with a focus on transferring useful and needed knowledge into the clinical setting. The text provides an overview of the anatomy and physiology of the central nervous system, analyzes mechanisms that can produce stroke and stroke syndromes, and examines how stroke interrupts normal functioning. Research studies on treatment modalities and care techniques are incorporated throughout the text and specific assessment and intervention strategies are discussed to assist the caregiver in providing the highest quality care.

The goals in developing this book on research-based stroke care are to provide advanced education and clinical content to those nurses and caregivers with basic understanding of stroke along with assisting nurses to recognize and apply research findings in the clinical setting. Ultimately, the focus is to enhance and improve the quality of care received by stroke victims. As nurses, we care for stroke patients at all phases of the illness continuum, from acute and postacute to rehabilitation and community reentry. Because of this continuity of nursing care throughout the recovery process, the nurse is the single most important person in planning, coordinating, and implementing care interventions that incorporate both short- and long-term needs and goals. This book can assist with both planning and intervention strategies and will facilitate nurses' identifying the unique aspects of care related to each stroke patient.

In order to be a useful clinical manual this book specifically addresses nursing interventions related to patient care situations. To provide such a clinical guide, the text is organized in several categories that will enable the reader to:

- understand the process of stroke including basic anatomy and physiology, typical stroke syndromes with their clinical presentations, common medical and surgical treatment approaches and nursing implications.
- find information, research literature and intervention strategies essential to providing care to the stroke patient including assessment criteria and care techniques.
- plan individualized comprehensive care from admission to discharge, acute illness to rehabilitation based on alterations in basic functions such as mobility, communication, and sensation.
- access information and community resources to enable patients and families to gain knowledge and assistance.
- coordinate care and communicate with other health team members to deliver organized care and plan for discharge.
- facilitate patient adaptation throughout the illness by incorporating current theories and research on coping.

This reference book is primarily intended for practicing nurses and student nurses who are providing care to stroke patients. Because of its comprehensive approach incorporating both acute care and rehabilitation issues, it can enhance care in both the hospital and rehabilitation setting. In addition, the information may assist family members in understanding the stroke process and provide insight and ideas for delivering care by significant others. Of particular interest to families may be the community resources information.

The book is divided into three major sections. The first section discusses the incidence and demographics of stroke, physiological mechanisms that cause stroke and stroke syndromes, and medical and surgical approaches to treatment. The second section focuses on alterations in normal functioning that commonly occur in stroke. Each of the chapters addresses normal anatomy and physiology of the function, how a stroke may alter the function, assessment techniques for identifying functional parameters, and nursing intervention strategies based on altered function. The chapters conclude with care plans developed from nursing diagnoses. The last section centers on discharge planning, home assessment, and community resources.

Throughout the entire book research findings are incorporated to support clinical knowledge and intervention plans. This approach is unique and distinguishes it from other nursing texts on the subject. It is the authors' hope that through such research utilization this book will foster quality care for the stroke patient and will become a reference manual for nurses caring for these patients.

We gratefully acknowledge the contributions of several people who provided guidance and expertise in the preparation of this manuscript. These include Dr. Rosemary Camilleri, for her collaboration and editorial expertise; Mary Mulrow for her comments on specific chapters; Linda Kernick, Melissa Cagle, and Ellen Stimac, for their timely assistance with reference materials. We thank our photographer Linda Bassi and our medical illustrator Lydia Johns for her fine artwork. We are also appreciative of the expertise and feedback of our reviewers. A special thanks goes to Mosby–Year Book, Inc., particularly to our editors William Brottmiller and Winifred Sullivan for their ongoing encouragement and expertise. We are also grateful to members of the production staff Mark Spann and Daniel J. Johnson and to designer Gail Morey Hudson.

Finally, we thank our colleagues, families, and friends. Without their support, understanding, and encouragement, this book would not have been possible. A special thanks goes to Dr. Kathryn Christiansen, Xavier Smith, Constance Jarvis, Carol Boyd, Martha Smith, Russell Bozian, Cheryl Johnson, and Colleen Ernst for their undaunted support and the hope they inspired. Additionally, we thank Marty Bronstein and Thomas Amidei, whose endurance and patience are unsurpassed; and Richard Schofield, whose experience with stroke personalized the need for this book.

Kathryn Schofield Bronstein
Judith M. Popovich
Christina Stewart-Amidei

Contents

Section I

Overview of Stroke

Chapter 1

Mechanisms of Stroke

HISTORICAL PERSPECTIVES

The first detailed description of stroke appeared in the writings of Hippocrates (460-370 BC). He used the broad term *apoplexy* to denote the syndrome of loss of speech, paralysis of parts of the tongue, and weakness or paralysis of parts of the body (McHenry, 1969). At that point in time the level of understanding of anatomy and physiology was limited, thus apoplexy encompassed many etiologies that could have produced signs and symptoms similar to stroke. Apoplexy means "struck with violence" in Greek, an apt term for the sudden change in physical well-being experienced by stroke victims. Early thoughts on the causes of stroke attributed them to "the hand of God" striking down people for wrongdoing. From the early accounts of stroke until the seventeenth century, physicians sought to identify parts of the brain; they made crude guesses about the functions of sections of the brain and attempted to identify the course of blood through the vessels.

As knowledge of anatomy advanced, Wepfer (1620-1695) identified bleeding within the brain as one of the primary causes of apoplexy. He also singled out as being the most susceptible obese individuals whose faces were often red and who had erratic heart beats (McHenry, 1969). In addition, he recognized the clinical syndrome of transient ischemic attacks in which persons would have brief episodes of apoplexy and then, shortly after, return to normal (Hill and others, 1984). Morgagni (1761) went further and described the neuropathologic findings after hemorrhage, correlating lesion site with symptomatology. He identified nonhemorrhagic apoplexy based on observations made during autopsy, of changes that were present within the brain parenchyma in people who had apoplexy but were not present in the brains of people without apoplexy.

Throughout this period there was growing recognition that stroke was not caused by the hand of God but by changes in blood flow and brain substance. Classifications of stroke similar to what we now use were delineated by Abercrombie (1928). He divided apoplexy into cerebral hemorrhage with massive infarction, subarachnoid hemorrhage, and cerebral vascular insufficiency. Clinical investigations subsequent to this led to the concept of vessel disease as a cause of apoplexy and that changes in cerebral circulation could cause "cerebral accidents," thus leading to usage of the term *cerebral vascular accidents* to denote stroke. Later in the 1900's, vascular disease was found to be only one of many mechanisms responsible for stroke. More recent observations have identified changes in the blood itself, alteration in cardiac function, and certain genetic disorders as also being responsible for causing disruption in brain functioning. As more mechanisms have been identified that can cause a decrease in brain perfusion it is no longer considered an "accident." The current accepted terminology—*stroke*—is a step back into the past. This term, in the sense of cerebral vascular disease, was initially coined in a reference from the sixteenth century referring to the "stroke of God's hand." Many words that are used to describe various aspects of stroke, such as *plegia*, are derived from the word *plesso*, a Greek verb meaning stroke (Sweeny and Furlan, 1986).

INCIDENCE

Trends in the incidence of stroke have been measured for several decades. *Incidence* refers to the number of new cases of a disease per year in a defined population. Numerous studies have been carried out to determine the incidence of stroke at both the national and local level (Broderick and others, 1988). Perhaps the most complete reports on national statistics are included in the *National Survey of Stroke* (Robins and Baum, 1981) and *Cerebrovascular Survey Report* (McDowell and Caplan, 1985), funded by the National Institute of Neurological and Communicative Disorders and Stroke. Based on the number of patients hospitalized during 1975 and 1976, the incidence of initial stroke was estimated at 594,000 for the two year period, averaging to 297,000 per year. The incidence rate was higher in older segments of the population and greater in men than women. In addition, approximately 117,000 persons who had a history of one or more previous strokes were hospitalized during this period, indicating that subsequent strokes are not uncommon. Recent efforts to better identify stroke incidence and prevalence have greatly increased the amount of data available to estimate national statistics. Incidence rates in the United States are currently thought to be between 1 and 2 per 1000, while prevalence rates are between 5 and 6 per 1000.

Several other studies have examined the incidence of stroke based on a limited population-based sample. For example, the incidence of stroke in Rochester, Minnesota, has been followed for many years (Garraway and others, 1979 and 1983a,b; Anderson and Whisnant, 1982; and Davis and others, 1987). Because this region has a relatively defined population that uses a limited number of health care institutions, the data from this study are believed to be reflective of general trends in epidemiology. The findings from this ongoing study show a declining incidence of stroke in Rochester, Minnesota, over the past 35-year period from 192 per 100,000 in the years between 1945

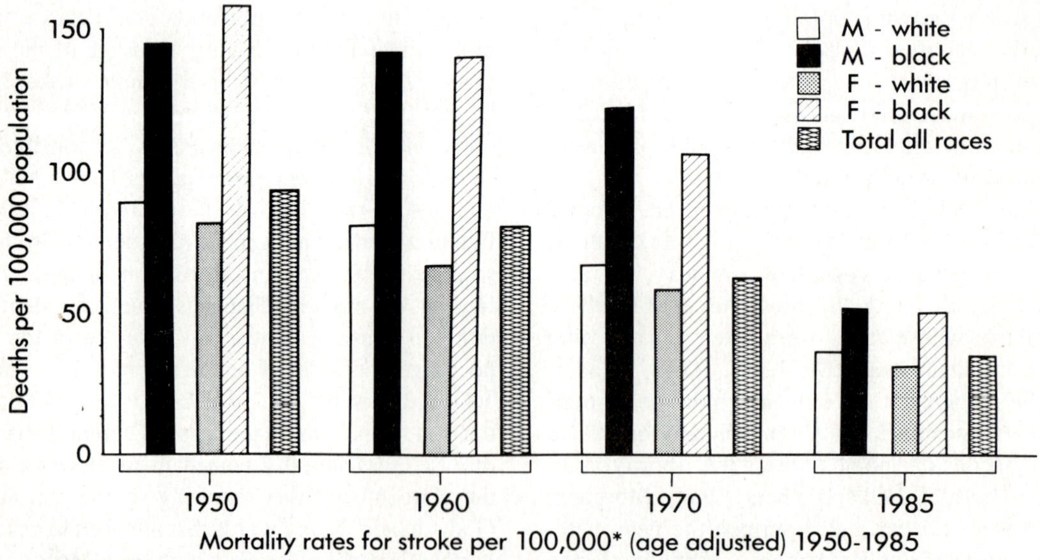

Fig. 1-1 Mortality rates for stroke from 1950-1985 per 100,000* *(Total refers to all ages, all races.)*

and 1949 to 89 per 100,000 in the years 1975 to 1979. A primary theory about the reason for the decline relates to the introduction of antihypertensive medications during this period.

Stroke incidence was also assessed prospectively in the population of southern Alabama (Gross and others, 1984). The incidence rate was found to be 109 per 100,000 for whites and 208 per 100,000 for blacks. This difference in incidence rate by race has been further examined and is believed to be related to the higher incidence of hypertension correlated with stroke that is found in the black population (Gillum, 1988). Other racial trends have been identified within the Japanese population, where the incidence of intracranial hemorrhage has been reduced in conjunction with the treatment of hypertension.

While the overall incidence rate of stroke has been declining (Whisnant, 1984), so too has the mortality rate. According to the National Center for Health Statistics (1988), stroke was the seventh leading cause of death in 1900, but by 1950 it had moved to third place. As of 1985, it was still ranked third, but the overall number of deaths attributed to stroke has declined significantly. Fig. 1-1 reflects the changing mortality rates associated with stroke. As indicated, stroke-related mortality has dropped dramatically; however, blacks between 45 and 54 years of age continue to have three times the death rate of whites of the same age. The reasons for the overall change in mortality from stroke have not been clearly identified. The fact that hypertension, a major risk factor for stroke, has been treated aggressively since the advent of antihypertensive medications in the 1950's may account for some of the decline. Another factor may be the emphasis placed on lifestyle changes following publication of the Surgeon General's *Report on Heart Disease*. This report encouraged Americans to reduce their intake of fatty foods, increase the amount of fish in their diet, and increase their level of exercise. These events, coupled with the decrease in smoking and the improved medical treatment of acute stroke, have probably had the greatest impact in decreasing mortality from stroke.

PATHOPHYSIOLOGY OF THE DISEASE PROCESS

Hemorrhage

Stroke pathology can be divided into two distinct categories: hemorrhage and ischemia. Hemorrhage within the brain can result from either a primary intracerebral hemorrhage or a subarachnoid hemorrhage. When blood is released into the brain, pressure is exerted on the brain tissue by the expanding volume of blood. Primary intracerebral hemorrhage is caused by extravasation of the blood from the vessels into the brain. When blood escapes from the cerebral vessels it first follows the path of the axons of the central nervous system neurons, which constitute the white matter of the brain. Occasionally, blood is released into the ventricles of the brain, causing dissemination of the blood within the subarachnoid space. After the acute bleeding ceases, the blood clots within the tissue and is gradually broken down by macrophages. Eventually the clot is reabsorbed, leaving a vacant area of the brain, often filled with serous fluid. This extravasation occurs most commonly in hypertensive patients who have damage to the small arterioles within the cerebral circulation. The damage allows blood to seep out of the vessels and form clots within the brain parenchyma. Brott and others (1986) found in reviewing charts of patients with intracerebral hemorrhage that 54% had a history of hypertension or left ventricular hypertrophy. They estimated the relative risk of middle-age adults having an intracerebral hemorrhage was 3.9 times greater in those patients who had hypertension than those who did not.

Another cause of intracerebral hemorrhage is from alterations in the normal clotting mechanisms within the blood. Several diseases known to be associated with cerebral hemorrhage include: disseminated intravascular coagulation, thrombocytopenia, and hemophilia.

Subarachnoid hemorrhage from either an aneurysm or arterial venous malformation also distributes blood within the subarachnoid space. In these cases, in addition to bleeding there can be vasospasm of the cerebral blood vessels, leading to tissue ischemia. This contributes to the ischemia already being caused by increased intracranial pressure. The goals in managing intracerebral and subarachnoid hemorrhage are to minimize the amount of initial bleeding, reduce intracranial pressure, and maintain perfusion to viable brain cells.

Ischemia

Ischemia, lack of blood perfusing brain tissue, occurs whenever the blood supply to tissue is interrupted or totally obstructed. Ultimate survival of the ischemic areas is dependent on the length of time the brain tissue must survive without blood and thus oxygen, and the degree of brain metabolism. In the immediate ischemic area there is influx of sodium and water into the cells, with a build up of toxic metabolic wastes as cells die. In the area surrounding the ischemic region, cells may be marginally surviving. Their survival depends on the amount of collateral circulation and their metabolic needs. In this critical region it is vital to preserve neurologic functioning; therefore many of the interventional techniques available focus on maintaining these marginally surviving cells.

Many factors can cause ischemia within brain tissue. Embolism from the heart, aorta, or carotid or vertebral vessels can lodge in cerebral vessels obliterating blood flow to the distal portion of the vessel. Types of cardiac disease known to have an association with embolic stroke include mitral valve prolapse, mitral valve stenosis, infectious endocarditis, cardiac myopathy, rheumatic heart disease, and arrhythmias, especially atrial fibrillation (Halperin and Hart, 1988). In fact, atrial fibrillation has been estimated to increase the risk of stroke by up to five times the average. The elderly seem particularly prone to stroke from this source as documented by the Framingham Heart Study, which estimates that more than one third of strokes in this age group occur in persons with atrial fibrillation (Kannel and others, 1981).

Thrombotic stroke also produces ischemia within the brain. The mechanism by which thrombosis occurs starts with damage to the lining of the vessel walls. Most often atherosclerosis is the primary culprit that causes endothelial damage within the vessel lining; it propagates fatty materials that cluster and form plaques on the vessel wall. These plaques accumulate within the vessel, resulting in changes in the normal pattern of blood flow. As blood swirls around the region, platelets and other clotting materials adhere to the plaque. Eventually the vessel becomes obstructed. Also, pieces of the plaque and clots that form on the plaque can break away, obstructing distal vessels and producing ischemia.

RISK FACTORS IN STROKE

The role hypertension plays in causing stroke has been known for several years; however, its magnitude has only recently been identified (Wolf, 1975; Wolf and others, 1983). Several investigations, including the Framingham Heart Study, have shown an association between increased systolic and diastolic blood pressure and stroke in both men and women. The concept of stroke from hypertensive causes is multifactoral because of the close relationship among increased blood pressure, cardiac changes, and blood vessel damage. In the Harvard Stroke Registry, 55% of thrombotic stroke patients and 75% of lacunar stroke patients had a history of hypertension, while in the Michael Reese Stroke Registry the figures were reversed, with 75% of the thrombotic stroke patients and 55% of the lacunar stroke patients having a hypertensive history (Caplan and others, 1986). Lacunar strokes result from disease of the very small perfusing vessels deep within the brain, most often in the motor pathways or thalamus. In these regions minute atheromatous deposits occur in persons with hypertension, eventually obstructing the vessel. Examination of the resulting abnormality reveals small lesions, usually less than 1 cm, frequently looking like irregular shaped cavities.

Diabetes also contributes to the development of stroke. The Harvard and Michael Reese Stroke Registries documented between 26% and 28% of stroke cases in the thrombotic and lacunar categories had diabetes. Diabetes contributes to the incidence of stroke in a twofold manner. First, diabetes produces vascular changes in both the systemic and cerebral circulation. These changes result in vascular occlusive disease and narrowing of the vessels. Second, diabetics tend to have an increased risk of hypertension, so this combined with the vascular changes produced by the disease itself lead to a significantly higher incidence of stroke among diabetics. Recently a population-based study followed persons in California for an average of 12 years (Barrett-Conner and Khaw, 1988). They found that diabetics, especially female diabetics, had higher blood pressures. Further analyses were conducted to determine if high blood pressure was the primary risk factor for stroke or if having diabetes added an additional risk. By statistically controlling the data for the effects of blood pressure, the researchers found that diabetic persons still had higher rates of stroke, indicating that diabetes contributes additional risk for stroke occurrence.

Changes within red blood cells can also produce stroke. Severe sickle cell disease is the primary case in point (Rothman and others, 1986). In patients with this disorder, blood viscosity is very high, with sickled erythrocytes clumping together and reducing blood flow. Ischemia results from poor tissue perfusion, leading to regional acidosis, which causes further sickling. Most of the ischemia in these patients occurs in the microcirculation, although there have been arteriographic reports of narrowing of the carotid arteries, possibly caused by vessel wall ischemia leading to intimal changes in the vessel (Grotta and others, 1982). Often on CT scanning these patients have multiple areas of minute infarcts that have previously gone undetected. Any stroke in a young black person should warrant investigation into the possibility of sickle cell disease being the causative mechanism.

Substance Abuse and Stroke

A tragic and avoidable cause of stroke has been identified in the past ten years. With the growing use of drugs, there has been an increase in the incidence of drug-induced stroke. Heroin abuse is a prime example. Because heroin is rarely pure, intravenous use of the substance causes both serologic changes and possibly the development of an immune response to the drug. Users of heroin are known to suffer from ischemic strokes either soon after injection of the drug or within 24 hours after injection.

Injection of other drugs, such as methylphenidate and pentazocine (Talwin), has led to stroke from undissolved particles in the solution acting as emboli. If the carotid artery is the site of injection, these emboli can become lodged in smaller cerebral vessels, leading to occlusion and subsequent stroke. Strokes in drug users are compounded by the high incidence of hepatitis, infective endocarditis, acquired immunodeficiency syndrome (AIDS), and fungal infections found in this population, all of which can produce cerebral vasculitis, infection, or more emboli.

Drug usage can lead to both ischemic stroke and intracranial hemorrhage. Caplan and others (Caplan and others, 1982; Levine and Welch, 1988; and Cahill and others, 1981) have documented the association of amphetamine use with the abrupt onset of headache, seizures, and confusion marking the beginning of bleeding within the brain. More recently, cocaine-induced hemorrhagic stroke has been identified. Theories about why these substances cause stroke are varied. One theory is that the transient increase in systemic blood pressure caused by certain drugs leads to vessel rupture, especially in people who have underlying vessel pathologic conditions, such as cerebral aneurysms, arterial venous malformations or drug-induced vasculopathy. Cocaine use may also be responsible for ischemic strokes. Since 1977, several series of case reports have shown infarction after cocaine use in patients who had no other stroke risk factors (Kessler and others, 1978; Golbe and Merkin, 1986; Wojak and Flamm, 1987). Apparently, drug-induced vasoconstriction of the cerebral vessels produced the brain ischemia.

Alcohol Consumption and Smoking as They Relate to Stroke

Chronic ingestion of alcohol has known effects on both the heart and brain (Gorelick, 1987; Taylor, 1982). It appears that moderate drinking (fewer than two drinks per day) does not increase the risk of cardiovascular disease. However, cardiac arrhythmias, hypertension, and cardiac myopathy are associated with the habitual use of large amounts of alcohol. In alcoholics, effects of alcohol on the liver lead to the development of cirrhosis, which in turn produces changes in blood clotting ability that are due to decreased platelet function (Weisberg, 1988). In chronic excessive alcohol ingestion, there is a propensity for intracranial hemorrhage. Acute withdrawal from alcohol has been shown to affect a rebound increase in platelets and produces a hypercoagulable state (Hutton and others, 1981). When this happens there is an increased risk of ischemic events within the entire vasculature of the body. This changing picture within the blood's clotting mechanism results in alcoholics having a propensity for both intracerebral bleeding and ischemic strokes. For more moderate drinkers, several studies (Gill and others, 1986; Hillbom and Kaste, 1981; Hillbom and others, 1983a,b and 1985) have linked acute ingestion or intoxication to stroke. Studies conducted in Scandinavia have noted an increased incidence of stroke on weekends, frequently associated with drinking among young people. Conflicting reports exist concerning the magnitude of the acute alcohol intake-stroke risk relationship. Gorelick and others (1987) conducted a case-controlled study to identify the relative risk associated with acute alcohol ingestion leading to stroke in older people. Their results indicated that alcohol alone was not found to be an independent risk factor for ischemic stroke. The variables found to be highly associated with stroke were hypertension and smoking. Thus the effects of alcohol consumption may be masked by the overwhelming risk of stroke from these other factors. Of note is that this study included only persons over the age of 44, thus, alcohol consumption and stroke risk may be different in younger people.

Smoking continues to be associated with stroke risk. While reports differ as to the magnitude of the relationship and the role of smoking as a primary cause of stroke, most experts agree that smoking contributes some factor to the development of stroke. In a report of the Framingham Heart Study, smoking ranked third after age and hypertension as an independent contributor to stroke. Persons who smoked more were at higher risk, although the risk rapidly decreased after smoking cessation and approached the same level of risk for nonsmokers within 5 years after stopping smoking. Bonita (1987) identified a threefold increase in risk of stroke in smokers as compared with nonsmokers. This higher risk may be due to the fact that smoking increases hematocrit, a risk factor associated with stroke by itself. The combination of both smoking and hypertension increased this risk to twentyfold.

Prevention of Stroke

Numerous studies have strived to identify stroke risk factors with the concept behind them being that if risk can be delineated, then appropriate interventions can follow. There exists a parallel between previous efforts to reduce heart disease and the current efforts to reduce stroke. For years the Surgeon General of the United States and the American Heart Association have pushed public awareness programs emphasizing the factors that lead to heart disease (such as high cholesterol diets and obesity) and how Americans can respond to improve their cardiac health. Such programs for stroke are still in their infancy. Unlike the warning signs of heart attack, which are common household knowledge, most people do not know the warning signs of stroke. In a survey of 1253 people conducted by the American Heart Association's Stroke Subcommittee, few knew that weakness on one side of the body may be a sign of stroke and fewer than half thought that stroke was the third leading cause of death in the United States. This lack of knowledge regarding stroke presents a major challenge to health care professionals.

Hypertensive persons certainly have a higher rate of stroke than normotensive persons (Wolf and others, 1983; LaRue and others, 1987). For the borderline hypertensive person the risk is twice as great, and for the person with blood pressures greater than 160/95 the risk is four times as great (Wolf, 1986). Hypertension is the most significant risk factor for stroke over which a person has some control (McGill, 1988; Perry and others, 1989). Certainly weight control and exercise programs help to reduce hypertension, but even these may not completely reduce high blood pressure (Masserli, 1982). For those persons who have hypertension, despite their efforts to control it by lifestyle modification, medical intervention is essential. Antihypertensive drugs have been found to adequately control blood pressure when taken consistently and according to a plan prescribed by a person's physician (Spence, 1986). For blood pressure control to be of benefit in preventing stroke, such intervention must be initiated early in the disease process and not several years after hypertension has resulted in major vascular changes.

Although diabetes is also a major risk factor in stroke, there is a paucity of data reflecting that control of blood sugar decreases risk of stroke. Certainly, adequate management of diabetes reduces complications, such as venous stasis ulcers and peripheral neuropathy, frequently seen in poorly controlled diabetics. At best, such control may decrease the magnitude of risk that diabetes contributes to the development of cerebral vascular disease.

Certainly smoking, alcohol consumption, and use of drugs are risk factors that are controllable by the individual. In the case of smoking, quitting has been shown to decrease the risk of both stroke and cancer. For alcohol, moderate intake is cited as being beneficial in preventing heart disease. It is the chronic ingestion of large amounts of alcohol and binge drinking that are associated with stroke occurrence. The growing use of drugs in the general population and the high rates of drug abuse in the adolescent segment have fostered massive efforts by the government, medical organizations, civic groups, and individuals to speak out against drugs. Until the hazards of drug abuse are recognized, the rate of stroke from this cause will be associated with the overall rate of drug use.

Other factors, such as advancing age and race, are not directly under an individual's control but have been shown to increase stroke risk. Some studies have shown that certain races have a higher rate of stroke; however, in most instances this has been correlated with hypertension, which is more prevalent within certain populations. Thus control of hypertension may negate the influence of race on stroke incidence statistics. Other risk factors, such as cardiac arrhythmias, problems with blood clotting, and high hematocrits, cannot be prevented but may be controlled by adequate medical intervention once diagnosed.

PROMOTION OF HEALTH SEEKING BEHAVIORS

Perhaps the greatest contribution to stroke prevention that can be made by health professionals in general and nurses specifically, is to educate the public about the causes of stroke and the risk factors that may be altered to help prevent stroke. Several steps are involved in educating people about preventing stroke. An assessment of current knowledge, knowledge deficits, and readiness to learn will help in planning an individualized program. Formal or informal teaching methods incorporating the family into the process can enhance learning. This is especially important in changing behaviors rooted in culture for which the entire family may need to modify their lifestyles to reduce risk. Such individualized teaching of the person who is at high risk may enable behavior changes that are needed to prevent stroke. (Individual patients can also see Community Resources in Chapter 15 of this book for many sources of informational literature.)

But education is not enough; merely informing people about risk will not reduce their chances of stroke. Nurses must intervene and assist people in changing their risk profile. Preventative health care, including weight control, smoking cessation,

NURSING CARE PLAN

Nursing Diagnosis	Interventions	Expected Outcomes
Health Seeking Behaviors: related to stroke prevention **Defining Characteristics:** ■ Expressed or observed desire to seek higher level of wellness ■ Concern about present health status ■ Unfamiliarity with behaviors needed to improve health and reduce risk	**Ongoing Assessment** ■ Assess current health behaviors ■ Assess knowledge related to stroke risk and weight, diet, exercise, smoking, blood pressure control **Therapeutic Interventions** ■ Promote efforts to improve patient and family health ■ Provide access to health promotion literature ■ Reinforce health seeking behaviors	■ A higher level of wellness is attained for both patient and family ■ Patient experiences a reduction in risk factors for stroke

Patient Education:
- Educate patient and family about risk factors and behavior modification related to specific risks
- Provide booklets and information on risk reduction (see Chapter 15, Community Reintegration)
- Reinforce attempts at learning and alterations in lifestyle to reduce stroke risk

management of antihypertensive regimens set up by physicians, and moderation of alcohol intake can be facilitated by interested nurses. Becoming actively involved in such programs that are aimed at health improvement not only sets an example for the clients we interact with but also makes a statement about the nursing profession's commitment to the prevention component of health care delivery.

REFERENCES

Anderson GL and Whisnant JP: A comparison of the trends in mortality from stroke in the United States and Rochester, Minnesota, Stroke 13:804, 1982.

Barrett-Connor E and Khaw KT: Diabetes mellitus: an independent risk factor for stroke, Am J Epidemiol 128:116, 1988.

Bonita R: Cigarette smoking and risk of premature stroke in men and women, Stroke 18:305, 1987.

Broderick JP, Phillips SJ, Whisnant JP and others: Stroke

incidence in Rochester, Minn. 1945-1984: The end of the decline in stroke? Neurology 38(3), Supp 1: 146, 1988.

Brott T, Thalinger K, and Hertzberg V: Hypertension as a risk factor for spontaneous intracerebral hemorrhage, Stroke 17:1078, 1986.

Cahill DW, Knipp H, and Mosser J: Intracranial hemorrhage with amphetamine abuse, Neurology 31:1058, 1981.

Caplan LR, Hier DB, and Banks G: Stroke and drug abuse, Stroke 13:869, 1982.

Caplan LR and Stein RW: Stroke: A clinical approach, Boston, 1986, Butterworth Publishers.

Davis PH, Dambrosia JM, Schoenberg BS and others: A prospective study in Rochester, Minnesota, Ann Neurol 22:319, 1987.

Garraway WM, Whisnant JP, Furlan AJ and others: The declining incidence of stroke, N Engl J Med 300:499, 1979.

Garraway WM, Whisnant JP, and Drury I: The continuing decline in the incidence of stroke, Mayo Clin Proc 58:520, 1983a.

Garraway WM, Whisnant JP, and Drury I: The changing pattern of survival following stroke, Stroke 14:699, 1983b.

Gill JS, Zezulka AV, Shipley MJ and others: Stroke and alcohol consumption, N Engl J Med 315:1041, 1986.

Gillum RF: Stroke in blacks, Stroke 19:1, 1988.

Golbe LI and Merkin MD: Cerebral infarction in a user of free-base cocaine ("crack"), Neurology 36:1602, 1986.

Gorelick PB: Alcohol and stroke, Stroke 18:268, 1987.

Gorelick PB, Rodin MB, Langenberg P and others: Is acute alcohol ingestion a risk factor for ischemic stroke?: results of a controlled study in middle-aged and elderly stroke patients at three urban medical centers, Stroke 18:359, 1987.

Gross CR, Kase CS, Mohr JP and others: Stroke in south Alabama: incidence and diagnostic features—a population-based study. Stroke 15:249, 1984.

Grotta J, Ackerman R, Corrcia J and others: Whole blood viscosity parameters and cerebral blood flow, Stroke 13:296, 1982.

Halperin JL and Hart RG: Atrial fibrillation and stroke: new ideas, persisting dilemmas, Stroke 19:937, 1988.

Hill EG, McHenry LC, and Freyman JM: Wepfer's view of apoplexy: the first basis for the modern understanding of cerebrovascular disease, Neurology 34, Suppl 1:109, 1984.

Hillbom M and Kaste M: Ethanol intoxication: a risk factor for ischemic brain infarction in adolescents and young adults, Stroke 12:422, 1981.

Hillbom M, Kaste M, and Rasi V: Ethanol intoxication a risk factor for ischemica brain infarction, Stroke 14:694, 1983a.

Hillbom M, Kaste M, and Rasi V: Can ethanol intoxication affect hemocoagulation to increase the risk of brain infarction in young adults?, Neurology 33:381, 1983b.

Hillbom M, Kangasaho M, Kaste M and others: Acute ethanol ingestion increases platelet reactivity: is there a relationship to stroke?, Stroke 16:19, 1985.

Hutton RA, Fink FR, Wilson DT and others: Platelet hyperaggregability during alcohol withdrawal, Clin Lab Haematol 3:223, 1981.

Kannel WB, Wolf PA, McGee DL and others: Systolic blood pressure, arterial rigidity and risk of stroke: The Framingham Study, JAMA 245:1225, 1981.

Kessler JT, Jortner BS, and Adapan BD: Cerebral vasculitis in a drug abuser, J Clin Psychiatry 39:559, 1978.

LaRue L, Alter M, Lai SM and others: Acute stroke, hematocrit, and blood pressure, Stroke 18:565, 1987.

Levine SR and Welch KAM: Cocaine and stroke, Stroke 19:779, 1988.

Masserli FH: Cardiovascular effects of obesity and hypertension, Lancet 2:1165, 1982.

McDowell F and Caplan L, editors: Cerebrovascular Survey Report for the National Institute of Neurological and Communicative Disorders and Stroke, 1985.

McGill HA: Cerebral artery atherosclerosis and diet, Stroke 19:801, 1988.

McHenry LC, editor: Garrison's History of Neurology, Springfield, 1969, Charles C. Thomas.

National Center for Health Statistics: Health, United States, 1987, Pub no (PHS)88-1232, Public Health Service, Washington, DC, 1988, US Government Printing Office.

Perry HM, Smith WM, McDonald RH and others: Morbidity and mortality in the systolic hypertension in the elderly program (SHEP) pilot study, Stroke 20:4, 1989.

Robins M and Baum HM: The National Survey of Stroke: incidence, Stroke 12 (Suppl 1):45, 1981.

Rothman SM, Fulling KH, and Nelson JS: Sickle cell anemia and central nervous system infarction: a neuropathological study, Ann Neurol 20:684, 1986.

Spence JD: Antihypertensive drugs and prevention of atherosclerotic stroke, Stroke 17:808, 1986.

Sweeny PJ and Furlan AJ: "Stroke"–origin of the term, Stroke 3:559, 1986.

Taylor JR: Alcohol and strokes, N Engl J Med 306:1111, 1982.

Weisberg LA: Alcoholic intracerebral hemorrhage, Stroke 19:1565, 1988.

Whisnant JP: The decline of stroke, Stroke 15:160, 1984.

Wolf PA: Hypertension as a risk factor for stroke. In Whisnant JP and Sandok B, editors: Cerebral vascular disease, New York, 1975, Grune and Stratton.

Wolf PA, Kannel WB, and Verter J: Current status of risk factors for stroke, Neurol Clin 1:317, 1983.

Wolf PA, Kannel WB, and McGee DL: Prevention of ischemic stroke: risk factors. In Barnett HJM, Mohr JP, Stein BM and others, editors: Stroke: pathophysiology, diagnosis, and management, New York, 1986, Churchill-Livingstone.

Wojak JC and Flamm ES: Intracerebral hemorrhage and cocaine use, Stroke 18:712, 1987.

Chapter 2

Stroke Syndromes

In the previous chapter, mechanisms of stroke, such as ischemia and hemorrhage, were outlined. While the pathophysiology of the disease process affects the vessels specifically, the signs and symptoms vary according to the region of the brain the affected vessels perfuse. Traditionally, strokes have been classified according to impairment related to vascular distributions within the brain. Using this method, the majority of stroke syndromes of vascular origin can be described. For nurses this classification enhances assessment and planning of nursing care because patients with stroke in similar vascular distributions should have similar presentations. Individual variations may occur because of variations in vessel size, flow patterns, or extent of disruption in flow of blood to the brain, but in general strokes have typical patterns.

The tempo of stroke onset and the pace of development of deficits are important in understanding pathophysiology. There are four categories in which to group symptoms and temporality of stroke onset.

Transient Ischemic Attack (TIA). TIAs are brief periods of focal cerebral ischemia and dysfunction. The onset is rapid and lasts anywhere from several minutes to hours. As the episode resolves, the patient returns to normal neurologic functioning. Common symptoms of TIA include: weakness or numbness in an arm or leg, alterations in speech patterns, and decreased vision in one eye.

Reversible Ischemic Neurologic Deficit (RIND). Although similar to a TIA, RIND can last for 24 to 48 hours, after which the patient returns to normal functioning.

Stroke in Evolution. Also called progressing stroke, stroke in evolution is a pattern of increasing neurologic deficits over a period of hours to days, indicating that the patient has the potential to become more severely impaired. The frequency of clinical worsening is estimated to occur in 20% to 35% of all patients admitted to a hospital, with the diagnosis of stroke. This worsening typically occurs within the first 7 days after the onset of symptoms.

Completed Stroke. Completed stroke is the stabilization of neurologic function in a person with stroke.

ANTERIOR CIRCULATION SYNDROMES

Middle Cerebral Artery (See Fig. 2-1)

The middle cerebral artery (MCA) supplies a major portion of the lateral cerebral hemisphere. Occlusion within this vessel is the most common type of stroke, with the incidence being highest in both the black and oriental populations as compared with the white population (Gorelick and others, 1984 and 1985).

Many patients with a stroke in this region report previous transient attacks of weakness, aphasia, or that the symptoms have gradually developed over several days. These episodes of increasing deficits may reflect gradual narrowing of the vessel or periods of low flow. When these situations occur, the brain is not perfused well enough to function normally, and the patient experiences changes in neurologic functioning. When the flow to the brain is improved, the neurological deficit resolves.

Complete occlusion of the middle cerebral artery (usually caused by an embolism) has the following characteristics:

Motor: In relationship to the site of the stroke, there is contralateral hemiplegia with the face and arm displaying greater weakness than the leg.

Sensory: Contralateral sensory impairment that ranges from mild to severe.

Vision: Blindness in the right or left halves of the visual fields (homonymous hemianopia).

Gaze: The patient's eyes are deviated toward the side of the brain where the lesion is located, and she has difficulty in turning her eyes to look at the paralyzed side (cerebral gaze palsy).

Speech: If the lesion is in the left MCA, then the patient will have severe aphasia.

Neglect: If the lesion is in the right MCA, the patient will have severe neglect, poor motivation, apathy, and constructional apraxia (the inability to carry out purposeful movements in the absence of paralysis). In this case, she cannot draw or copy, cannot read a map, and easily gets lost, even in familiar environments.

Denial: The patient neglects or denies (anosognosia) the affected body part and is unable to recognize her own arm or leg.

The person who suffers from a complete middle cerebral artery occlusion is incapacitated. While some recovery of function may occur, the level of functional ability usually remains poor.

Upper Trunk, MCA (See Fig. 2-2)

If the middle cerebral artery is not completely occluded, the patient may have a partial occlusion of the upper or lower portion of the vessel. An upper trunk occlusion has features similar to a complete MCA occlusion but is not as extensive. This portion of the artery supplies the frontal and superior parietal lobes of the brain. Signs and symptoms include:

Motor: Contralateral hemiplegia greatest in the face and arm. The leg is generally not affected.

Sensory: Contralateral sensory loss in the same distribution as the weakness.

Gaze: Cerebral gaze palsy in which the patient looks toward the side of the brain where the lesion is located and has difficulty in turning his eyes to the other side.

Speech: If the lesion is in the left MCA upper trunk, the patient is usually aphasic. Sometimes patients may be able to nod their heads correctly to simple "yes" or "no" questions. Comprehension may be affected, and there is little if any verbal output. This type of speech impairment is commonly referred to as Broca's aphasia, after the person who identified the pattern.

Neglect: If the lesion is in the right MCA, there is denial of the physical impairment. Some of these patients leave out the left side of pages when reading and are not aware of things happening in the left side of space. These patients often cannot figure out why they are in the hospital.

Lower Trunk, MCA (See Fig. 2-3)

The lower trunk of the middle cerebral artery brings blood to the temporal and inferior parietal lobes. Signs and symptoms include:

Motor: No motor impairment.

Sensory: No sensory impairment.

Vision: Patient has either contralateral hemianopia or upper quadrantanopia.

Speech: If the problem is in the left MCA, the patient has fluent speech but his words make no sense. Language comprehension is poor, and repetition is impaired. Interestingly, these patients can often read without a problem and communication with them can be enhanced

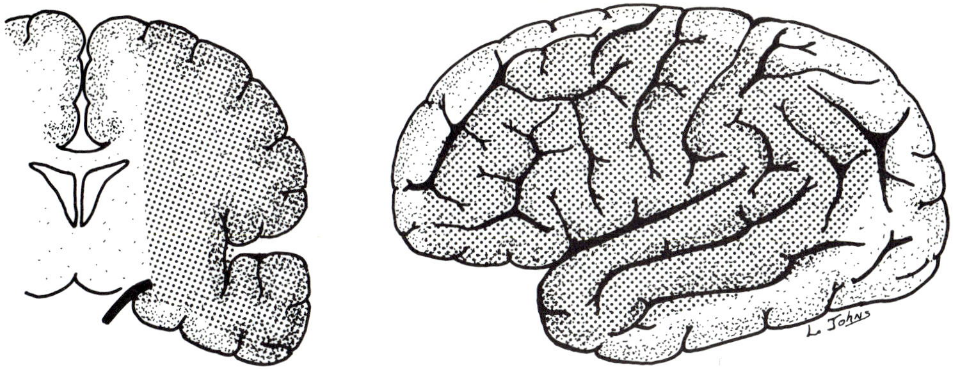

Fig. 2-1 Complete middle cerebral artery occlusion.

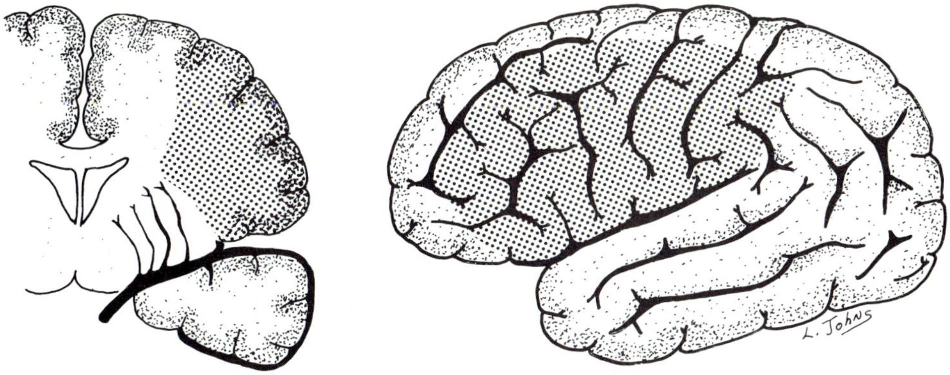

Fig. 2-2 Upper trunk middle cerebral artery occlusion.

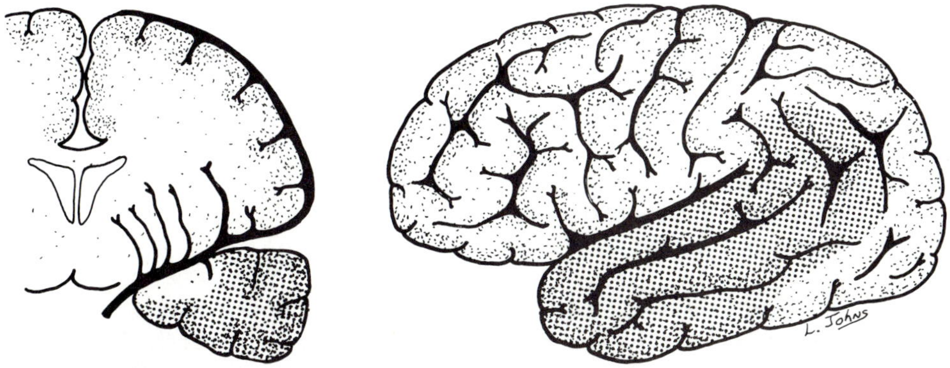

Fig. 2-3 Lower trunk middle cerebral artery occlusion.

by writing instructions or information and by giving visual cues. Of note is that these patients are often agitated and may be physically violent.

Apraxia: If the problem is in the right MCA, constructional apraxia may exist in which the patient cannot draw, copy, or read a map and gets lost in familiar surroundings. If able to get out of bed, these patients may wander out of their rooms and are unable to find their way back.

Deep MCA (See Fig. 2-4)

This portion of the vessel supplies blood deep within the hemispheres in the lenticulostriate branches. Often there is enough collateral circulation for the cortical region of the brain to receive blood, limiting the ischemia to the deep gray matter called the basal nuclei. These patients have the following presentations:

Motor: Varying degrees of contralateral weakness of the face, arm, and leg.

Sensory: Little or no sensory impairment but, if present, it follows a hemisensory pattern, with the contralateral half of the body being affected.

Speech: If the stroke is on the left, a transcortical sensory aphasia may be present in which the lesion interrupts the pathway between the speech center and the rest of the brain.

Neglect: If the lesion is on the right, there may be temporary visual and sensory neglect that gradually dissipates with time.

Anterior Cerebral Artery (See Fig. 2-5)

The anterior cerebral artery supplies the paramedian frontal lobe superior to the corpus callosum. It also supplies the caudate nucleus deep within the brain. Complete obstruction of this vessel is the least common cause of stroke (Caplan and Stein, 1986).

Motor: Contralateral paralysis greatest in the foot and thigh. The patient may have foot drop. In the upper extremity, shoulder muscles may be weak while the arm and hand have normal strength.

Sensory: Sensory loss follows the pattern of the weakness but is usually mild. The patient may have tactile extinction in which only the stimuli on the unaffected side of the body are recognized.

Speech: If the lesion is on the left, transcortical motor and sensory aphasia may be present. The patient has abulia with decreased speech output, but his ability to repeat is preserved. He may have a flat affect and be easily distracted. Accompanying such findings are personality and behavioral changes.

Apraxia: If the lesion is on the right there can be apraxia of the left arm because of the inability of the commands to cross the corpus callosum from the left language center to the right frontal motor area. The result is the inability to do tasks with the left arm and correctly name objects placed in the left hand. If the object is switched into the right hand, the patient can easily identify the object correctly.

In rare instances, a patient may have bilateral anterior cerebral artery occlusions. These patients have both bowel and bladder incontinence resulting from their inability to control elimination. This occurs in spite of the intact sensory components that retain the ability to detect the urge to urinate or defecate. This finding may also be seen in unilateral lesions in some patients.

POSTERIOR CIRCULATION SYNDROMES

The posterior circulation supplies blood to the brainstem and the cerebellum. Atherosclerosis is the most common culprit responsible for stroke in this region, affecting both the vertebral and basilar arteries, especially at the junctions or divisions of vessels (Caplan, 1986).

Vertebral Artery (See Fig. 2-6)

Rarely do lesions of one vertebral artery result in neurologic symptoms. The reason for this fortunate situation is that the two vertebral arteries unite to form the basilar artery distally. If for some

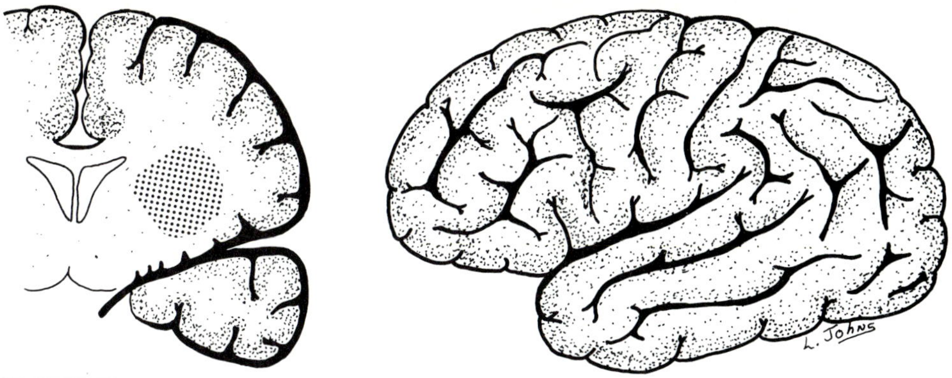

Fig. 2-4 Deep middle cerebral artery occlusion.

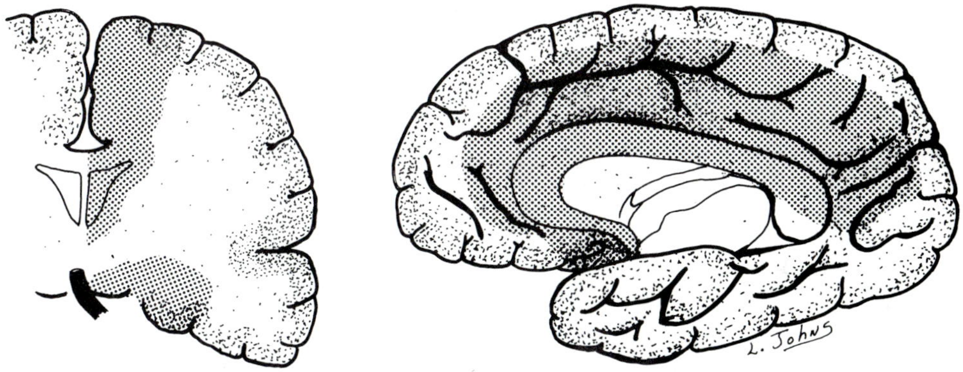

Fig. 2-5 Anterior cerebral artery occlusion.

reason there is decreased flow in one vessel, blood from the other vertebral artery can easily cross over via the basilar artery and provide retrograde flow to fill the sections where there is poor perfusion.

Basilar Artery (See Fig. 2-7)

The basilar artery is the continuation of the fusion of the two vertebral arteries. It supplies blood to the brainstem, specifically the pons. Occlusion of this artery may spare damage to the medulla and cerebellar hemispheres.

Motor: The patient usually has quadraparesis or quadraparalysis (bilateral) with flaccidity of tone in the limbs and loss of reflexes (areflexia). This situation gradually changes to increased tone with stiffness of the limbs and hyperreflexia.

Sensory: Normal sensation.

Cranial Nerves: Impairment of the cranial nerves that supply the face leaves the patient with her face, mouth, palate, and tongue paralyzed on one or both sides. The patient may have difficulty swallowing and phonating. Facial reflexes, such as jaw and gag, are increased in tone, and the patient may exhibit emotional outbursts of laughing or crying at inappropriate times.

Gaze: The patient may not be able to move her eyes in any direction because of involvement of cranial nerves III, IV, and VI. Most com-

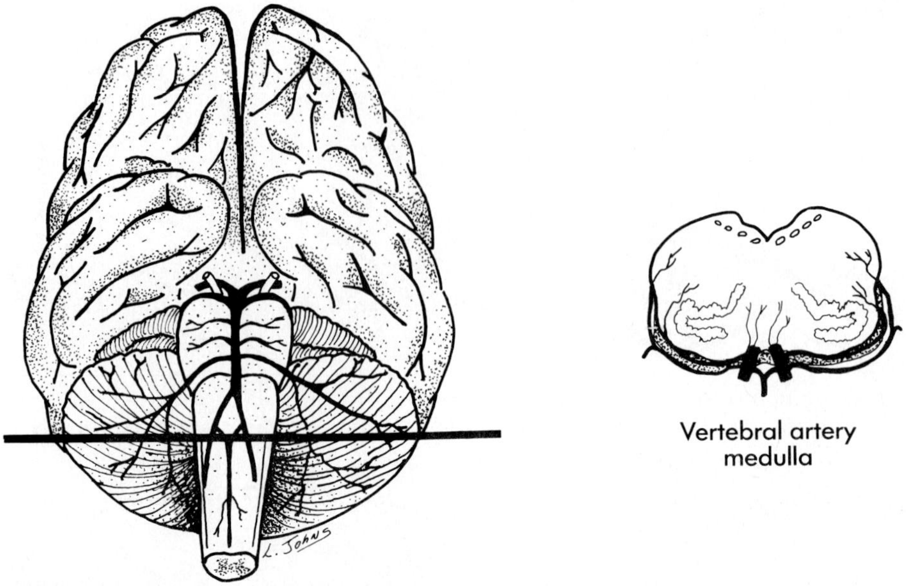

Fig. 2-6 Vertebral arteries, medulla.

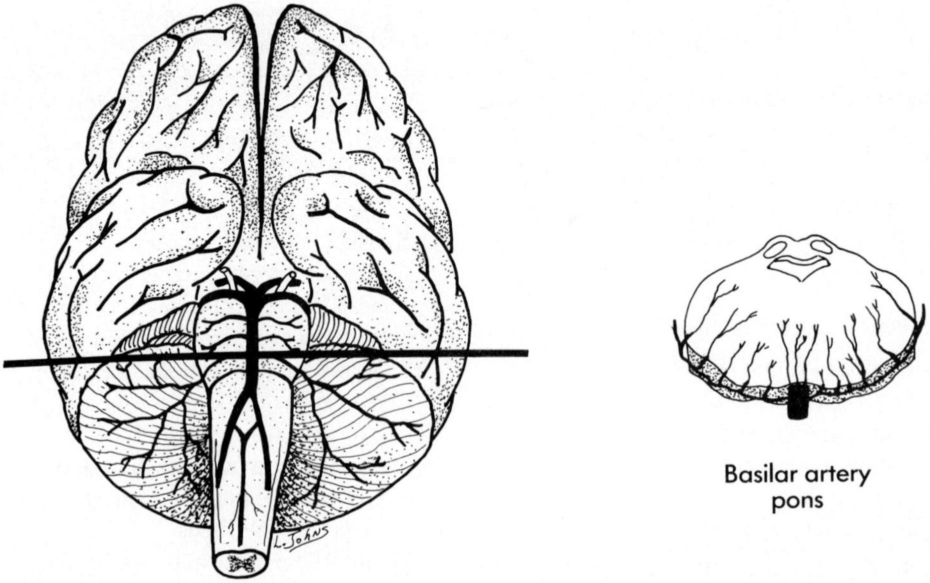

Fig. 2-7 Basilar artery, pons.

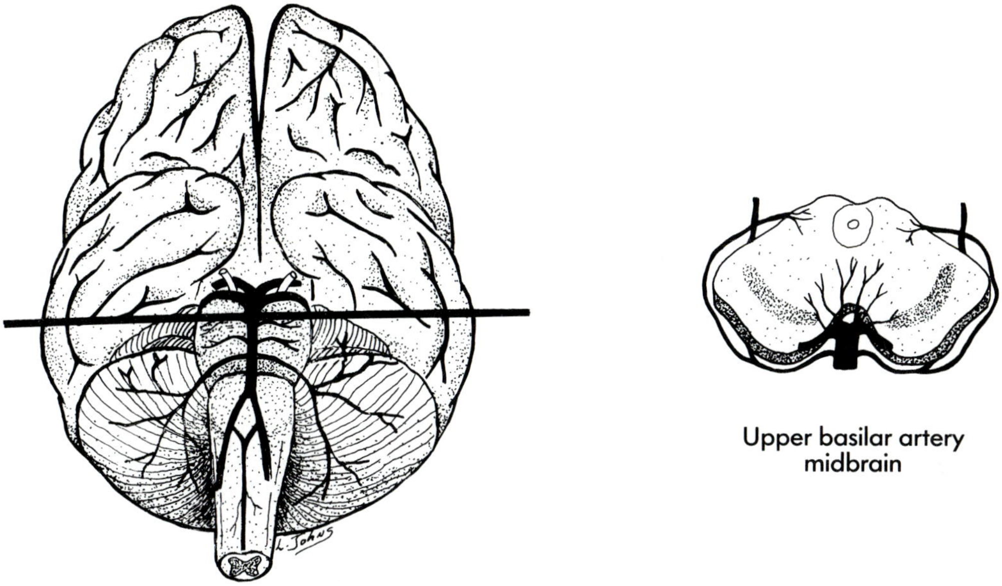

Fig. 2-8 Upper basilar artery, midbrain.

monly seen is internuclear ophthalmoplegia in which the ipsilateral eye cannot be adducted and the contralateral abducting eye demonstrates nystagmus or rhythmic beating when moved.

Alertness: Some patients exhibit a decreased level of consciousness that is due to bilateral damage of the medial pontine tegmentum. Some patients who have a pontine infarction are termed "locked-in" because of their inability to move their legs, arms, or face. They also cannot vocalize. Often their only remaining function is the ability to blink. While these patients are motionless, they are totally aware of the environment and can hear and understand spoken language.

Upper Basilar Artery (Distal)
(See Fig. 2-8)

The upper basilar artery supplies the midbrain and diencephalon. It then branches off to form the right and left posterior cerebral arteries. Signs and symptoms of occlusion include:

Alertness: Patients suffer coma caused by alteration in function of the reticular activating system, which runs through the brain system. This structure is responsible for maintaining alertness and is often referred to as the "on-off" switch for the brain.

Memory: Both short-term and long-term memory may be impaired as may the ability to make new memories.

Gaze: The patient often cannot move his eyes either up or down. On examination his eyes may appear skewed or deviated from normal position.

Pupils: Changes in pupil size are common, with the most frequent findings being either very small or dilated pupils. The pupil itself may not look round and has a decreased light reaction.

Posterior Cerebral Arteries
(See Fig. 2-9)

The basilar artery bifurcates to form the left and right posterior cerebral arteries. The posterior cerebral arteries feed three types of smaller vessels:

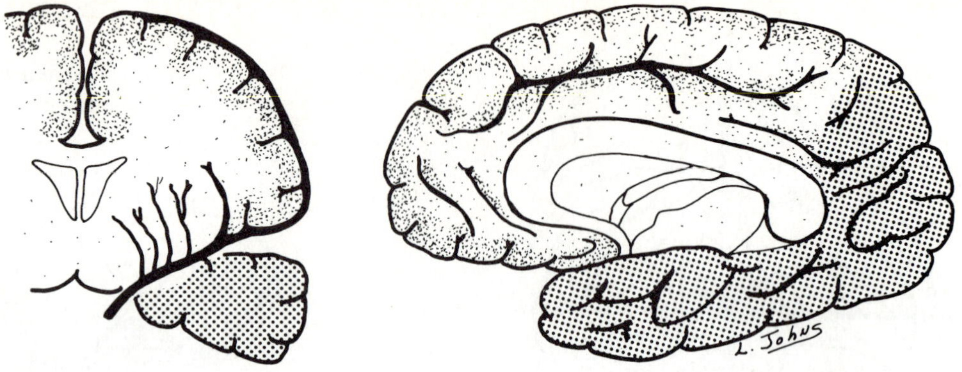

Fig. 2-9 Complete posterior cerebral artery occlusion.

paramedian penetrating, short circumferential, and long circumferential. Through these vessels the midbrain and thalamus receive their blood supply. The incidence of occlusion from intrinsic vessel disease in these vessels is quite rare, while the incidence of emboli is much higher (Mohr, 1986). Emboli traveling in the posterior circulation pass through the vertebral and basilar arteries and lodge in the posterior cerebral arteries. Interruption of blood flow within these vessels results in devastating neurological deficits. Because emboli may occlude the upper portion of the basilar, both posterior cerebral arteries may be involved. Signs and symptoms include:

Motor: Hemiplegia is present, which gradually improves with time. The resulting movement of the arm is usually uncoordinated and the arm may exhibit choreic patterns typified by involuntary, rapid, jerking movements.

Sensory: Hypesthesia or anesthesia results from dysfunction within the thalamus. The patient reports his arm feels like "dead weight" or very cold with tingling or discomfort upon stimulation of the affected extremity.

Vision: Common visual patterns found are macular sparing, in which the visual field is limited to the central portion of the normal visual field, or hemianopia. If there is bilateral occlusion of the PCA, then a variety of visual field patterns may be encountered.

Alertness: With bilateral infarctions the patient may present with a decreased level of consciousness and impairment in memory.

Other: A number of syndromes can be seen in these patients. Prosopagnosia, or the inability to recognize familiar people, is one. Alexia is another in which the alphabet is no longer familiar and the ability to read is lost.

SMALL VESSEL DISEASE
(See Fig. 2-10)

Infarction in the small penetrating vessels of the brain most commonly occurs in the region of the basal ganglia. Known as lacunes (small holes deep within the brain) various pathologic processes account for their development. Several authors attribute lacunar strokes to microatheroma, which leads to arterial stenosis (Mohr, 1986). Risk factors associated with lacunes include hypertension and diabetes, two diseases known to increase the development of atheroma. Patients who have a lacunar infarct frequently report a gradual onset of symptoms over a period of several hours. The following represent the most common types of lacunar strokes.

Pure Motor Stroke

This presentation is thought to be the most common type of lacunar stroke (Mohr and others, 1984). In these cases the area of insult is frequently located in the internal capsule of the brain, most commonly in the posterior portion. Recovery from

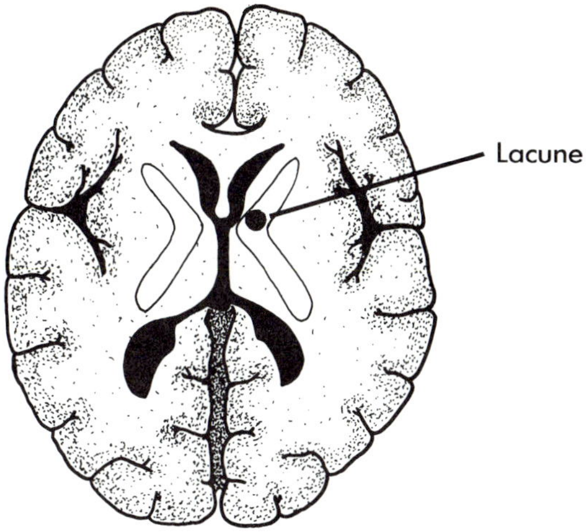

Fig. 2-10 Common site of small vessel disease (lacune).

this type of stroke may occur over time following the insult. Usually those people with the least deficit improve the most.

Motor: Hemiparesis or hemiplegia that affects the face, arm, and leg equally, although the pattern may vary according to the exact location of the infarct.

Sensory: Normal sensation.

Cranial Nerves: Normal cranial nerves.

Dysarthria—Clumsy Hand Syndrome

The anterior limb of the internal capsule is most often involved in this syndrome.

Motor: The upper extremity has uncoordinated movement (ataxic) with weakness of varying intensity. The face is also weak.

Speech: Dysarthria is present in which the patient's speech seems as if he is stammering. Patients are very susceptible to aspiration because of weakness of the muscles of deglutition and, if dysphagia is present, special precautions should be instituted for feeding the patient.

Ataxic Hemiparesis

The exact location of the lesion in these cases is varied, but lesions have been reported in the pons and posterior limb of the internal capsule in autopsied cases.

Motor: Varying degrees of weakness can be found in the leg, with the greatest weakness in the foot and ankle. While there is no weakness in the arm, it is usually extremely ataxic, as is the leg. Patients have uncoordinated movements of the arm and leg when voluntary movements are attempted.

Pure Sensory Stroke

The lesions in these patients are usually found in the thalamus. Sensory findings are the hallmark of the problem with the intensity varying with each person.

Sensory: Partial or complete sensory loss involving the face, arm, trunk, and leg. The uniqueness of the sensory loss is that it stops exactly at midline including the middle of the tongue. Most people experience loss of sensation, but some people have reported increased or unusual sensations ranging from pins and needles to severe pain.

HEMORRHAGE (See Fig. 2-11)

Supratentorial Intracranial Hemorrhage

The majority of intracranial hemorrhages occur in the deep structures of the brain or in the subcortical white matter in the lobes of the brain. Three major hemorrhagic syndromes have been identified within the basal ganglia: putaminal, caudate, and thalamic.

Putaminal Hemorrhage

Most hemorrhages in the putamen are large, with the initial presentation including both headache and vomiting. The patient has severe motor, sensory, and visual losses. Shortly after the bleeding occurs, there is a gradual decrease in the level of consciousness. Physical findings include the following:

Motor: Severe contralateral hemiplegia of the face, arm, and leg.

Sensory: Complete sensory loss in a distribution

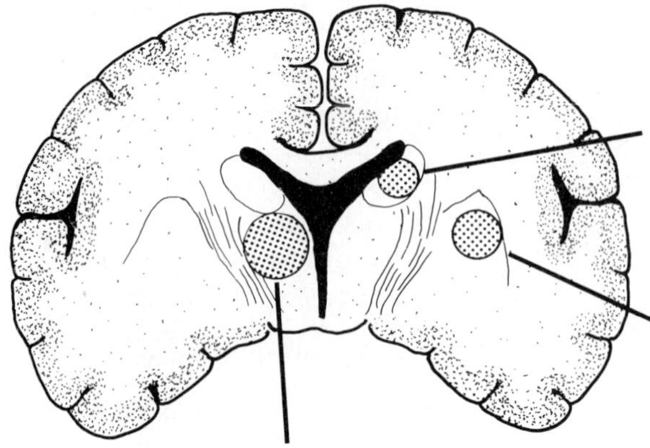

Fig. 2-11 Common sites of intracerebral hemorrhage.

similar to the motor deficits.

Vision: Homonymous hemianopia.

Gaze: The eyes are deviated to the side of the brain where the lesion is located.

If the patient has less severe neurologic findings, and is more alert, the chances of improvement are greater.

Thalamic Hemorrhage

Hemorrhage within the thalamus may extend to other nearby regions of the brain, or blood may enter the cerebral spinal fluid system via rupture in the third ventricle. The onset of hemorrhage and resulting symptomatology is usually abrupt, accompanied by vomiting. Unlike putaminal hemorrhage, most people do not experience a headache.

Motor: Hemiparesis or hemiplegia that is equal in both the upper and lower limb.

Sensory: Hemisensory loss in the same pattern as the motor deficits. If the hemorrhage occurs in the region of the posterior cerebral artery, the patient may report pain in the affected extremities.

Vision: There may be a transient homonymous hemianopia.

Gaze: The patient has unique eye findings in which there is an upward gaze palsy resulting in her being able to look only downward, and the pupils becoming small and unreactive. Occasionally a patient may have horizontal eye deviation in which she looks toward the side of the brain opposite to where the lesion is located. This is the reverse of eye deviation, caused from hemispheric lesions, in which the patient looks toward the side of the brain where the lesion is located.

Hemispheric Hemorrhage

Hemorrhage within the lobes of the brain mainly occurs in the parietal, temporal, or occipital lobes. Many mechanisms may be responsible for the hemorrhage, such as an arteriovenous malformation, clotting abnormalities, or tumors. Interestingly, hypertension is a less common etiology of hemorrhage in these regions than in the basal ganglia. Presentation of lobar hemorrhage consists of headache, seizure, and neurologic findings correlated with the region of insult. A hallmark of hemorrhage is the sudden onset of the symptoms.

Patients with a lobar hemorrhage may recover much of their functional abilities. Since the blood courses along the white matter fibers and compresses the nerve tracts in these types of hemorrhages, when the blood is reabsorbed over the course of several weeks, the pathways are again able to function.

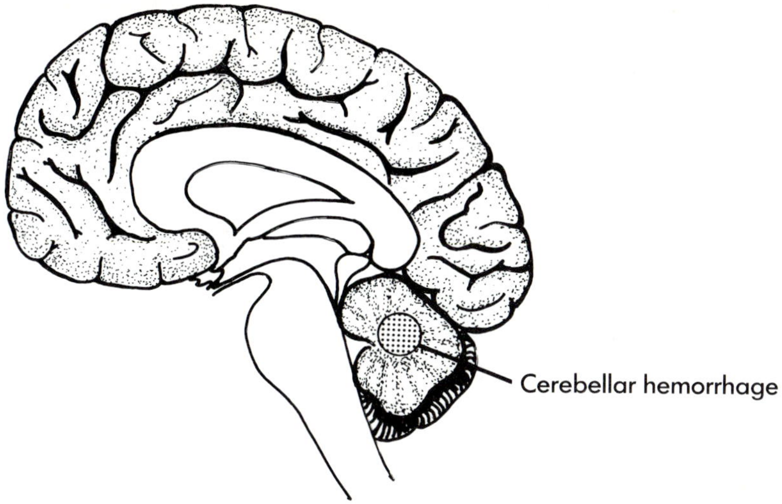

Fig. 2-12 Cerebellar hemorrhage.

Cerebellar Hemorrhage (See Fig. 2-12)

Cerebellar hemorrhages frequently occur in one side of the cerebellum and may extend into the fourth ventricle. The three key symptoms associated with a hemorrhage in this region are the inability to walk, headache, and vomiting. Neurologic findings are distinct and include ataxia or incoordination, gaze palsies, nystagmus in which the patient exhibits a rhythmic beating motion of the eyes on lateral gaze, hemiparesis, and nuchal rigidity. The prognosis in these patients is varied. Frequently, surgical evacuation of the hematoma is necessary to prevent pressure on the brainstem, which could lead to death. Whether treated surgically or not, many of these patients improve tremendously over the months after hemorrhage; however, not all patients are this lucky. Some patients have a gradual downhill course with a deteriorating level of consciousness eventually leading to coma and death.

Major findings on examination include:

Motor: Incoordination of muscle movement with inability to perform finger-to-nose and heel-to-shin testing. If walking is attempted, the patient cannot support his own weight and cannot coordinate the movement required to propel himself forward. While incoordination is the prominent finding on muscle testing, hemiparesis can also be found in some patients.

Gaze: Horizontal gaze palsy on the ipsilateral side accompanied by loss of the corneal reflex.

Cranial Nerves: Patient loses his gag reflex and is prone to aspiration. Numerous unusual eye findings can be seen, including skewing of the eyes and nystagmus.

Brainstem Hemorrhage (See Fig. 2-13)

The majority of brainstem hemorrhages occur in the pons although hemorrhage in the midbrain and medulla has been reported. Hemorrhage in the pons results from bleeding in arteries branching off the basilar artery and is usually hypertensive in origin. Patients may complain of severe headache that is rapidly followed by depressed level of consciousness and coma. Respiratory abnormalities include changes in rhythm or loss of respirations totally. Commonly called apneustic respirations, there is lack of patterning in the respirations and there can be long periods of apnea. Central neurogenic hyperthermia is also found with the patient's tem-

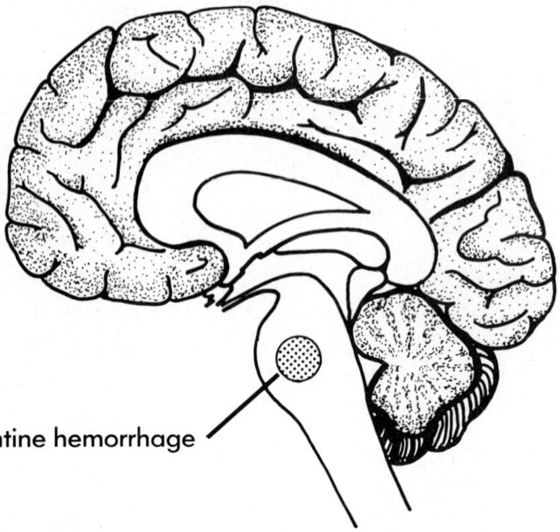

Fig. 2-13 Pontine hemorrhage.

perature rapidly rising to above 40°C. Other findings include:

Motor: Complete quadraplegia with decerebrate posturing. This posturing consists of extension and internal rotation of the arms and legs with stimulation. Weakness is also found in the facial muscles, with puffing of the cheeks seen on expiration. This lack of facial and oral tone makes the patient susceptible to aspiration.

Pupils: Small pupils that may react to intense light.

Eye Movements: Complete lack of horizontal eye movements that cannot be overcome by "doll's eyes" testing. The eyes can also bob within the orbits with rapid downward movement and a gradual return to midposition.

Hemorrhages in this location are fatal. Patients remain in a coma with a gradual, overall downhill course. If the patient does not succumb in the initial phase, then infection in the respiratory or urinary systems, causing sepsis, soon leads to death.

REFERENCES

Caplan LR: Vertebrobasilar occlusive disease. In Barnett HJM, Mohr JP, Stein BM and others, editors: Stroke: pathophysiology, diagnosis and management, New York, 1986, Churchill Livingstone.

Caplan LR and Stein RW: Stroke: a clinical approach, Boston, 1986, Butterworth Publishers.

Gorelick PB, Caplan LR, Hier DB and others: Racial differences in the distribution of anterior circulation occlusive disease, Neurology 34:54, 1984.

Gorelick PB, Caplan LR, Hier DB and others: Racial differences in the distribution of posterior circulation occlusive disease, Stroke 16:785, 1985.

Mohr JP: Lacunes. In Barnett HJM, Mohr JP, Stein BM and others, editors: Stroke: pathophysiology, diagnosis and management, New York, 1986, Churchill Livingstone.

Mohr JP, Case CS, Wolf PA and others: Lacunes in the NINCDS pilot stroke data bank Ann Neurol 12:84, 1984 (abstract) .

Chapter 3

Trends in Stroke Management

Until the mid-twentieth century, little treatment was available for stroke patients. This was in part due to limited understanding of the mechanisms of stroke and in part due to the lack of medical or surgical options available for patients. As understanding of stroke mechanisms grew so too did the sophistication of pharmacologic and surgical intervention needed for managing the complex situations often evidenced by these patients. Many treatment options are now available, and medical and nursing care is based on the type of stroke, site of stroke, cerebral vascular dynamics, and the general medical status of the patient. The importance of early and accurate treatment cannot be over-emphasized and the role of the nurse in this process is to educate the public so that people seek appropriate stroke treatment. Once treatment plans are established, the nurse can implement and monitor treatments, assess for side effects, and develop the patient's understanding of his illness and how to manage ongoing medical therapy.

Options for treatment revolve around five concepts that maintain or improve blood flow to the brain, increase oxygenation of the brain, or reduce pressure. Concepts include noninvasive approaches to improving blood flow; medical therapies to improve blood flow; protecting the brain from ischemia; controlling cerebral edema; and hypervolemic hemodilution of the blood. These concepts will be discussed from both a medical and nursing standpoint, and related nursing interventions are incorporated in the treatment plan.

NONINVASIVE APPROACHES TO IMPROVING BLOOD FLOW

Patient Position

One of the most basic elements in improving cerebral circulation is the position of the patient. In ischemic strokes, tight stenotic vessels need adequate blood flow to perfuse surrounding tissues. Most healthy people are easily able to adjust cardiovascular output and cerebral perfusion in response to changes in position. The stroke patient, however, has more difficulty in maintaining cerebral perfusion during position changes and, often, going from a lying position to a standing position will increase the neurologic symptoms exhibited by the patient. A supine position, with the head flat, allows blood to flow more easily toward the brain without the additional influence of gravity. Caplan and Sergay (1976) documented such ischemic changes related to position in four patients. The recommendation for care for these patients with fluctuating signs and symptoms is to keep them in a flat position, with gradual mobilization after the acute phase has passed. Ischemic stroke patients should lie flat in bed initially, and any elevation of the head of the bed or movement of the patient to an upright position should increase the nurse's monitoring of the patient for changes in blood pressure or increased signs and symptoms. The opposite is true for patients with hemorrhagic strokes. These patients have increased intracranial pressure and congestion within the cerebral vessels. The head of the bed should be maintained at a 30 degree elevation (without flexion of the patient's neck) to promote venous drainage of the cerebral vessels.

Blood Pressure

Maintaining blood pressure is one key factor in maintaining cerebral perfusion. Pressure should be neither too high nor too low. In an ischemic stroke, chronic hypertension was often a factor in its development. People with these types of strokes are admitted to the hospital with blood pressures well above the "normal" range. While blood pressure must be lowered, it should be done gradually.

There must be a balance between high blood pressures, which can lead to hemorrhage in the stroke region and congestive heart failure, and low blood pressures, which can cause further ischemic infarction. Most physicians want the blood pressure of a patient with chronic hypertension kept in the high range of normal. The patient who is being managed with antihypertensive medications should be monitored for rapidly decreasing blood pressure because a severe decrease in blood pressure can lead to poor cerebral perfusion. Wallace and Levy reported in 1981 that the blood pressures of stroke patients decreased spontaneously without antihypertensive treatment while they were hospitalized. With this in mind, blood pressure control should proceed with caution and be closely monitored.

In hypertensive intracranial hemorrhages, an extremely rapid rise in blood pressure has often been the cause of the hemorrhage. To decrease the force and the amount of bleeding, the rampant hypertension must be brought under control. Antihypertensive medications are given to these patients, and careful monitoring is needed because rebound hypotension can occur with intravenous administration of such drugs.

Another factor that influences blood pressure is the hydration status of the patient. Diuretics and lack of fluid intake contribute to decreased blood pressure, especially in older, debilitated patients. The nurse should maintain careful intake and output records, especially in the early phase of hospitalization.

Activity Level

During the initial period after a stroke all patients should be prescribed bedrest. This ensures adequate blood flow to the brain and also reduces the risk of potential injury to the patient because of her unfamiliarity with the neurologic deficits. As the patient's cerebral blood flow is stabilized, activity can be gradually increased. As the patient becomes more active, the nurse should perform ongoing assessment of neurological status and blood pressure. Activities such as toileting, transfers, and ambulation require close supervision.

MEDICAL THERAPIES TO IMPROVE BLOOD FLOW

In patients with atherosclerosis there is a disequilibrium between the patient's hemodynamics and vessel structure. In areas of high flow and turbulence platelets can aggregate and, with the addition of fibrin, develop into arterial thrombi ("white platelet plugs"). In low flow situations, thrombi can also form but are composed of red blood cells, platelets, and fibrin and are referred to as "red clots" (Caplan and Stein, 1986). Besides clot formation, sluggish flow and severe stenosis can lead to vessel occulusion. Higher flow dynamics, or when low flow changes to high flow, can result in small pieces of thrombi becoming dislodged and then being carried by the moving blood stream, eventually being stopped by small diameter distal vessels.

Several situations can promote the development of thrombi within vessels: disruption of the endothelium in the lining of the vessel; stasis of blood; increased clotting; and stimulation of platelet aggregation (Barnett and others, 1986). It is by modifying these factors that an attempt is made at stroke prevention. In those patients who already have ischemic changes within the brain, alteration in blood components may limit the extent of infarction.

Anticoagulation

Many drugs have recently become available for treating the blood itself to increase blood flow to the brain. If a red clot has been the cause of stroke, or if cardiac abnormalities, such as myocardial infarction, atrial fibrillation, cardiac myopathies, or prosthetic valves, are a cause of cerebral emboli, then treating the clotting factors of the blood is indicated. Anticoagulation may be indicated in progressing stroke, multiple transient ischemic attacks (TIAs), partial stroke in the vertebrobasilar system (especially if there is a risk of progression), and cardioembolic stroke.

For short-term use, heparin is the drug of choice to prevent the conversion of prothrombin to thrombin within the blood and thus clot formation. It is mainly given intravenously, with an initial loading dose followed by continuous infusion. While there are many ways to prepare the medication for administration, generally, a loading dose of 5000 to 10,000 units is given and 5000 units of heparin are mixed in 500 ml of D5W and administered at a rate of 1000 to 2000 units per hour. Depending on the fluid status of the patient, if fewer fluids are indicated, the solution can be mixed at higher concentrations; however, the IV bag should be clearly labeled so that an inadvertent overdose can be avoided. Use of an IV pump helps ensure accurate fluid delivery and is recommended when giving heparin. For heparin to be considered effective the patient's partial thromboplastin time (PTT) value should be maintained between one and a half to two times the normal. While the initial dosing is being accomplished, PTT levels should be drawn every 4 to 6 hours. Once dosage is stabilized, a PTT is usually drawn twice a day until the patient is stable and then daily. Patients receiving heparin therapy should be observed closely for bleeding. Gums should be checked for bleeding during oral care, and evidence of bruising of the skin should be documented. Testing urine and stool for blood should be done routinely.

For longer anticoagulant treatment, warfarin is the drug of choice. Warfarin inhibits the mechanism of vitamin K in clotting. Most patients have already been taking heparin for a period of time before they are gradually switched over to warfarin. This process takes several days because the action of warfarin gradually changes the clotting process. The dosage of warfarin varies with each individual, but the range is from 2 to 10 mg per day. Adequate anticoagulation is achieved by day 5 or 6, at which time a daily dose for ongoing maintenance can be determined. Unlike heparin, a loading dose is not indicated for warfarin, since the mechanism of anticoagulation needs time to take effect. During this dosing period, clotting times are monitored with daily prothrombin times (PT). When PTs are one and a half to two times normal, then administration of heparin is stopped. Nursing care of these patients follows guidelines similar to those for heparin therapy. If patients are discharged to home and prescribed warfarin therapy, safety instructions should be given, including not shaving with a straightedge razor blade; avoiding the use of equipment where injury could occur; and taking special precautions when using sharp instruments, such as knives. Outpatient PTs are usually monitored at regular intervals for these patients.

Platelet Antiaggregants

The theory behind antiplatelet treatment is that by inhibiting platelet function there will be less chance of thrombi developing, especially in tortuous, stenotic cerebral vessels. The primary target for such treatment is ischemic strokes that are believed to be the result of stenosis or vascular disease within the carotid or cerebral vessels. Treating a patient with platelet antiaggregants is done to try to prevent any further thrombotic event from occurring and is not an attempt to treat the patient for a prior ischemic event.

Aspirin was the first drug to be tried for such effects. Aspirin prevents the synthesis of prostaglandins and thromboxane and, as a result, decreases platelet aggregation. While aspirin is beneficial in treatment, one drawback is that aspirin also inhibits prostacyclin, a platelet antiaggregant that also facilitates vessel dilatation, an important factor when the goal of treatment is to improve cerebral perfusion. Even so, recent analysis of multicenter aspirin trials has demonstrated the benefits of aspirin in patients with transient ischemic attacks and mild strokes. There has also been a decrease in the risk of second stroke, myocardial infarction, and death resulting from vascular origin for patients taking aspirin for long-term maintenance (Antiplatelet Trialists Collaboration, 1988). Optimal dosage has been discussed extensively in the literature and current regimens can range from 2.5 grains to 20 grains a day. Nursing care of patients on aspirin therapy should include teaching the patient to observe or having the nurse personally observe for signs of increased bruising, bleeding gums when performing oral care, or longer bleeding times with small cuts. As always with aspirin ingestion, care should be taken to protect the stomach lining and prevent gastritis. Administering aspirin with milk or meals facilitates this prevention process.

Other drugs are also being tested for their effect on platelet aggregation. Dipyridamole (Persantine) also inhibits platelet function, but its effectiveness in stroke management is questionable. Several studies, including those with double-blind methodology, have demonstrated no difference in patients managed on aspirin and dipyridamole and those patients managed on aspirin alone (Bousser and others, 1983). One of the more promising drugs is ticlopidine. It inhibits platelet aggregation, prolongs bleeding time, and blocks platelet release action. Clinical trials are still underway to determine the efficacy and safety of ticlopidine (Gent and others, 1988).

PROTECTING THE BRAIN

Besides maintaining cerebral blood flow and modifying blood components, a thrust of recent research has been to try to protect the brain from the permanent effects of ischemia. This might prove beneficial to patients who have poor perfusion and marginal ischemia. Giving medications that prevent irreversible ischemia from occurring may allow time for the brain to develop adequate collateral circulation or for medical and surgical interventions to become effective.

Calcium channel blockers are a type of drug whose purpose is to prevent cellular influx of calcium that destroys the cell's viability. Normally, extracellular calcium concentrations are high compared with those within the cell. This dichotomy is maintained because the cell membrane is impermeable to calcium. As the cell is subjected to ischemic changes, the cell membrane breaks down, leading to an influx of calcium into the cell that causes its ultimate demise. Calcium channel blockers, such as nimodipine, have been used in clinical trials with mixed results. Gelmers and others (1986) reported that in a double-blind study of nimodipine vs placebo, there were fewer deaths from stroke and greater improvement in neurologic function in the nimodipine-treated group.

Another area of research is with opiate receptor antagonists, such as naloxone. While the exact mechanisms by which such drugs protect the brain from ischemia is unclear, it is postulated that it may be a combination of vasoregulation and calcium mediation. Several uncontrolled clinical trials have been done with naloxone but in much lower doses than in animal studies. Some patients showed temporary clinical improvement after receiving the drug. Estanol and others (1985) gave naloxone to a total of 48 patients with cerebral infarcts. Patients who had infarcts for more than 7 days before therapy and those with intracerebral hemorrhage showed no response. Seven of 20 patients with recent (less than 24 hours) infarcts showed long-lasting improvement in neurologic function. Three other patients who developed ischemia during angiography also showed dramatic improvement in neurologic status after injection with naloxone. Adams and others (1986) found transient sustained improvement in neurologic function in 13 of 27 patients enrolled in a dose-escalation study of naloxone. These drugs show promise in the treatment of stroke, but patients must be treated soon after the onset of symptoms for the drugs to be effective. Thus educating the general public—especially those with many stroke risk factors—about the warning signs of stroke is important so that if a stroke occurs they will seek treatment immediately.

CONTROLLING CEREBRAL EDEMA

When brain infarction occurs, blood flow immediately reduces in the vicinity of the stroke and cell death occurs. This initially produces cytotoxic edema or swelling of the cells and vascular congestion. Eventually, cell membranes rupture leading to the development of vasogenic edema or interstitial edema. All of these events lead to compromised circulation in the tissue surrounding the infarct. Blood flow in these regions can be reduced to a point where the cell is still alive but unable to function. Clinically, patients may show neurologic impairment, but, if edema is reduced and blood flow restored, there can be reversal of symptomatology.

Historically, steroids (dexamethasone) have been used to treat edema in patients with ischemic strokes. Dexamethasone is effective in vasogenic edema, not cytotoxic edema. Since ischemia primarily causes cytotoxic edema, the use of steroids is questionable. Numerous studies have shown the treatment of ischemic stroke with steroids to be ineffective (Fishman, 1982; Anderson and Cranford, 1979).

In contrast, hemorrhagic strokes produce large amounts of vasogenic edema. Corticosteroids can be used to reduce edema in these cases but, because their action is relatively slow, most physicians prefer to use hyperosmolar agents, which cause water to be drawn from the interstitial space into the blood stream. The kidney then filters and excretes the fluid. Mannitol is one drug used to achieve the rapid reduction of edema, which is especially important in the acute stage of hemorrhage. The usual dose is 1.5 to 2.0 g/kg of body weight infused intravenously over 30 to 60 minutes. Care of the patient receiving mannitol includes monitoring urine output, electrolytes, serum and urine osmolarity, blood pressure, and renal function. To aid in these efforts an indwelling urinary catheter is necessary and, if indicated, a central line is useful if central venous pressures are to be evaluated. The central line is especially important in patients who may develop congestive heart failure or who have impaired kidney function.

HYPERVOLEMIC HEMODILUTION

Hypervolemic hemodilution (HH) is a relatively new approach to the treatment of stroke. The overall purpose of HH is to augment cerebral blood flow (CBF), thereby reversing ischemic deficits or preventing infarction. Current research indicates a very narrow time frame during which CBF must be increased (probably 4 to 6 hours) to accomplish this purpose. Other interventions, particularly surgery, are difficult to implement within this time frame. The advantage to HH therapy is that it can be quickly and relatively safely implemented in the appropriate patient to improve outcome.

An understanding of normal CBF and alterations in CBF accompanying stroke is essential to implementation of HH therapy. *Cerebral blood flow* may be defined as *the amount of blood required to adequately perfuse the brain for ongoing neuronal function.* In this context, ischemia is a focal or diffuse reduction in CBF below what is required for normal neuronal function. Infarction results with CBF decreases below that required for neuronal survival.

Decreases in CBF may be caused by cerebral embolus, thrombosis, or vasospasm. The resulting ischemia decreases neuronal metabolic and electrical activity, which is manifest as a neurologic deficit. Should ischemia progress, neuronal death ensues. Duration and depth of ischemia are factors directly related to the severity of infarct. The longer the time of ischemia and the greater the extent, the more severe the deficit. Therapy is aimed at decreasing duration and extent of ischemia through improving CBF.

The Hagen-Pouiseille equation has been used to describe CBF.* The equation is:

$$Q = \frac{\Delta P \pi r^4}{8 L n}$$

where Q = Blood flow
P = The pressure gradient in the vessel (roughly, blood pressure)
r = Vessel radius
L = Vessel length
n = Blood viscosity

Obviously, from this equation, several factors influence CBF. Blood flow may also be manipulated through some of these factors. By increasing blood pressure (BP), CBF may secondarily increase; of-

*This is a general equation of blood flow rather than one specific CBF. It does not take into account unique aspects such as autoregulation.

ten hypertension is seen in response to cerebral ischemia. Pharmacologically induced hypertension may also achieve the same result. However, hypertension may lead to intracerebral hemorrhage, and increasing BP can be precarious in the presence of essential hypertension or cardiac compromise. Blood vessel radius may be increased by utilizing medications that relax or dilate cerebral vasculature. However, clinical studies have shown little benefit in improving CBF to date, possibly because vessels are already maximally dilated in ischemic areas. Vessel length is a factor that obviously cannot be manipulated. The last factor, blood viscosity, can be directly manipulated by utilizing hypervolemic hemodilution. Hypervolemic hemodilution decreases blood viscosity and secondarily increases or augments CBF.

Several factors contribute to blood viscosity, including erythrocyte aggregation and flexibility, platelet aggregation, plasma viscosity, hematocrit (Hct), and shear rate. Of these factors, Hct is the main determinant of blood viscosity and is the easiest factor to manipulate. By decreasing Hct, CBF may be subsequently increased.

Hct may be lowered by using hypervolemic or normovolemic hemodilution. Hypervolemia refers to an iatrogenic increase in total blood volume. When hypervolemia is accomplished by use of a colloidal solution, hemodilution results, causing Hct to decrease. Colloidal solutions, such as albumin or dextran, or plasmanate solutions are used because the solution remains in the intravascular space rather than distributing itself throughout the fluid compartments. In contrast, normovolemic hemodilution may be accomplished by removal of up to 1 liter of blood followed by volume replacement with a colloidal solution. Hence, volume status remains unchanged while Hct is lowered.

The use of HH has been advocated in the treatment of patients with ischemic deficits. Positive results have been seen from early studies, including clinical improvement and improvement in regional CBF and electroencephalographic (EEG) activity. Questions remain, however, about who the most appropriate candidates are, how hemodilution should be accomplished, and how long the therapy should be used.

Indications

Most studies evaluating the benefit of HH therapy have included a small number of patients or patients with varying degrees of deficits or have not been double-blind studies. As a result, there are no clear guidelines to date for determining who might best benefit from the therapy. A culmination of information from prominent researchers in the area has suggested several indications. HH may be indicated as a therapy in any patient having evidence of acute ischemic neurologic deficit. However, since duration and extent of ischemia influence outcome, patients with deficits existing longer than 24 hours or those who are moribund or in coma will most likely not benefit from the therapy. Origin of the deficit is also important. Therapy appears to be most applicable to the patient with cerebral embolus, thrombosis, or vasospasm. Hypertensive intracerebral hemorrhage represents a contraindication to HH therapy, because hypervolemia may contribute to additional bleeding and worsening of the deficit. In addition, several studies have demonstrated HH benefit reliance on the existence of collateral circulation. For example, while patients with basilar artery stenosis showed improvement with HH therapy, those with basilar occlusion did not. These indications highlight the importance of detailed physical examination and appropriate diagnostic testing (usually through computed tomography (CT) and cerebral angiography) preceding patient selection for this therapy. Since hypervolemia may contribute to increased intracranial pressure (ICP) in the unstable patient, ICP should be normal before initiation of therapy; elevated ICP is a contraindication. Finally, patients must be medically stable to tolerate hypervolemia and hemodilution. Patients with cardiopulmonary compromise may not be able to tolerate the hypervolemia; normovolemic hemodilution may be utilized in this circumstance. Patients with a low baseline Hct may not be able to tolerate hemodilution until blood replacement is accomplished.

Any other situation in which hypervolemia or hemodilution compromises the patient's situation (such as renal failure) may preclude use of this therapy.

Preprocedural Nursing Management

The nurse plays an important role during HH therapy in establishing baseline function and preparing the patient for initiation of therapy.

The nurse must evaluate, in detail, the extent of deficit in the patient who is admitted with acute ischemia, because this serves as the basis for determining response to therapy. Specific attention is paid to level of consciousness, behavior, affect, and cognitive function. In addition, the patient is evaluated for deficit in motor strength, coordination, and tone. Any sensory or cranial nerve deficits are also noted; speech function should be evaluated. Patients should also be questioned about allergic history because infusates used for HH therapy may produce an anaphylactic response. If available, ICP should be monitored, with any ICP value above 15 mm Hg reported. Baseline Hct and other laboratory values as ordered (hemoglobin, total blood volume, blood viscosity, arterial blood gases, etc.) are monitored and a baseline Hct of less than 33 mg/dl is reported. Baseline volume status should be determined because this serves as one of the adjustment parameters during therapy. Central venous pressure (CVP) or pulmonary capillary wedge pressure (PCWP) are utilized because peripheral measures are less reliable. The nurse is expected to be involved in insertion of these invasive monitoring devices. An elevated CVP or PCWP must be reported before initiation of therapy because this represents a potential contraindication to HH. Baseline BP is also determined. Evidence of hypertension is reported as an additional contraindication. The physician may order additional baseline parameters, such as blood glucose, cardiac index, etc., with the nurse reporting any abnormalities.

Before initiation of HH therapy, detailed diagnostic evaluation is essential. The nurse's role during this time focuses on explaining to the patient and/or family the purpose of the diagnostic testing ordered, what to expect during testing, and the patient's role following each procedure. Anticipated diagnostic testing includes CT scanning and cerebral angiography. Additional testing, such as EEG, regional CBF monitoring, and others may be ordered as indicated. However, since all diagnostic testing must be completed promptly, usually within a few hours, little time may be available for such explanations. Since invasive monitoring most likely will be utilized, the purposes of the devices and associated discomforts should be explained. Also, patients and families must be informed of the need for frequent neurologic assessments, ongoing monitoring, and repeat diagnostic testing. Physician explanations of the purpose and procedure of HH therapy, along with expected outcomes, should be reinforced.

Procedural Aspects

Once diagnostic evaluation has been completed, baseline assessments determined, and the patient deemed an appropriate candidate, HH therapy is begun. Several solutions are currently available for clinical use, but the most widely used is 5% albumin. The albumin is usually administered intravenously (IV) in a 250 ml loading dose over 30 minutes and repeated every 4 hours. Low molecular weight dextran infused continuously or intermittently has also been used. Synthetic plasma volume expanders, such as hetastarch and pentastarch, have recently been developed at a lesser cost with fewer adverse effects. Fresh frozen plasma has also been used. Any of these infusates may be used for normovolemic hemodilution.

Continuing dosage of the infusate is adjusted on an individual basis according to a number of parameters:

- *Neurologic status*—improvement in neurologic function is anticipated within hours of initiation of therapy. Evidence of neurologic deterioration warrants immediate discontinuation of the infusion and further diagnostic evaluation
- *Hematocrit*—normal Hct ranges from 37 to 45 mg/dl with a therapeutic Hct on HH of 30 to 33

mg/dl. This is considered to be the optimal Hct to offset blood oxygen content reduction that occurs as a result of hemodilution. Should the Hct be above the therapeutic parameter, dosage is progressively increased until Hct is sufficiently lowered. Should Hct be lower than 30 mg/dl, dosage is decreased

- *Volume status*—optimal hemodilution is individually defined. Generally, the CVP is maintained at 12 cm H_2O or less, and PCWP is maintained at 20 mm Hg or less. However, at times a PCWP of 25 to 30 mm Hg may be necessary to achieve adequate hemodilution. Desmopressin may be used to promote hypervolemia. In contrast, should volume status become unstable, mannitol or furosemide may be used. Objective and subjective assessment of cardiopulmonary status should be performed; any evidence of cardiopulmonary compromise warrants discontinuation of the infusion
- *Blood pressure*—BP should be monitored closely, preferably continuously via an indwelling arterial catheter. BP should be maintained within 20 mm Hg of the patient's baseline or normal systolic BP. Increases in BP above this point must be reported immediately because of the danger of intracerebral hemorrhage or additional ischemia. Control of BP may be accomplished with sodium nitroprusside; hydralazine and propanolol should be avoided because they potentially decrease CBF. Vasopressor medications may be administered should hypotension occur
- Other parameters may be ordered by the physican including regional CBF measurements, cardiac index, arterial blood gases, blood glucose, and ICP. Decline in any of these parameters should be reported immediately; discontinuation of the infusion may be warranted.

No single parameter should be used for dose adjustment. Rather, the entire clinical picture should be evaluated and dose individualized to the patient.

Timing of the therapy is important. As previously mentioned, HH therapy should be initiated within the first 24 hours of onset of ischemic deficit; benefit after this point is questionable. Length of therapy is variable but usually continues for 72 hours, with each dose adjusted as necessary. The patient should be slowly weaned by gradually decreasing the dose to prevent rebound declines in CBF resulting from abrupt volume changes. Weaning is generally accomplished over several days. Some patients become infusion-dependent, with neurologic deterioration accompanying weaning attempts. Therefore, the HH may be continued from 5 days up to several weeks; however, the average time is about 5 to 7 days.

Nursing Management During Therapy

Since it is the nurse who administers the therapy and performs bedside assessments, the role of the nurse during therapy is extremely important. Not only must the nurse be knowledgeable about the pathophysiology of stroke and its relationship to blood flow, but the nurse must also have an understanding of HH principles.

The nurse is intimately involved in dosage adjustment through frequent bedside assessments. Frequent, ongoing assessment of neurologic status, volume status, BP, and other necessary parameters is vital. These assessments are usually performed and documented hourly, with any adverse alterations being reported immediately. Sudden or severe changes in any parameter warrants immediate discontinuation of the infusion and physician notification along with further diagnostic testing. Hct and other lab values may be monitored every 4 to 6 hours. Since the therapy requires intensive care and often enforced bed rest, nursing measures to promote rest and to prevent the hazards of immobility should be instituted.

Patient and family education and support during this time is important. HH appears to be a passive therapy to the family or patient who may perceive little is being done to help them. The pathophysiology of stroke and rationale for HH should be explained. Physical, occupational, or speech therapies may be started during this time as indicated, and families should be involved in the patient's physical care. Patients or families may resent frequent assessments or the invasiveness of monitoring, especially if dramatic improvement in their status has occurred. Therefore the need for the assessments and monitoring should be explained and reinforced. Any other patient or family questions or concerns should be addressed as they arise.

Once HH therapy has been discontinued, no follow-up specific to the therapy is necessary. However, deficits may still be present that warrant treatment. The patient should be evaluated by all members of the rehabilitation team and appropriate therapies initiated. A discharge plan, initiated upon admission, is implemented. The patient may be discharged to an in-patient rehabilitation facility, extended care facility, or home with therapy depending upon the patient's exact situation.

Outcome

Reports in the literature indicate HH and normovolemic hemodilution do improve stroke outcome in certain patients. However, the studies involve small numbers of patients with various deficits; previous studies have not been randomized or double-blind approaches. Therefore, additional study in this area is warranted. To date, reports have shown improvement in neurologic function within 15 minutes to 14 hours of initiation of therapy. In a high percentage of patients, neurologic deficit was completely reversed. In addition, HH therapy was associated with improvements in regional CBF measurements and background EEG activity. Finally one study reported decreased hospitalization and rehabilitation time for patients treated with normovolemic hemodilution. Safety of hypervolemic hemodilution has been evaluated in several studies with researchers concluding that the therapy is not harmful, but frequent assessments, especially of hemodynamic status, are essential.

Any therapy has potential complications. Those reported in the literature focus on complications related to hypervolemia, the infusate, circulatory access, medical complications, and the disease state itself. Incidence of complications overall is thought to be less than 5%. Specific complications are listed in the box above.

COMPLICATIONS OF HYPERVOLEMIC HEMODILUTION THERAPY

COMPLICATIONS RELATED TO HYPERVOLEMIA

Congestive heart failure
Pulmonary edema
Cerebral edema: confusion, decreased level of consciousness

COMPLICATIONS RELATED TO THE INFUSATE

Anaphylaxis
Infusate rebound
Transmission of infection: hepatitis, AIDS
Liver dysfunction
Coagulopathy
Hyponatremia

COMPLICATIONS RELATED TO CIRCULATORY ACCESS

Bacteremia
Sepsis
Pneumothorax

REFERENCES

Adams HP, Olinger CP, Barsan WG and others: A dose-escalation study of large doses of naloxone for treatment of patients with acute cerebral ischemia, Stroke 17:404, 1986.

Anderson D and Cranford R: Corticosteroids in ischemic stroke, Stroke 10:68, 1979.

Anti-Platelet Trialists Collaboration: Secondary prevention of vascular disease by prolonged anti-platelet therapy, Br Med J 296:320, 1988.

Barnett HJM, Mohr JP, Stein BM and others: Stroke: pathophysiology, diagnosis and management, New York, 1986, Churchill Livingstone.

Bousser MG, Eschwege E, Haguenau M and others: "AICLA" controlled trial of aspirin and dipyridamole in the secondary prevention of athero-thrombotic cerebral ischemia, Stroke 14:5, 1983.

Caplan LR and Sergay S: Positional cerebral ischaemia, J Neurol Neurosurg Psychiatry 39:385, 1976.

Caplan LR and Stein RW: Stroke: a clinical approach, Boston, 1986, Butterworth Publishers.

Estanol B, Aguilar F, and Corona T: Diagnosis of reversible cerebral ischemia by the intravenous administration of naloxone, Stroke 16:1006, 1985.

Faden AI: Opiate antagonists in the treatment of stroke, Stroke 15:575, 1984.

Fishman R: Steroids in the treatment of brain edema, N Engl J Med 306:359, 1982.

Gelmers HJ, Gorter K, de Weerdt CJ and others: Effect of nimodipine on clinical outcome in patients with acute ischemic stroke, Stroke 17:145, 1986.

Gent M, Blakely JA, Easton JD and others: The Canadian American Ticlopidine Study (CATS) in thromboembolic stroke: design, organization and baseline results, Stroke 19:1203, 1988.

Wallace JD and Levy LL: Blood pressure after stroke JAMA 246:2177, 1981.

BIBLIOGRAPHY

American-Canadian Cooperative Study Group: Persantine-aspirin trial in cerebral ischemia: end-point results, Stroke 16:406, 1985.

Cerebral Embolism Study Group: Immediate anticoagulation of embolic stroke: a randomized trial, Stroke 14:668, 1983.

Fallis RJ, Fisher M, and Lobo RA: A double-blind trial of naloxone in the treatment of acute stroke, Stroke 15:627, 1984.

Fields WS, Yatsu F, Conomy J and others: Persantine-aspirin trial in cerebral ischemia: the American-Canadian cooperative study group, Stroke 14:97, 1983.

Gent M, Blakely JA, Hachinski V and others: A secondary prevention, randomized trial of suloctidil in patients with a recent history of thromboembolic stroke, Stroke 16:416, 1985.

Gilroy J, Barnhart MI, and Meyer JS: Treatment of acute stroke with Dextran-40, JAMA 210:293, 1969.

Grotta J, Ackerman R, Correia J and others: Whole blood viscosity parameters and cerebral blood flow, Stroke 13:296, 1982.

Heiss WD, Prosenz P, Tschabitscher H and others: Effect of low molecular dextran on total cerebral blood flow and on regional flow within ischemic brain lesions, Eur Neurol 8:129, 1972.

Henriksen L, Paulson OB, and Smith RJ: Cerebral blood flow following normovolemic hemodilution in patients with high hematocrit, Ann Neurol 9:454, 1981.

Hint H: The pharmacology of dextran and physiologic background for the clinical use of Rheomacrodex and Macrodex, Acta Anaesthesiol Belg 19:119, 1968.

Jabaily J and Davis JN: Naloxone administration to patients with ischemic stroke, Stroke 15:36, 1984.

Kee DB and Wood JH: Rheology of the cerebral circulation, Neurosurg 15:125, 1984.

Krepp HP, Beez M, and Bock P: Treatment of acute cerebral infarction by hypervolemic hemodilution with 10% Hydroxyethyl starch 200/0.5 and 10% dextran 40, Klinikarzt 13:597, 1984.

Miller VT and Hart RG: Heparin anticoagulation in acute brain ischemia, Stroke 19:403, 1988.

Pritz MB, Giannotta SL, Kindt GW and others: Treatment of patients with neurologic deficits associated with cerebral vasospasm by intravascular volume expansion, Neurosurg 3:364, 1978.

Rosenberg B and Wulff K: Hemodynamics following normovolemic hemodilution in elderly patients, Acta Anaesthesia Scan 25:402, 1981.

Stewart-Amidei C: Hypervolemic hemodilution, Heart Lung 18:590, 1989.

Strand T, Asplund K, Erickson S and others: A randomized controlled trial of hemodilution therapy in ischemic stroke, Stroke 15:980, 1984.

Tohgi H, Yamanouchi H, Murakami M and others: Importance of the hematocrit as a risk factor in cerebral infarction, Stroke 9:369, 1979.

Wood JH, Simeone FA, Fink EA and others: Correlative aspects of hypervolemic hemodilution: low molecular weight dextran infusions after experimental cerebral arterial occlusions, Neurology 34:24, 1984.

Wood JH, Polyzoidis KS, Epstein CM and others: Quantitative EEG alterations after isovolemic hemodilutional augmentation of cerebral perfusion in stroke patients, Neurology 34:764, 1984.

Wood JH, Simeone FA, Kron RE and others: Rheologic aspects of experimental hypervolemic hemodilution with low molecular weight dextran: relationships of cortical blood flow, cardiac output, and intracranial pressure to fresh blood viscosity and plasma volume, Neurosurg 11:739, 1982.

Wood JH: Hypervolemic hemodilution: rheologic therapy for acute cerebral ischemia, Contemporary Neurosurgery 21:1, 1982.

Wood JH and Fleischer AS: Observations during hypervolemic hemodilution of patients with acute focal cerebral ischemia, JAMA 248:2999, 1982.

Wood JH, Simeone FA, Snyder LL and others: Hemodilutional and nonhemodilutional hypervolemia in treatment of focal cerebral ischemia, J Cereb Blood Flow Metab 1(Suppl):S178, 1981.

Wood JH and Kee DB: Clinical rheology of stroke and hemodilution. In Barnett HJ, Stein BM, Mohr JP and others, editors: Stroke: pathophysiology, diagnosis, and management, New York, 1986, Churchill Livingstone.

Chapter 4

Surgical Alternatives for Stroke

Although stroke has been a fairly well-defined phenomenon for many years, surgical treatment options for stroke are relatively new developments. A number of factors have converged, leading to the development of surgical alternatives for stroke. First, a more recent emphasis on stroke prevention has evolved, leading clinicians to search out effective preventive measures rather than deal with the aftereffects of stroke. It is important to note that the goal of any surgical intervention is to prevent or minimize the risk of developing an ischemic deficit of the brain; surgery is not effective in reversing deficits. Second, diagnostic advances, such as digital venous subtraction angiography, selective vessel angiography, positron emission tomography, and others, have afforded a more precise diagnosis of the underlying lesion. As result, it is possible to better define those who might benefit from surgical intervention. Third, advances in surgical technology have made surgical intervention technically feasible. Such advances include improved surgical instrumentation, development of the operating room microscope, and advanced technical skills of the surgeon. Yet, despite these advances, surgery remains a preventive measure, applicable as a treatment option in a limited number of cases. The exact nature of the problem determines the precise type of surgery and the timing of intervention. In this chapter several surgical alternatives for stroke will be presented, including indications, procedural aspects, preoperative and postoperative nursing management, and patient outcomes.

CAROTID ENDARTERECTOMY

The carotid endarterectomy (CE) procedure was first introduced in 1953 by Robb. The procedure involves incising the carotid artery to remove obstructing and embolizing plaque from the intima of the common carotid artery (CCA) at the bifurcation of the external carotid artery (ECA) and internal carotid artery (ICA). The purpose of this procedure is to prevent the occurrence or worsening of an ischemic neurologic deficit caused by a carotid lesion. The CE is the second most commonly performed vascular procedure, second only to coronary artery revascularization. Yet despite the decreasing incidence of stroke, the frequency of CE performance continues to increase. In the last 15 years, over 300 reports on the procedure have appeared in medical literature. Yet, controversy remains about the efficacy of the procedure, since these reports either conflict or are incomplete. Specific questions relating to patient selection, efficacy in preventing stroke, and maximum acceptable morbidity and mortality rates remain to be answered.

Indications

The primary indication for CE is evidence of carotid artery stenosis and one or more corresponding transient ischemic attack (TIA) episodes. In addition, those persons with limited, stable deficits who demonstrate a lesion on angiogram (such as a high-grade carotid stenosis) that places them at a high risk for recurrent stroke may be advised by the surgeon of potential benefit from CE. Controversy surrounds other indications for the procedure. In studies that have examined CE in the population with progressive or unstable neurologic deficit, some patients have demonstrated remarkable neurologic improvement. However, surgical mortality rates are often quite high. Therefore, the patient with a progressive deficit is usually considered a poor surgical candidate. Morbidity and mortality rates are also high for those patients with moderate to severe fixed neurologic deficits; therefore, CE is not advocated in this population. However, patients with completed strokes may benefit from CE, if they have evidenced good recovery and have lesions on angiogram (ICA ulceration, carotid stenosis greater than 80%) that place them at risk for recurrent stroke. Perhaps the greatest controversy surrounds the asymptomatic patient who, during evaluation of a carotid bruit, is found to have greater than 75% stenosis of the carotid artery. Providing the patient is medically stable, morbidity and mortality rates following CE in this population are low. Most importantly, stroke incidence and carotid occlusion have been demonstrated to be lower in the CE population when compared with the medically managed population. In contrast, other studies have shown no change in stroke incidence in the operated patient. Consequently, there remains disagreement about appropriateness of surgery in patients with asymptomatic bruit. Overall, these indications highlight the importance of CE as a preventive procedure.

Other contraindications to the procedure exist. Patients with multiple vascular lesions are considered poor risks. Such lesions might include contralateral ICA occlusion or stenosis above the siphon, vertebral stenosis or occlusion, contralateral carotid artery occlusion, and evidence of aortic arch arteriosclerosis. Medical risks include ischemic heart disease (especially recent myocardial infarction), poorly controlled hypertension, chronic obstructive pulmonary disease, obesity, and age over 70 years.

Preprocedural Nursing Management

Preoperative nursing management focuses on assessment of baseline function, facilitation of the patient's transition through testing, and patient education. (Refer to this section under Extracranial-Intracranial Bypass on p. 42.)

If the patient was asymptomatic before surgery, symptoms referable to the lesion should be explained to the patient along with the importance of reporting such symptoms. For example, a patient with asymptomatic stenosis of the left carotid artery should be told to report symptoms of right hand, arm, and/or leg numbness, tingling or weakness, speech difficulties, or any change in vision.

Additional testing unique to the CE population may include high resolution ultrasound duplex real-time imaging with transcranial Doppler sonography. In addition, ophthalmodynamometry and oculopneumoplethysmography (OPG) testing may be ordered. These tests are commonly performed on an outpatient basis but may be incorporated into the patient's preoperative evaluation during hospitalization.

Procedural Aspects

The carotid endarterectomy procedure is designed to improve or restore blood flow through the carotid system by removal of artherosclerotic plaque from the carotid bifurcation. Plans for the specific approach or any special needs (such as a graft) are established before the patient's arrival in the operating room (OR). There are many variations to the procedure but it is usually performed as follows.

The patient is taken to the OR and placed under general anesthesia. Arterial pressure is monitored via an indwelling catheter; other hemodynamic monitoring devices are placed as necessary. The neck area is shaved as necessary, and skin is prepped in the manner customary to the institution. The patient is placed in the supine position with her head turned lateral to allow adequate exposure to the operative side of the neck. The head is then stabilized. If additional monitoring techniques are used (such as intraoperative electroencephalogram (EEG) or regional cerebral blood flow monitoring (rCBF)), detectors are placed at this time. If a saphenous vein graft is planned, the operative leg is also positioned, shaved, and prepped.

A linear incision is made along the anterior border of the sternocleidomastoid muscle (Fig. 4-1), and the carotid bifurcation is exposed (Fig. 4-2). The CCA, ECA, and ICA are gently dissected,

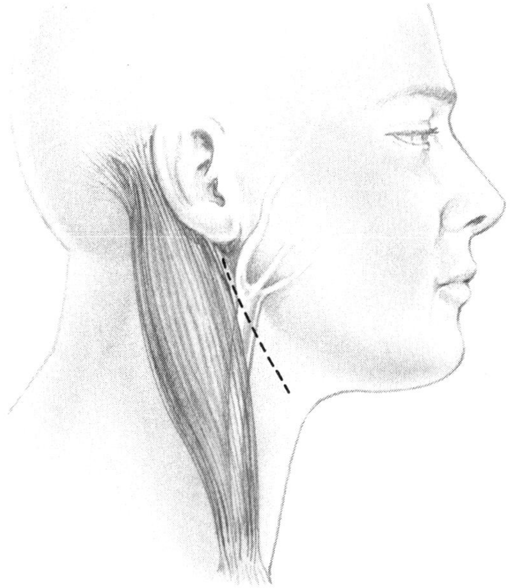

Fig. 4-1 Line of skin incision in relationship to sternocleidomastoid muscle and underlying carotid arteries.*

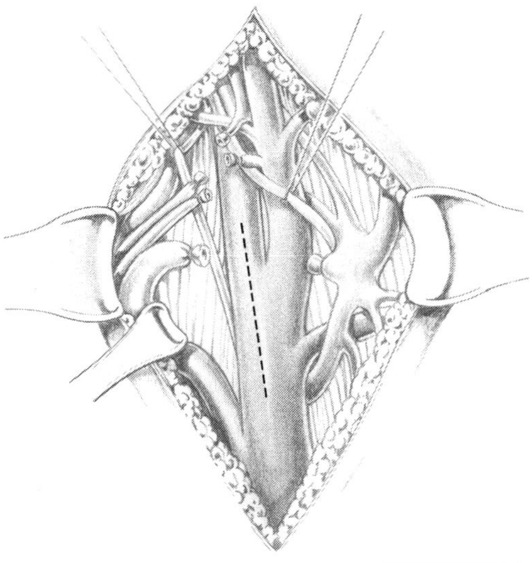

Fig. 4-2 Carotid artery branches are exposed and widely mobilized; facial vein and small veins in region of bifurcation are ligated. Incision is indicated by dotted line.

avoiding manipulation of the carotid sinus. The sinus may be injected with 1% xylocaine to avoid blood pressure fluctuations. Heparin (7000 units) is administered intravenously. The ECA, CCA, and ICA are occluded with noncrushing clamps above and below the stenotic or occluded area. Should any change in EEG activity or rCBF occur, a temporary shunt may be placed to preserve blood flow by creating a temporary carotid bypass. Blood pressure must be closely controlled during clamping to promote adequate cerebral perfusion.

Using loupes or magnifying glasses, an incision is made into the ICA and CCA. Plaque material is gently dissected out of the intima, usually in one piece (Fig. 4-3). Any plaque extending into the ECA will also be dissected. Plaque extending proximally toward the aorta may be dissected using special instruments. The vessels are then irrigated with a 1:100 heparin solution and any fragments are washed out. Should the vessels be unusually small or appear to be weakened, a saphenous vein, Gortex or Dacron graft may be sutured into place to allow for greater vessel diameter (Fig. 4-4). A thin teflon sheath may be used for vessel reinforcement. The remaining arterial incision is then sutured (Fig. 4-5). Clamps are removed from the CCA, ECA, and ICA, respectively, restoring flow. Usual duration of occlusion is 15 to 20 mintues. If a graft is placed, occlusion may last up to 40 minutes. Muscle and skin are then approximated and closed with a fine running suture (Fig. 4-6). A small Penrose drain may be left in place to minimize fluid accumulation in the wound. The incision is then dressed and the patient sent to the recovery room.

Variations in this procedure may be performed according to the patient's unique situation. When an occluded ICA is serving as a source of embolization through the ECA, ICA stump angioplasty with ECA endarterectomy may be peformed. Occlusion or stenosis of the ICA distal to the bifur-

*Figs. 4-1 through 4-10 are from American Association of Neuroscience Nurses: Core curriculum for neurosurgical nursing in the operating room, Chicago, 1980, The Association.

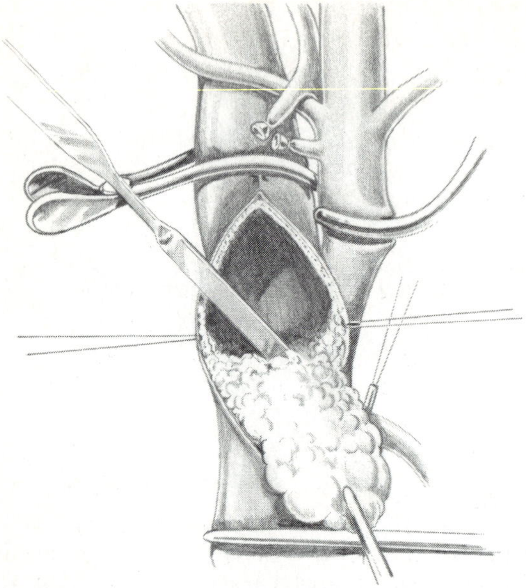

Fig. 4-3 Plaque is carefully dissected free of underlying media.

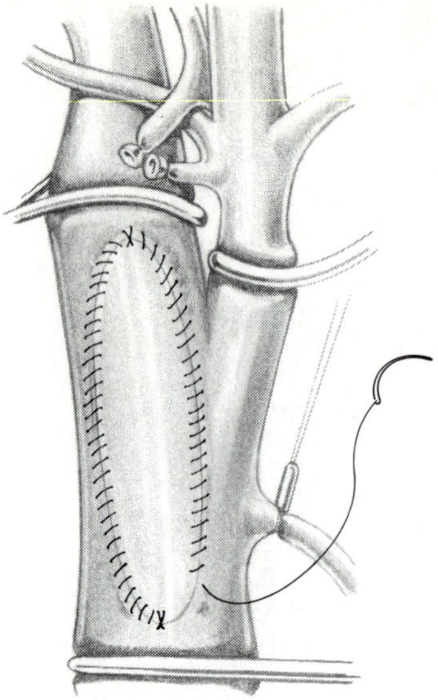

Fig. 4-4 Incision may be closed with a patch.

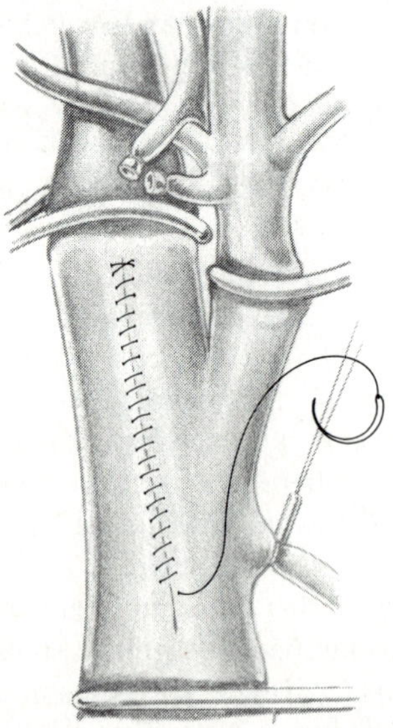

Fig. 4-5 Incision may also be closed directly with running polypropylene sutures.

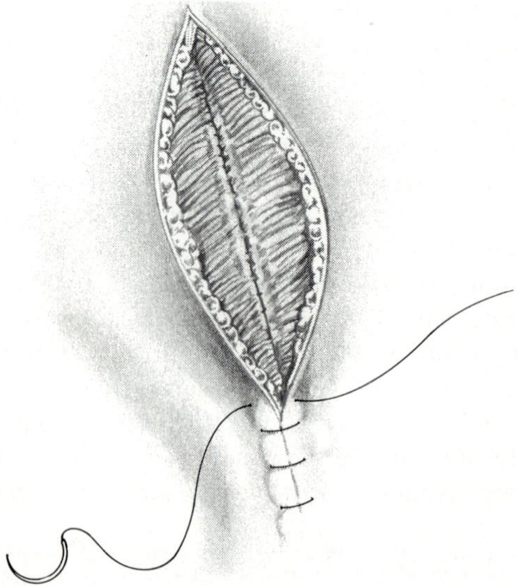

Fig. 4-6 Platysma and skin are closed with suture.

cation may be treated by threading a Fogarty balloon catheter into the area and inflating the balloon in an attempt to restore flow through this area. Endarterectomies have been performed on other vessels with lesser frequency and greater risk. Other vessels include the middle cerebral artery (MCA), and vertebral-basilar system.

Postprocedural Nursing Management

During the postoperative period, nursing care is focused on close monitoring for any change in baseline function, institution of measures to prevent any complications, and provision of patient education in preparation for discharge.

Neurologic function, as previously described, should be monitored at least every 2 hours for the first 24 hours after surgery, then every 4 hours for the next 24 hours, then every shift until the patient is discharged. Observations are compared with the patient's baseline, with specific attention paid to any subtle changes. In particular, any symptoms referable to the operative side should be noted and reported immediately. In addition, because of the close proximity of several cranial nerves to the carotid bifurcation, the facial, vagus, spinal accesory, and hypoglossal nerves on the operative side should be closely evaluated and any deficits reported immediately. Blood pressure should be monitored closely and maintained within 20 mm Hg of the patient's preoperative norm. Carotid sinus manipulation may cause lability in blood pressure. Any hypotension or hypertension should be reported immediately because of the danger of carotid occlusion or hemorrhage at the operative site, respectively. Monitoring ECG pattern is advocated for 24 hours after surgery because of the possibility of preexisting cardiac disease contributing to the patient's situation. Patients should also be encouraged to report any subjective cardiac symptoms. Cardiac complaints or ECG abnormalities should be reported immediately.

Respiratory status must be monitored closely because edema or hematoma in the operative site might cause tracheal deviation and subsequent respiratory distress. Any difficulty in swallowing or respiratory distress should be reported immediately. Some physicians recommend frequent measurements of neck circumference to determine the presence of an expanding hematoma. However, bleeding may occur internally without change in neck circumference. Bleeding or hemorrhage may be a concern because administered intraoperative heparin is not reversed. Therefore, in addition to being alert for signs of obvious bleeding from or inside the operative site, the nurse should closely monitor the patient's clotting values, hematocrit, and hemoglobin. Wound integrity should be assessed at least every shift. Any evidence of frank bleeding or decline in those laboratory values should be reported immediately. Preexisting medical problems should be monitored closely during the postoperative period. Oral temperature should be monitored at least once each shift, and any temperature over 37.5°C should be reported.

Preventive nursing measures are important during this time. Bed rest is usually enforced for 24 hours after surgery. The patient should be encouraged to lie on his back or nonoperative side with his head slightly elevated. If a pillow placed under the head causes neck kinking, the pillow may be removed. Turning and deep breathing while in bed should be encouraged. Intermittent positive pressure breathing (IPPB) treatments may be ordered. Once mobility restrictions are lifted, ambulation should be encouraged but with caution to avoid postural hypotension and fatigue. Some physicians order medications (such as heparin, warfarin, aspirin, or dipyridamole) to promote carotid patency. These and other preoperative medications ordered during the preoperative period should be administered as ordered while the patient is observed for any adverse effects. Although the incidence of seizures is low in the CE population, seizures may occur during the postoperative period. Any patient with a history of seizure should have seizure precautions available at the bedside. Nutritional status may be a concern. A clear liquid diet may be started once bowel sounds have returned and the patient's abilty to swallow adequately has been assessed.

Diet is then advanced as tolerated. Constipation is not unusual during the postoperative period. Fluids, diet, and activity may prevent or alleviate this problem; laxatives may be necessary.

Preparing the patient for discharge through adequate patient education is essential. (Education should include expectations during the hospital stay and patient responsibilities following discharge.) Length of hospital stay is usually 2 to 5 days. Sutures may be removed on the seventh day or earlier, with steri-strips applied at the physician's discretion. Once sutures are removed, no special wound care is required. Should a hematoma be present, it may persist for a month or even longer; patients should not be concerned because this will gradually reabsorb. Driving is usually restricted until the first follow-up visit. Fatigue is normal and rest is required. Pain is usually not a problem but, if necessary, the physician will usually recommend acetaminophen. Blood pressure control is important. The patient should be encouraged to monitor BP at home and continue antihypertensive medications as ordered. The purpose, dose, frequency, and potential adverse effects of all discharge medications should be reviewed with the patient and family. The need for follow-up care with the physician and therapy (if applicable) should be discussed. Return to work should be discussed on an individual basis with the physician but, generally, it is allowed 4 to 6 weeks after surgery. Any other activity restrictions should be reviewed. The importance and types of symptoms to report should be reviewed in detail. Written information to supplement teaching and a contact phone number for questions should also be given.

Outcome

Outcome can be measured in a variety of ways. In spite of the numerous reports evaluating outcome in this population, efficacy is yet to be agreed upon by clinicians.

Mortality from the procedure generally ranges from 1% to 2.1%. However, ranges reported in the literature are 0% to 51%, depending on the condition of the patient and the lesion involved. Permanent morbidity rates generally range from 1% to 3.5%. The lowest morbidity and mortality rates are reported in patients who had stable TIAs or were asymptomatic before surgery. Patients with progressive strokes or recurrent strokes during one admission who were subsequently operated on had much higher morbidity and mortality rates. In addition, timing of surgical intervention appears controversial. Based on results from older studies, physicians waited 4 to 6 weeks after an ischemic episode to operate. However, it was found that patients whose surgery was delayed longer than 3 weeks had not only an increased risk of recurrent stroke but also higher postoperative morbidity and mortality rates. Therefore, surgery is often recommended for the stable patient 1 to 2 weeks after an ischemic episode. Other factors that appear to influence postoperative morbidity and mortality include the surgeon's technical expertise and evidence of other preexisting disease.

Specific complications reported in the literature range from operative to medical complications as follows:

- **Hypotension resulting from manipulation of the carotid bulb**—could lead to potential carotid artery thrombosis and subsequent stroke
- **Hypertension**—could lead to potential hemorrhage at the operative site or to intracranial hemorrhage
- **Intracranial hemorrhage**—thought to be related to a hyperperfusion syndrome that follows restoration of blood flow to an ischemic area
- **Wound hematoma**—if sufficiently large can cause tracheal deviation and respiratory distress; usually avoided by placement of a Penrose drain
- **Cranial nerve injury**—resulting from the proximity of cranial nerves to the carotid bifurcation (cranial nerves possibly affected with related deficits are listed in Table 4-1.)
- **Recurrent stenosis**—reported incidence is less than 2%
- **Medical complications**—including myocardial infarction and pulmonary embolus

The true benefit of CE in preventing stroke or reducing stroke incidence remains controversial.

Table 4-1 Cranial nerve deficits following carotid endarterectomy

Involved cranial nerve	Type of deficit
Facial (7th CN)	Facial weakness (usually affecting lower face and mouth)
Vagus (10th CN)	Dysphagia Loss of gag reflex Dysarthria Hoarseness
Spinal acessory (11th CN)	Shoulder droop Difficulty turning head, shrugging shoulder, or raising arm horizontally
Hypoglossal (12th CN)	Dysarthria Dysphagia Tongue weakness Upper airway obstruction

Several studies have demonstrated no decrease in stroke incidence in the operative vs nonoperative group and, at times, have even demonstrated an increase in stroke incidence. Operated patients with carotid lesions and corresponding TIAs have a significantly lower stroke incidence (2%) as compared with the stroke incidence in the TIA population (6%). In addition, patients who underwent prophylactic CE for asymptomatic high-grade carotid stenosis had minimal incidence of stroke after 10 years of follow-up and a long-term survival rate similar to a healthy age-matched population. Further research is warranted in this area. Despite the controversy, the procedure continues to be performed.

EXTRACRANIAL-INTRACRANIAL BYPASS

The extracranial-intracranial (EC-IC) bypass procedure was introduced in 1967 by Yasargil. The surgery creates a bypass of an occluded or stenotic vessel that is inaccessible by a direct surgical approach. Lesions involving the internal carotid, middle cerebral, or vertebral arteries may be bypassed. Even though the surgery is technically feasible and carries a low morbidity and mortality rate, controversy remains regarding exact indications and the benefit of the procedure. To date, the EC-IC bypass is the most widely used method of cerebral circulatory augmentation.

Indications

The primary indication for the EC-IC bypass is occlusion of the ICA or stenosis of the siphon of the ICA and clinical evidence of corresponding ischemia. For example, the patient demonstrating a TIA involving the right arm and hand in addition to expressive aphasia, who on angiography demonstrates a left ICA occlusion, may be considered a surgical candidate. Patients with symptomatic MCA stenosis or occlusion are also potential candidates. Generally, the extent of ischemic deficit is an important factor. Patients with TIAs or a mild completed stroke are considered good candidates, whereas those with severe or progressive deficits are considered poor candidates. An additional requirement is the presence of inadequate collateral circulation. Surgery is not advocated, even in the presence of symptomatic high grade stenosis or occlusion, when collateral circulation appears angiographically adequate. Other contraindications to surgery include medical risks (such as recent myocardial infarction or other serious cardiac disease); severe, uncontrolled hypertension or diabetes; renal failure; or progressive malignancy.

It has been suggested, in light of the recent EC-IC Bypass Study (Awad and Spetzler, 1986), that indications for the bypass be revised. Recommendations include evidence of ICA occlusion with subsequent symptoms following the initial episode; persistence of symptoms with adequate medical management; and angiographic progression of the lesion.

Other less common indications for the bypass procedure exist. Posterior circulation bypass may be indicated in the presence of vertebrobasilar junction or distal basilar stenosis when corresponding symptoms are present. In situations in which intentional occlusion of the ICA is planned, the bypass may be performed before the intentional occlusion to provide adequate collateral circulation. Such situations include carotid cavernous malformations fed by the ICA.

Preprocedural Nursing Management

Preoperative nursing management focuses on assessment of baseline function, facilitation of the patient's transition through testing, and patient education.

In establishing baseline status, the nurse focuses on evaluating neurologic function. Evaluation includes assessment of motor, sensory, and cranial nerve function; level of consciousness; cognitive function; and speech with specific attention paid to deficits in any of these areas. Also, a detailed history of the ischemic event experienced should be obtained. This history should include a description of specific deficits experienced, warning symptoms, duration of symptoms, and residual effects. Since patients may be unfamiliar with which symptoms are important to report, specific questions to elicit this information should be asked. Multiple ischemic episodes may have occurred; each episode should be described. Recording this information on the chart is essential for comparison of future events. The patient should be questioned about preexisting medical diseases, in particular, cardiac, renal or pulmonary disease, hypertension, or diabetes. A baseline picture of the patient's blood pressure (BP) and cardiac status, usually through an ECG, should be established.

Additional testing may be accomplished during the preoperative period. The nurse's role focuses on informing the patient of the testing scheduled, what the testing involves, and the patient's role in the testing. Specific testing that might be indicated includes cerebral angiography, computerized axial tomography (CT) scan, magnetic resonance imaging (MRI), and electroencephalogram (EEG). If available, regional cerebral blood flow (rCBF) measurements may be ordered. Some institutions incorporate neuropsychologic evaluations as part of the baseline assessment. Additional testing may be ordered, depending on the patient's situation. For example, detailed cardiac studies, pulmonary function studies, or other laboratory work may be ordered.

Patient and family teaching during the preoperative period is essential in promoting an optimal outcome. Information provided clarifies the underlying disease process while reinforcing the rationale for surgery. In addition, the nurse must reinforce the purpose of the surgery and the anticipated outcome, emphasizing that present deficits are not expected to improve. Information should also be provided on what the surgical procedure involves, the length of the surgery, and anticipated postoperative discomforts and restrictions. During this time, patients and families should be given the opportunity to ask questions and express concerns or fears. It may be helpful to have a patient who has completed the surgery talk to the patient and family. Any unusual fears or concerns should be relayed to the surgeon.

Procedural Aspects

An EC-IC bypass procedure revascularizes the brain, bypassing an occluded or stenotic vessel by diverting blood supply from a scalp artery to a superficial cortical artery. Plans for the specific approach are established before the patient's arrival in the operating room (OR). The procedure is usually accomplished as follows.

The patient is taken to the OR and placed under general anesthesia. Arterial pressure is monitored via an indwelling catheter; other hemodynamic monitoring devices are placed as necessary. The head is shaved and skin prepped in the manner customary to the institution. The patient is placed in the supine position with the head turned lateral to maintain the operative site in the uppermost position. The head is stabilized by applying a head frame.

An incision is made alongside of the scalp artery selected, usually the superficial temporal artery (STA), a branch of the external carotid artery (Fig. 4-7). (Although diversion of blood supply from this artery may impair scalp circulation, collateral circulation is usually more than adequate to prevent any circulatory compromise.) The artery is care-

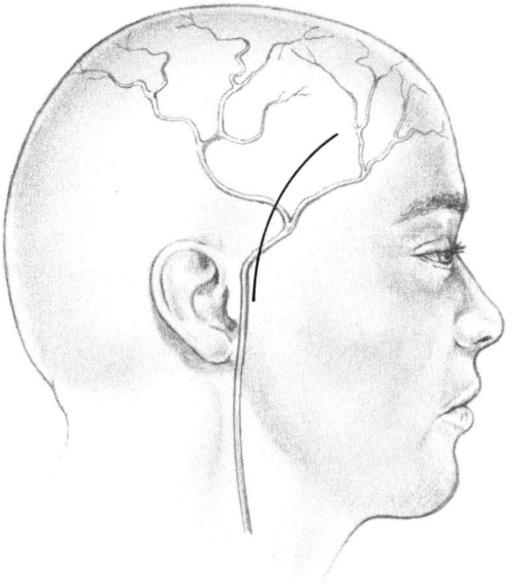

Fig. 4-7 Gently curving skin incision near superficial temporal artery. Craniectomy is performed over Sylvian fissure.

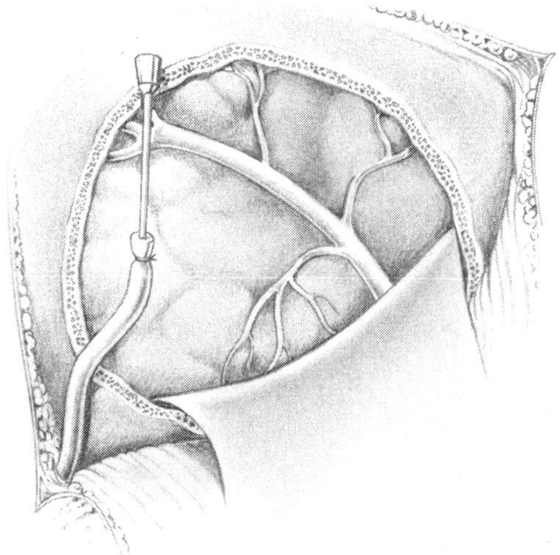

Fig. 4-8 Skin and dura retracted. Superficial temporal artery and pedicle dissected from skin flap and distended with heparinized saline.

fully dissected away from the scalp (Fig. 4-8). Underlying muscle is incised and the cranium is exposed. A small burr hole, up to 7 cm in diameter, is made and the dura opened, exposing the cortex and superficial cortical vessels.

The OR microscope is brought into place to examine the cortical surface and vessels, and an appropriate artery for anastomosis is selected. The angular or posterior branches of the MCA are usually selected because of their size and accessibility. Preparation of the arteries for anastomosis is also performed under the microscope. Branches of the scalp artery are ligated and a noncrushing temporary clip is applied to the distal end. The artery is cut diagonally to maximize anastomotic area; the artery is then mobilized. Two noncrushing temporary clips are then applied to the cortical artery, one proximal and one distal to the anticipated anastomotic site (Fig. 4-9). The cortical artery is then incised between the clips and blood is drained from the clamped arterial segment. The segment is irrigated with a heparinized solution and a silastic stent inserted to maintain patency and facilitate suturing. The scalp artery is approximated over the cortical artery and sutured into place (Fig. 4-10). The stent is removed before final suturing is completed. The clips are removed and blood flow is restored. The anastomotic site is examined for adequacy of flow and hemostasis.

The dura is loosely approximated to allow adequate room for the scalp artery. Fascia and the temporalis muscle are approximated separately, then the scalp is carefully sutured to avoid pressure on the anastomosis. Pulsation of the scalp artery (STA) can be palpated to provide a rough indication of anastomotic patency. The incision is then dressed and the patient is sent to the recovery room.

Occasionally, unusual circumstances preclude the procedure from being performed as described. Should the STA or other branches be inadequate, a superficial vein from the leg or arm may be harvested and incorporated as a graft between a branch

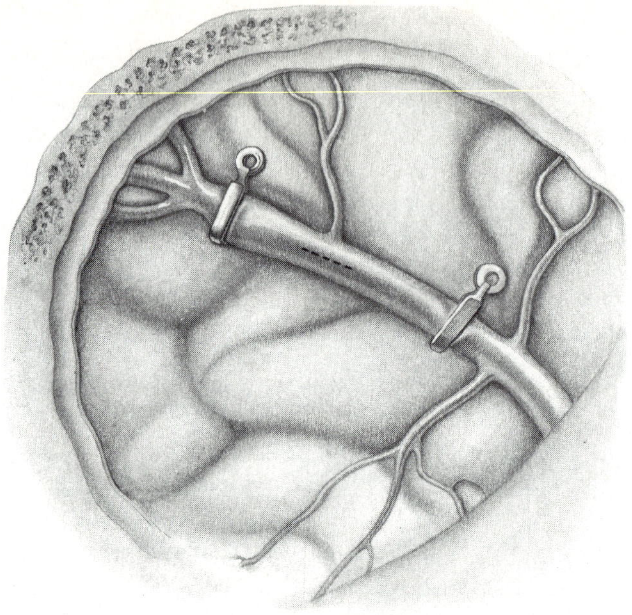

Fig. 4-9 Middle cerebral artery is clamped. Dotted line indicates incision for anastamosis.

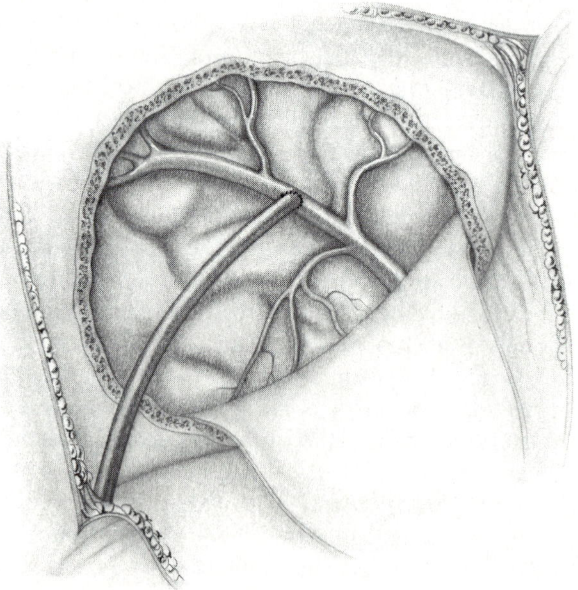

Fig. 4-10 The anastamosis is completed with a needle on monofilament nylon suture.

of the external carotid artery (ECA) and a branch of the MCA. Branches of the occipital artery have also been used for MCA anastomosis. Although posterior fossa revascularization has been performed in fewer cases, it is technically feasible. In the first posterior circulation procedure (performed by Ausman), the occipital artery was anastomosed to the posterior inferior cerebellar artery (PICA). Other posterior revascularization procedures have since been performed, including occipital to anterior inferior cerebellar artery (AICA) anastomosis, and STA to superior cerebellar artery anastomosis.

Postprocedural Nursing Management

During the postoperative period, nursing care focuses on close monitoring for any change in baseline function, institution of measures to prevent any complications, and provision of patient education for discharge planning.

Neurologic function (as previously described) should be monitored every 2 hours for the first 24 hours after surgery, then every 4 hours for 48 hours, then every shift until the patient is discharged. Neurologic status is compared with the patient's baseline, with particular attention paid to any subtle changes. New deficits should be reported immediately to the surgeon. It is important for the nurse to know about the patient's previous ischemic episodes to determine whether new deficits correspond to them. Blood pressure must be closely monitored. As a general rule, postoperative BP should be within 20 mm Hg of the patient's preoperative norm. Hypertension or hypotension may occur during the postoperative period, leading to hemorrhage or occlusion of the anastomosis. Any deviation in BP should be reported immediately. Since cardiac arrhythmias may contribute to morbidity and mortality, ECG monitoring is advocated for 24 to 48 hours after surgery. Patients should also be encouraged to report any subjective cardiac symptoms, such as chest pain or shortness of breath, especially when a past history of cardiac symptoms is reported. Cardiac symptoms or ECG changes should be reported immediately.

Other preexisting problems should also be closely monitored during the postoperative period. The STA pulse quality should be assessed at least once each shift (on the side of operation) as a rough measure of anastomostic patency. In addition, the wound should be assessed a minimum of once each shift. Any evidence of infection, bleeding, or other drainage should be reported. Swelling in the operative area is not unusual and may peak 72 hours after surgery. Ecchymosis is not unusual in the operative area. Any other change in incisional or scalp coloration should be reported because this may indicate early necrosis of the skin flap. Oral temperature is monitored at least once each shift, with the nurse reporting any temperature over 37.5° C. Finally, patients should be informed about the necessity of monitoring all of these aspects during the postoperative period, especially if they feel well or their status is stable.

Preventive measures are important during this time. Bed rest is usually enforced for 24 to 48 hours after surgery. The patient should be encouraged to lie on her nonoperative side or back with her head elevated for comfort, avoiding pressure on the bypass site. If the head is dressed, the dressing may need to be loosened (should edema occur) to avoid constriction of the bypass. Turning and deep breathing while in bed should be encouraged. IPPB treatments may be ordered. Once bed rest is eliminated, early mobilization is advocated but with caution to avoid hypotension and fatigue. Some physicians incorporate medications (such as antiplatelet aggregates) into the patient's postoperative regime to promote and maintain bypass patency. Preoperative medications will most likely be continued during the postoperative period. Medications should be administered as ordered while the patient is observed for any adverse effects. Although the incidence of seizures is low following mild stroke, seizures may occur in the susceptible patient during the postoperative period. Any patient with a history of seizures should have seizure precautions available at the bedside. Nutritional status may be a concern. Clear liquids are started as bowel sounds return, and diet is advanced as tolerated.

INSTRUCTIONS FOR THE PATIENT AFTER CEREBRAL BYPASS SURGERY

Your physician has established the following guidelines to aid in your recovery. Take time to review this information before leaving the hospital. We will be happy to answer any further questions you might have.

1. Avoid driving a car for the first week after discharge from the hospital. If you have any visual problems, these should be evaluated by an eye doctor before you resume driving.
2. Your activity is limited only by how you feel. Be as active as you like but avoid contact sports or other strenuous activity until advised by your doctor. Avoid heavy lifting (over 20 lbs.) for 1 month. Walking is excellent exercise and can help improve your strength and endurance. Stair climbing is acceptable.
3. It is normal to feel tired for the first few weeks after surgery. Gradually increase your activity while allowing time for rest and the tiredness will disappear.
4. Sexual relations are permitted.
5. Medications may not be necessary; however, if medications are necessary, take only those prescribed by your doctor.
6. A mild headache is to be expected occasionally for the first few weeks after surgery; you may take aspirin or acetaminophen (Tylenol) for this. Report persistent or severe headaches to your physician.
7. Once the sutures (stitches) have been removed, you may wash your scalp and hair as you please. Avoid rubbing the incision until it is well healed; pat it dry after bathing. Itching around the incision is a normal part of the healing process. It is also normal to have unusual sensations in the scalp during healing. Once your hair is grown out, you may comb or brush your hair as usual. A permanent wave may be used on the hair as long as the scalp is healed.
8. You will notice a small depression in your scalp and skull bone; this is where the bypass was done and is normal. This area will not close up but does not represent any danger to you. Avoid prolonged pressure near the bypass site. This includes anything that leaves an indentation in the skin, such as eyeglasses, hats, etc.
9. Report any unusual symptoms to your physician, especially symptoms similar to those you experienced before surgery.
10. If you work, you should expect to return to work 4 to 6 weeks after surgery. Specific return-to-work dates will be discussed at your follow-up visit.
11. Any other follow-up care will be discussed as necessary.

Printed with permission of the Department of Neurological Surgery, Loyola University Medical Center, Maywood, IL.

Constipation is not unusual during the postoperative period. Fluids, diet, and activity may prevent or alleviate this problem; laxatives may be necessary.

Preparing the patient for discharge through adequate patient education is essential. Length of hospital stay is usually 5 to 8 days. Sutures are usually removed on the seventh postoperative day unless there is a concern about scalp healing. Once the sutures are removed, no special wound care is required. Driving may be restricted for 1 week and lifting restricted for 1 month. Because the patient may experience fatigue, rest is necessary. Mild headache is not unusual and may be relieved with acetaminophen. Blood pressure (BP) control remains important; patients should be encouraged to monitor BP while at home and continue antihypertensive medications. The purpose, dose, frequency, and potential adverse effects of all discharge medications should be reviewed with the patient and family. The necessity for follow-up care, including physician and therapy follow-up, should be discussed. In addition, follow-up angiography is often necessary to determine bypass patency. Measures to avoid pressure around the bypass site should also be discussed. By the time of discharge, the patient may sleep on the side of the bypass. However, any constriction around the ear (e.g., eyeglasses with a tight ear piece, tight hats, or wigs, etc.) should be avoided. Return to work should be discussed on an individual basis with the physician, but generally is allowed 4 to 6 weeks after surgery. The types of symptoms to report and their significance should be reviewed in detail, particularly in light of the lack of knowledge about symptoms documented in previous studies. Written information could be offered to supplement teaching (an example is included in the box on p. 46). Finally, a contact phone number should be given to provide a postdischarge source of information as necessary.

COMPLICATIONS OF EC-IC BYPASS

Occlusion of anastomosis
Superficial wound infection
Scalp necrosis
Subdural hygroma
Hematoma: subdural or intracerebral
Systemic complications: pneumonia, myocardial infarction, pulmonary embolus, septicemia

Outcome

Patient outcome following EC-IC bypass can be measured in a variety of ways. Although a number of studies have evaluated the outcome following this procedure, efficacy of the procedure is yet to be agreed upon by clinicians. Specific outcome aspects evaluated are as follows:

- **Morbidity and mortality**—Statistics have led most clinicians to conclude that the procedure is relatively safe. Thirty-day mortality rates are reportedly 2% to 4%. Specific complications reported are listed in the box above.
- **Stroke incidence**—Since the bypass is designed as a preventive procedure, stroke incidence following surgery is an important factor in outcome. A number of studies have reported a favorable decrease in stroke incidence. Chater (1983), Sundt (1985), and others report a 0.9% per year stroke incidence following surgery as compared with a 6% per year stroke incidence in patients with TIAs. Others have reported similar results. However, in the most extensive prospective randomized study in this population, the EC-IC Bypass Study Group reported a 20.3% stroke incidence in the bypass population, as compared with a 13.8% stroke incidence in the medically treated group. This has led some to conclude that until further investigation occurs, payment for the procedure should be eliminated and performance of the procedure restricted. Those critical of this study cite lack of information on collateral circulation, patient selection, lack of control of extraneous variables and criteria for stenosis, observer bias, and other reasons for the Bypass Study Group's findings. Additional study of efficacy is, of course, recommended. Despite the controversy, the procedure continues to be performed.
- **Neurologic function**—Neurologic function has been found to be preserved or improved following surgery. When neuropsychological function was evaluated, no change in status was noted up to 9 months after surgery, indicating that patients with deficits did not experience improvement. Decline in neuropsychologic function is not the norm following this procedure. Further research is indicated in this area with respect to identifying those whose neuropsychologic status might improve with the surgery.
- **Technical success**—Success of the procedure may be evaluated by examining bypass patency and cerebral blood flow. Patency rates for the anastomosis have been reported at 95% to 99%, indicating that surgery is technically feasible. Significant improvements have also been reported in local and overall rCBF following surgery; however, the exact relationship to ischemic symptoms is unclear.
- **Quality of life**—Any surgical procedure should be undertaken in part to improve quality of life. Yet few studies evaluate this particular aspect. In a study by Stewart-Amidei and Penckofer (1988), quality of life was assessed retrospec-

tively in the post-bypass population. Objectively, a decrease in the frequency and number of ischemic symptoms was reported following surgery. Also, patients working before ischemic symptoms and surgery were able to return to work after surgery. Subjectively, patients reported increased satisfaction with life, social activity, and body image after surgery. Other subjective and objective indicators were found to be insignificant. It appears the bypass procedure may be of value in improving overall quality of life, an important aspect to consider when planning and evaluating the outcome of this procedure.

CRANIOTOMY FOR REMOVAL OF INTRACRANIAL HEMATOMA

Hypertensive intracranial hematomas (ICH) may occur supratentorially or subtentorially; common locations are the thalamus and the cerebellum. These patients are usually seriously ill with moderate to severe neurologic deficits, increased intracranial pressure (ICP), and unstable blood pressure. Hence, surgical intervention is a precarious proposition and carries a high mortality rate. However, prompt surgical intervention may not only save the patient's life but also restore neurologic function.

Indications

Surgery is usually indicated when the hemorrhage is large enough to act as a space-occupying lesion, contributing to mechanical compression and increased ICP. Other factors to consider are anatomic location and clinical status. Hemorrhages located more superficially in the cerebral hemispheres or cerebellum are more easily approached. The more stable the patient, the better the prognosis. Patients with severe deficits or those who are moribund often have a poor outcome and do not do well with surgery. Studies have shown patients with hypertensive ICH appear to have the same benefit from conservative medical therapy as from surgery. Surgery involves entry into and manipulation of brain tissue, which may contribute to additional damage, whereas, if the patient survives the initial bleeding, eventually it will resolve, although permanent deficits are expected. Each case must therefore be considered on an individual basis.

Preprocedural Nursing Management

Since craniotomy is most commonly performed as an emergent procedure, the nurse's preoperative role focuses on establishing a baseline assessment and preparing the patient for surgery. A baseline assessment should include detailed evaluation of level of consciousness, motor, sensory and cranial nerve function, and reflex activity. Baseline blood pressure, cardiopulmonary status, and temperature are also determined. Routine surgical preparation proceeds as customary to the institution. During this time, the nurse plays an important role in administering treatments as ordered to stabilize the patient's situation. For example, medications might be ordered to control blood pressure and decrease ICP. Because these patients usually have a decreased level of consciousness, the nurse's presence provides reassurance for the patient and support and communication for the family.

Procedural Aspects

Craniotomy for removal of an intracranial hematoma is an invasive procedure. Surgical approaches for ICH based on involved anatomy are summarized in Fig. 4-11. The procedure is usually accomplished as follows.

The patient is taken to the OR and placed under general anesthesia. Arterial pressure is monitored via an indwelling catheter; other hemodynamic monitoring devices are placed as necessary. The head is shaved and the skin prepped in the manner customary to the institution. For an intracerebral bleed, the patient is placed in a supine position with his head turned lateral to maintain the operative site uppermost. For a cerebellar hemorrhage, the patient is placed in the sitting position. The head is stabilized by applying a head frame.

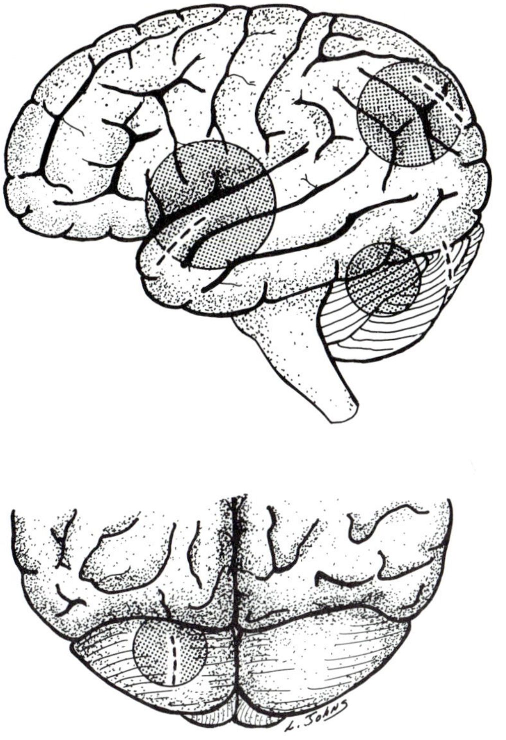

Fig. 4-11 Common sites for intracerebral hemorrhage with surgical approach indicated.

An appropriate scalp incision is made and the craniotomy performed to remove the bone over the site of hemorrhage. Craniectomy (removal of a smaller piece of bone that will not be replaced) is performed for cerebellar hemorrhage. The dura is opened and brain tissue entered or retracted to reach the site of the hemorrhage. Then the hematoma is evacuated, the dura is closed, and the bone flap replaced. Skin and underlying muscle are approximated and sutured. If the surgeon is concerned about recurrence, a drain may be left in place for 24 to 48 hours. The incision is dressed and the patient sent to the recovery room.

New developments in the neurosurgical realm offer some promise to the patient with ICH. Specifically, a stereotactic approach to the hemorrhage in its early stages, with the patient under local or general anesthesia, appears to have a better outcome. The procedure is less invasive and often requires less time. It can hold superior results to medical treatment because the brain can begin its recovery process immediately rather than waiting weeks to months for the hematoma to resolve. This procedure is expected to be performed with increasing frequency as stereotactic equipment and expertise become more readily available.

Postprocedural Nursing Management

Postcraniotomy care focuses on close monitoring for any change in baseline function, institution of measures to prevent complications, and preparation for discharge.

Neurologic function is monitored frequently as previously described. Improvement or decline in neurologic function should be reported immediately. Blood pressure monitoring is essential during the immediate postoperative period because hypertension may contribute to recurrent hemorrhage. Cardiac rhythm should be monitored and any arrhythmias reported. Airway and respiratory status are also closely observed, with interventions implemented as appropriate. Preexisting problems should be closely monitored.

Wound integrity is monitored each shift. Any evidence of unusual edema, bleeding, drainage, or infection should be reported immediately. Preventive measures are also important during this time. The patient should be positioned with her head elevated in a neutral position to assist in control of ICP and minimize edema. Because seizures are possible, seizure precautions should be available at the bedside. Often, prophylactic anticonvulsants are ordered. Fluids and nutritional support are provided as necessary. Measures to promote skin integrity may be instituted. Other nursing measures may be necessary, depending on the patient's particular situation.

Preparation for discharge can be quite complex. Since these patient's usually have deficits, early planning for rehabilitation is essential. Patients deemed to be poor rehabilitation candidates may be discharged to an extended care facility or home, depending on available resources. Patients with persistent coma may benefit from discharge to a coma program. Even those patients with radical improvement may require some type of outpatient rehabilitation program. During this time, patients and family alike should be informed of the patient's situation and likely outcome and involved in the patient's care and plan for discharge. When death is anticipated, the family should be afforded both time and privacy for grieving. In this situation, involving the family in the patient's care may ease the loss.

Outcome

Numerous complications may occur following craniotomy for removal of an intracerebral hemorrhage. Problems related to manipulation of intracranial tissue may occur and include cerebral edema, increased intracranial pressure, seizures, and hydrocephalus. Reaccumulation of the hematoma may also occur. Infection is possible, in the form of brain abscess, meningitis, or wound infection. Complications may occur related to surgical position, type of anesthetic used, and preexisting medical problems. Systemic complications may also develop.

The overall incidence of postoperative complications is generally higher for the patient undergoing craniotomy for removal of an ICH than it is for the patient undergoing carotid endarterectomy or EC-IC bypass surgery. This is probably because the craniotomy patient tends to be more critically ill at the time of surgery. Several factors that contribute to a poor postoperative outcome in this population are coma, presence of abnormal brainstem signs, and cerebellar (vs cerebral) hemorrhage.

OTHER SURGICAL CONSIDERATIONS

Various other surgical interventions have been implemented in an attempt to improve neurologic status and outcome. Some of these have been mentioned as new developments in relation to currently performed procedures. Other procedures include embolectomy and recanalization.

Embolectomy

Usually performed on the middle cerebral artery, the purpose of this procedure is to restore blood flow in an attempt to reverse the deficit. The procedure involves a craniotomy and is quite invasive. To have some benefit, it should be performed within a few hours of onset of ischemia. This usually limits the indication to those patients who develop an embolic insult in a hospital setting.

Recanalization

Although recanalization has been attempted more frequently in vessels other than those supplying the brain, the technique holds some promise for carotid or even intracranial lesions. At present, techniques have been studied only in animals and cadavers. In one technique, a catheter is inserted into a stenotic or occluded vessel, then a balloon is inflated into the plaque to flatten it and open the vessel. In another technique, a catheter is threaded into the stenotic or occluded area and laser (argon or carbon dioxide) is used to vaporize the plaque, and reopen the vessels. Early technical feasibility has been determined but obviously further research is necessary.

New surgical techniques, indications, and equipment are likely to be developed, just as present surgical techniques and indications will most likely be revised. This is expected for as long as stroke remains a problem and prevention remains an issue.

REFERENCES

Amano K, Kawamura H, Tanikawa T and others: Surgical treatment of hypertensive intracerebral hematoma by CT-guided stereotactic surgery, Acta Neurochir, Suppl 39:41, 1987.

American Association of Neuroscience Nurses: Core curriculum for neurosurgical nursing in the operating room, Chicago, 1980, AANN.

Auer LM, Auer T, and Sayama I: Indications for surgical treatment of cerebellar hemorrhage and infarction, Acta Neurochir 79:74, 1986.

Ausman JI, and Diaz FG: Critique of the extracranial-intracranial bypass study, Surg Neurol 26:218, 1986.

Awad IA, and Spetzler RF: Extracranial-intracranial bypass surgery: a critical analysis in light of the international cooperative study, Neurosurg 19:655, 1986.

Barnett HJ, Fox A, Hachinski V and others: Further conclusions from the extracranial-intracranial bypass trial, Surg Neurol 26:227, 1986.

Barnett HJM, Mohr JP, Stein BM and others, editors: Stroke: pathophysiology, diagnosis, and management, New York, 1986, Churchill Livingstone, Inc.

Binder LM: The effects of cerebrovascular surgery on behavior: what has been demonstrated?, Henry Ford Hosp Med J 31:145, 1983.

Chater NL: Results of neurosurgical microvascular extracranial-intracranial bypass for stroke: a decade of experience, West J Med 138:531, 1983.

Choy DS, Ascher P, Lammer J and others: Percutaneous laser catheter recanalization of carotid arteries in seven cadavers and one patient, AJNR 7:1050, 1986.

Day AL, Rhoton AL, and Little JR: The extracranial-intracranial bypass study, Surg Neurol 26:222, 1986.

Drinkwater JE, Thompson SK, and Lumley JS: Cerebral function before and after extra-intracranial carotid bypass, J Neurol Neurosurg Psychiatry 47:1041, 1984.

Fedun PC: Preoperative evaluation of patients undergoing microanastomosis for brain ischemia, J Neurosurg Nurs 12:46, 1980.

Fein JM, and Reichman OH: Microvascular anastomosis for cerebral ischemia, New York, 1974, Springer-Verlag.

Groeteboer J: Stroke, carotid endarterectomy, and the neurosurgeon, J Neurosurg Nurs 10:52, 1978.

Hopkins M, Valberg BM, and Robinson LM: A report on the EC-IC bypass study, J Neurosci Nurs 18:211, 1986.

Khanna HL, and Garg AG: 774 carotid endarterectomies for strokes and transient ischemic attacks: comparison of results of early vs late surgery, Acta Neurochir Suppl 42:103, 1987.

Mitchell SK, and Yates RR: Extracranial-intracranial bypass surgery, J Neurosurg Nurs 17:288, 1985.

Moneta GL, Taylor DC, Nicholls SC and others: Operative vs nonoperative management of asymptomatic high grade internal carotid artery stenosis, Stroke 18:1005, 1987.

Polhopek M: Stroke: an update on vascular disease, J Neurosurg Nurs 12:81, 1980.

Rosenthal D, Rudderman R, Borrero E and others: Carotid endarterectomy to correct asymptomatic carotid stenosis: ten years later, J Vasc Surg 6:226, 1987.

Rudy EB: Advanced neurological and neurosurgical nursing, St Louis, 1984, CV Mosby.

Sayner NC: The decision-making process in surgery for stroke prevention, Adv Nurs Sci 5:67, 1982.

Schwarts ML: Neuropsychological evaluation of the results of surgical treatment of cerebrovascular disease, Henry Ford Hosp Med J 31:150, 1983.

Sterpetti AV, Schultz RD, and Feldhaus RJ: External carotid endarterectomy: indications, technique and late results, J Vasc Surg 7:31, 1988.

Stewart-Amidei C and Penckofer S: Quality of life following cerebral bypass surgery, J Neurosci Nurs 20:50, 1988.

Sundt TM, Whisnant JP, Fode NC and others: Results, complications and follow-up of 415 bypass operations for occlusive disease of the carotid system, Mayo Clin Proc 60:230, 1985.

The EC-IC Bypass Study Group: Failures of extracranial-intracranial arterial bypass to reduce the risk of ischemic stroke, New Engl J Med 313:1191, 1985.

Weinstein PR, Rodriguez y Baena R, and Chater NL: Results of extracranial-intracranial arterial bypass for intracranial internal carotid artery stenosis: review of 105 cases, Neurosurg 15:787, 1984.

Whisnant JB, Sandok BA, and Sundt TM: Carotid endarterectomy for unilateral carotid system transient cerebral ischemia, Mayo Clin Proc 58:171, 1983.

Whisnant JP, Sundt TM, and Fode NC: Long term mortality and stroke morbidity after superficial temporal artery–middle cerebral artery bypass operation, Mayo Clin Proc 60:241, 1985.

Whittemore AD, and Mannick JA: Surgical treatment of carotid disease in patients with neurologic deficits, J Vasc Surgery 5:910, 1987.

Yasargil MG: Microsurgery applied to neurosurgery, Stuttgart, 1969, George Thieme.

Zeiger HE, Zampella EJ, Naftel DC and others: A prospective analysis of 142 carotid endarterectomies for occlusive vascular disease, J Neurosurg 67:540, 1987.

Zurbruegg HR, Seiler RW, Grolimund P and others: Morbidity and mortality of carotid endarterectomy, Acta Neurochir 84:3, 1987.

Section II

Physical, Psychologic, and Social Aspects of Caring for the Stroke Patient

Chapter 5

Alterations in Consciousness

The ability to interact with one's environment and respond to stimuli is an integral part of what makes each person unique. Many facets of the central nervous system govern this response, and any damage to either the primary pathways of consciousness or the secondary response centers may result in changes in the level of consciousness. When this occurs, the patient exhibits decreased responsiveness to the environment and may have abnormal or inappropriate responses. This situation places the patient at considerable risk because he cannot protect himself from harm or make his desires known. Care for such patients centers on protecting them from injury and compensating for their inability to adjust to environmental demands.

Strokes may cause impairment in consciousness, ranging from blunting of response to stimuli to lack of response to stimuli. Whenever there is impairment in consciousness, ongoing assessment of responses and appropriate interventions is essential for ensuring the highest potential of subsequent recovery. This chapter discusses the components of consciousness, how to assess the stroke patient who has actual or potential decreased responsiveness, and nursing care actions focused on prevention of permanent central nervous system damage and patient safety. For those patients who have prolonged decreased responsiveness and are surviving in some level of coma, interventions aimed at individualized stimulation of the sensory system are presented.

COMPONENTS OF CONSCIOUSNESS

The awareness of oneself and his or her surroundings is termed *consciousness*. Consciousness is considered to have two components: arousal and awareness. Both must be present for one to be conscious. The two components are mediated within the central nervous system by the reticular activating system (RAS) and the cerebral hemispheres.

The RAS runs throughout the brainstem and has projections into the hypothalamus and thalamus (Fig. 5-1). Fibers from all major sensory pathways feed into the RAS. Its primary function is to receive and relay sensory information from the environment surrounding a person to the hemispheres for interpretation. Wakefulness is determined by the RAS and damage to this system can produce a decreased state of arousal.

The second component, awareness, is much more complicated in its functioning. Once the RAS transmits sensory information to the cerebral hemispheres and cortex, the hemispheres must interpret and generate a response to the stimuli. The response can range from mere recognition of the stimulus to an attempt at withdrawal. A response may fall anywhere along the spectrum, from reflex action to higher level purposeful movement. Thus for awareness to be present, a person must have an intact cerebral cortex.

When both components are functioning normally, a person can maintain consciousness and

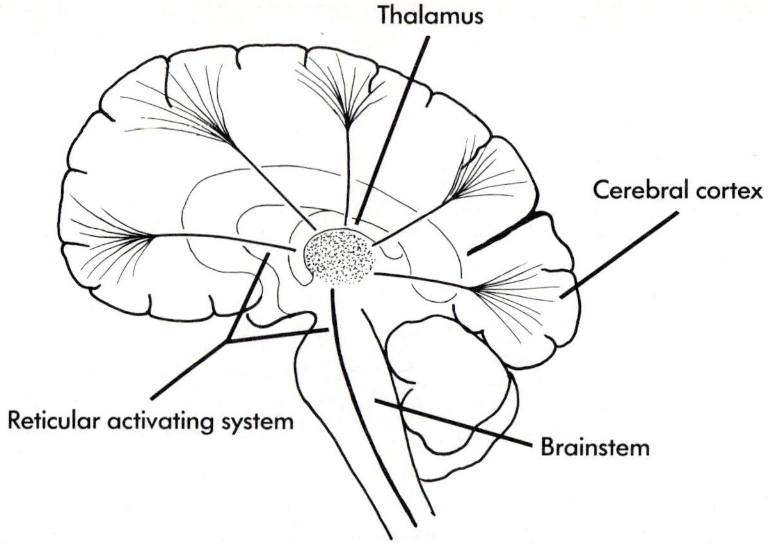

Fig. 5-1 Projections of the reticular activating system (RAS).

interact with the environment. It is this consciousness that makes each person unique.

Interruption or damage to these systems by a stroke is devastating, causing alteration in awareness and a decreased ability to respond to stimuli. Diffuse cerebral impairment can produce confusion, in which the person misinterprets stimuli and generates inappropriate responses, such as combativeness. Localized impairment, such as changes in speech or motor functioning, does not really impair awareness, but it does limit the degree or type of response a person can generate. In contrast to impairment of awareness, impairment of arousal decreases the person's wakeful state and produces an overall decrease in the level of consciousness. Strokes that interrupt brainstem functioning, such as with basilar or vertebral artery ischemia, may reduce consciousness. This change in functioning is usually not an all-or-none phenomenon. Depending on the site and extent of physiologic damage, the level of consciousness may vary. Because of this variation, numerous terms have been used to describe the clinical presentation of these patients. The most common terms follow:

Delirium—a change in cortical function characterized by restlessness and incoherence. The patient may have visual or auditory hallucinations. Metabolic or toxic events can produce this type of syndrome as diffuse cortical dysfunctioning occurs. Patients who are delirious have an intact RAS and a normal state of arousal, but dysfunctioning cerebral hemispheres are unable to interpret sensory information accurately and will generate inappropriate responses.

Obtundation—a blunting of consciousness. Patients with obtunded consciousness have a generalized reduced response to environmental stimuli and will drift in and out of sleep if not being aroused. Obtunded patients generally have more cerebral hemisphere impairment than delirious patients, but again the RAS is intact.

Stupor—severe impairment of awareness arising from hemispheric dysfunction. Unless a patient is constantly being aroused (often needing noxious stimuli to become aroused) he lapses back into deep sleep.

Semicoma—some impairment in arousal. There is no spontaneous movement, but with noxious stimulation the patient may groan and try to withdraw or localize the stimulus. Most reflexes remain intact.

Coma—severe impairment in arousal. Even noxious stimuli cannot produce a purposeful response. Reflexes remain intact and stimulation can produce extensor rigidity, accompanied by decorticate or decerebrate posturing. These primitive responses are evidence that the cerebral hemispheres can no longer respond to stimuli, and the reflex posturing is generated from the brainstem.

Deep coma—a truly unarousable, unresponsive state. Reflexes are lost and extremities remain flaccid.

Persistent vegetative state—a state in which the patient has periods of wakefulness and physiological sleep-wake cycles but is unaware of herself or the environment. The eyes may open at times, and breathing is spontaneous. These patients experience no pain or suffering. The patient is awake but unaware. Physiologically, the brainstem is intact and functioning, but there is complete loss of cerebral cortical functioning (American Association of Neuroscience Nurses, 1988). Another term that applies to this state is *apallic syndrome,* in which there has been severe anoxic injury resulting in bilateral cerebral hemisphere degeneration.

During assessment of the patient with an altered level of consciousness, the nurse must carefully observe for other states that can mimic coma. The most unusual, caused by infarction of the brainstem, is termed *locked-in syndrome*. Basilar artery occlusion with subsequent infarction of the pons produces the clinical presentation of paralysis of the extremities, paralysis of the muscles innervated by the cranial nerves, and changes in the ability to move the eyes, often accompanied by nystagmus. There is no alteration in consciousness except the inability to move. Patients may be able to move their eyes upward or blink to communicate. Sometimes these patients are mistakenly thought to be in coma because of their inability to move and talk, and inappropriate things are said and done in the patient's room because the patient is seemingly unaware. It is important when caring for such a patient to make all staff and ancillary personnel aware that the patient is alert and understands everything that is said to him.

Another state that has been identified is that of *akinetic mutism,* in which the patient has normal sleep-wake cycles, does not speak, is immobile, and has no outward signs of cerebral awareness. There may be some muscle movement or vocalizing with painful stimulation but no coordinated or purposeful actions. Several case studies have described such states, and the pathophysiology of the state is varied. At autopsy it was discovered that some patients had bilateral frontal lobe lesions while others had numerous lesions. All of these lesions seem to impair reticular formation to some extent but spare the adjacent corticospinal tracts.

MECHANISMS OF STROKE THAT CAUSE COMA

To directly alter the level of consciousness, a stroke must result in widespread damage to the cerebral cortex or focal damage to the brainstem. A supratentorial lesion (i.e., a large cerebral hemorrhage) produces a mass lesion that acts like a space-occupying lesion, which displaces the brain downward and eventually compresses the brainstem and reticular activating system. Clinical signs of gradually decreasing level of consciousness accompany respiratory and motor impairments. As cranial nerves are affected, the patient also shows abnormal extraocular eye movements and pupillary irregularities.

Subtentorial events affect the brainstem directly by compressing the reticular activating system or by primary ischemia or hemorrhage. Strokes within the brainstem cause destruction and necrosis of the nerve fibers. Infarction in the region of the midbrain and pons can result from vertebral or basilar artery insufficiency. Patients immediately lapse into coma and have accompanying clinical signs associated with the location of destruction. These patients are generally older and may have experi-

Table 5-1 Signs and symptoms related to coma-causing lesions

	Diencephalic late	Midbrain upper pons	Lower pons medulla	Uncal herniation third nerve impairment
Respiratory pattern	Cheyne-Stokes	Cheyne-Stokes or hyperventilation	Ataxic	Apneustic
Pupil size	Small	Midposition	Midposition	Ipsilateral dilated
Pupil reactivity	Small contraction	Fixed	Fixed	Ipsilateral does not constrict
Oculocephalic	Normal	Impaired	No response	Impaired
Oculovestibular	Normal (absent nystagmus)	Impaired (dysconjugate)	No response	Ipsilateral abnormal (contralateral full movement)
Motor response	Appropriate or decorticate	Motionless or decerebrate	Motionless and flaccid	Decorticate or decerebrate

enced transient ischemic attacks in the posterior circulation before the onset of infarction and coma. Hypertensive hemorrhages in the brainstem can also occur, mainly in the pons but sometimes extending into the midbrain. Patients demonstrate respiratory pattern changes, pinpoint pupils, and oculomotor changes. Motor involvement is evidenced by quadraparesis or quadraplegia. Body temperature is affected and the patient becomes hyperthermic.

Compression of the brainstem and the reticular activating system can also occur from cerebellar hemorrhages, causing pressure on the brainstem and resulting in ischemia. Because the rapidly expanding lesion is within the posterior fossa, which has little compensatory properties, the brainstem can be affected early in the course of the bleed. Symptoms vary because of the accompanying herniation of the brain, but oculomotor signs, such as ocular bobbing and gaze deviations, are common. Detailed descriptions of signs and symptoms related to lesions causing coma can be found in Table 5-1.

PHYSIOLOGIC RESPONSES IN COMA

Many physiologic changes can be experienced by the patient in coma. Pathways that mediate blood pressure and heart rate run from the spinal cord to the cerebral hemispheres. In addition, the areas responsible for respirations are located in the upper spinal cord and brainstem. Impairment of these structures by direct insult or by increased intracranial pressure results in instability of the mechanisms responsible for vital life functions. From a cardiac standpoint, the patient can have increases in blood pressure, changes in heart rate, and alterations in rhythm. If there is pressure on the brainstem or floor of the fourth ventricle from an expanding intracranial bleed, the classic Cushing response may develop, in which the blood pressure rises and the pulse slows. Acute intracranial hemorrhage can produce ventricular tachycardia and other cardiac arrhythmias as can large ischemic strokes; therefore, monitoring the acute stroke patient for ECG and blood pressure changes is important.

Respiratory changes are also produced in patients with stroke in the cerebral hemispheres or brainstem. Several classic patterns have been identified, based on the level of impairment. The patterns are based on progressive impairment, starting at the cerebral hemispheres and moving downward through the midbrain, pons, and medulla. Cheyne-Stokes respirations in stroke patients have a variety of causes (Fig. 5-2). Bilateral hemispheric lesions stimulate the patient to overbreathe and blow off carbon dioxide. As the level of CO_2 drops, the respiratory center is no longer stimulated and the patient stops breathing. As the level of CO_2 builds, the respiratory center is again stimulated and the patient takes a breath. Initially, the breaths are shallow, but subsequent breaths build until enough CO_2 has been blown off for the respiratory center to no longer be stimulated. This waxing and waning pattern of breathing is characteristic of Cheyne-Stokes respirations. Besides bilateral hemispheric lesions, rapidly expanding intracranial lesions and cerebellar hemorrhages have also been known to produce such patterns, but because the lesions have such profound pressure changes on the brainstem, the patterns are generally brief and the next lower level brainstem breathing pattern emerges rapidly.

Lesions in the midbrain and pons can produce primary *hyperventilation syndrome* (Fig. 5-3). This rare syndrome is characterized by a rapid respiratory rate and blood gases showing an elevated PaO_2 and a lowered $PaCO_2$ while the patient breathes room air. A similar clinical picture is found in patients who have pulmonary congestion. Aspiration and infection can contribute to the development of congestion, which stimulates afferent sensory nerves in the chest wall and lung. While similar to the tachypneic hypocapnic picture presented, most clinical evidence shows that these patients are experiencing pulmonary shunting. Whatever the cause, such breathing is an ominous sign and indicates a poorer prognosis.

Two other types of respiratory patterns may be observed in patients with brainstem stroke. Injury to the middle or lower pons by infarction produces *apneustic breathing* (Fig. 5-4). This pattern is characterized by a hesitation in breathing at the height of inspiration. Hemorrhage within the medulla or compression of this structure by cerebellar or pontine hemorrhag tends to impair the rhythm of respiration. Termed *ataxic respiration,* it is characterized by irregularities in rate and rhythm (Fig. 5-5). Pauses in breathing are interspersed with irregular breaths.

Pupillary Changes in Stroke

Structures responsible for controlling pupillary changes reside next to the RAS in the brainstem.

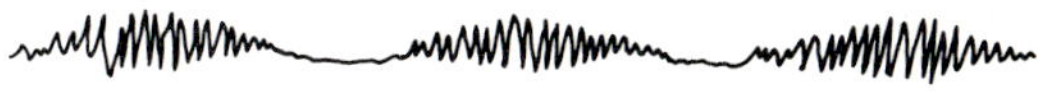

Cheyne-Stokes breathing

Fig. 5-2 The Cheyne-Stokes pattern is characterized by a regular alternation (crescendo/decrescendo) in the rate and depth of breathing.

Hyperventilatory breathing

Fig. 5-3 Primary hyperventilation syndrome may be caused by damage to the midbrain and pons.

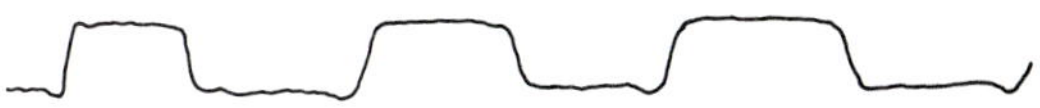

Apneustic

Fig. 5-4 The apneustic pattern is defined by a pause at the height of inspiration.

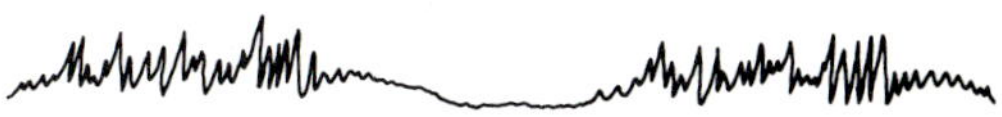

Ataxic breathing

Fig. 5-5 Ataxic respiration results in complete irregularity of breathing rate and rhythm.

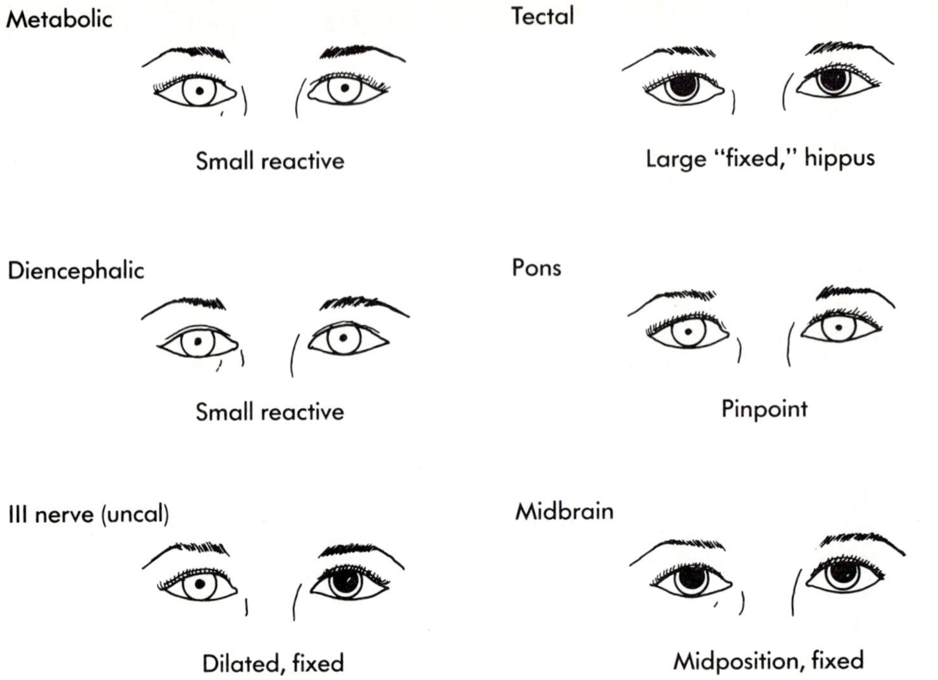

Fig. 5-6 Pupillary abnormalities in coma.

Because of this, changes in pupil function can serve as an indicator of lesion location. Horner's syndrome is perhaps the most widely recognized cluster of symptoms resulting from damage to the thalamus or hypothalamus. The classic presentation is ipsilateral pupillary constriction, ptosis, and lack of sweating, also on the ipsilateral side of the face. Other patterns of pupillary changes are also easily recognizable. Damage to the midbrain causes changes to the light reflex. Patients have midsize pupils that are round and do not react to the light. Pontine damage changes the size of the pupils. Pinpoint pupils bilaterally usually indicate pontine hemorrhage. Although the pupils still contract, the examiner may need to use a magnifying glass to observe the reflex because the pupils are so small. A summary of pupillary findings associated with cerebral hemisphere and brainstem lesions is found in Fig. 5-6.

Changes in Ocular Motility

Oculomotor reflex pathways also lie adjacent to the RAS and can serve as a guide to lesion location. Two ocular reflexes commonly impaired by brainstem lesions are the oculocephalic, or doll's eyes, and the oculovestibular, or caloric stimulation. In patients with intact brainstem functioning, the oculocephalic reflex is elicited by holding the patient's eyelids open and rotating the head from side to side. An intact reflex produces conjugate deviation of the eyes (Fig. 5-7). Strokes can produce damage in the medial longitudinal fasciculus (MLF), which decussates in the pons and is responsible for adduction of the ipsilateral medial rectus muscle controlling eye movement. Damage to this pathway results in the ipsilateral eye being unable to adduct, or turn in, toward the nose as the head is turned (Fig. 5-8). The term used for this phenomenon is *internuclear ophthalmoplegia*. If bilateral MLF

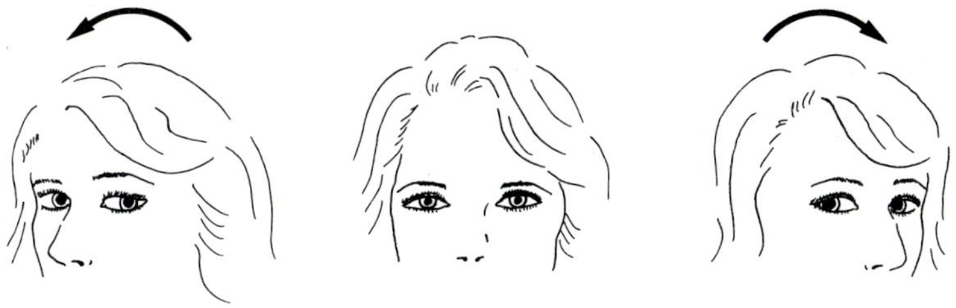

Fig. 5-7 An intact ocular reflex: conjugate deviation of the eyes.

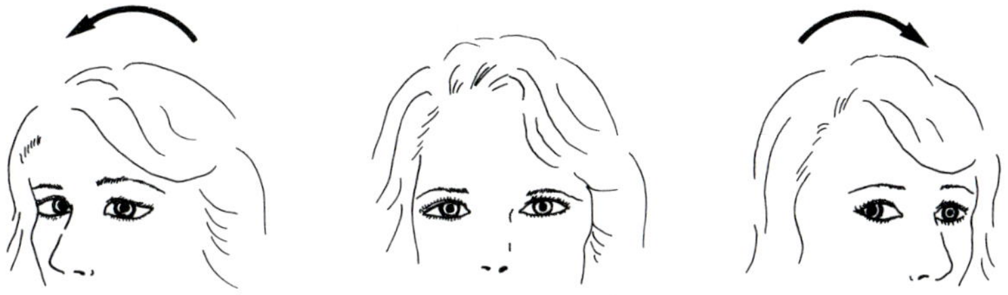

Fig. 5-8 An impaired ocular reflex: inability to adduct the eyes.

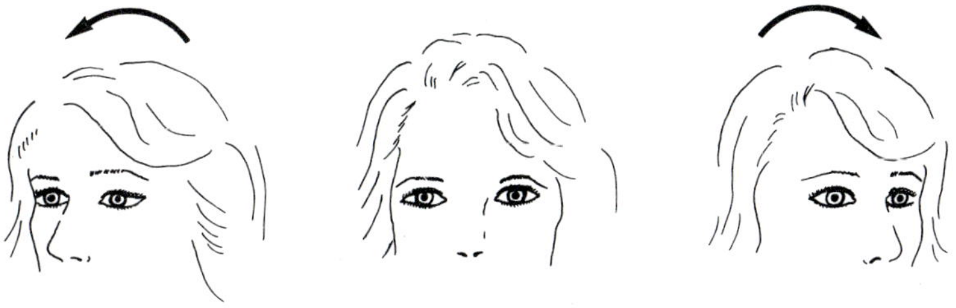

Fig. 5-9 Absent ocular reflex: inability to move the eyes.

function is destroyed, then both eyes are unable to turn toward the nose. Lower brainstem lesions result in the eyes being unable to adduct, abduct, or move vertically (Fig. 5-9).

The oculovestibular reflex is tested by instilling cold water into the ear canal and observing for subsequent eye movement. An intact reflex produces movement of the eyes toward the side of the ear being irrigated. Reflexes should be tested on both sides. Damage to the MLF produces movement of the ipsalateral eye toward the ear being irrigated, with the contralateral eye remaining midposition. Lower brainstem lesions result in both eyes remaining midposition when irrigation is attempted (Fig. 5-10).

Several other abnormal eye movements can be encountered in patients with stroke. Some patients who have damage to the frontal lobes can have interruption in the frontal eye fields. These patients have eyes that are deviated toward the side of the cerebral hemispheric lesion. Testing of oculocephalic and oculovestibular reflexes reveals that the eyes do move to the contralateral side, thus verifying an intact brainstem.

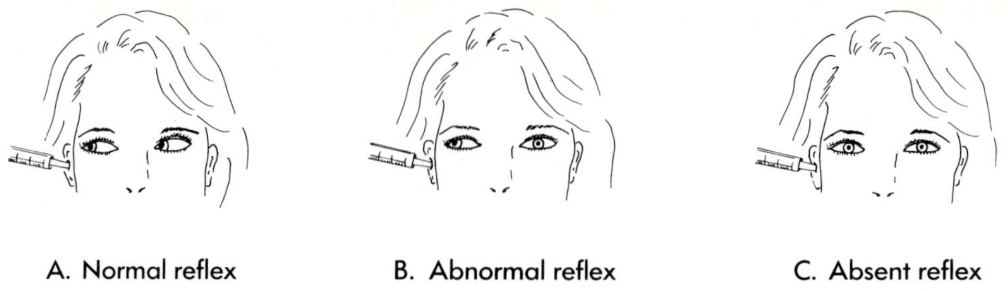

Fig. 5-10 Oculovestibular reflexes.

Some patients who are comatose have roving eye movements. Their eyes move horizontally and vertically at random and are often disconjugate. Others will demonstrate nystagmus and ocular bobbing. In the former, the eyes move quickly back to midposition after eye movement or show a rhythmic jerking. The latter term refers to the downward, repetitive movement of the eyes, after which they return to midposition. Lesions responsible for such bobbing most often are located in the pons.

ASSESSMENT

Unlike other system assessments, assessment of consciousness has many facets. First, the examiner must fully arouse the patient and then test all components of the neurologic system. Patients must have a baseline assessment made in the acute stage and then ongoing assessments made, as indicated by the severity of the stroke and the potential for further deterioration. Many attempts have been made to develop scales for assessing the unconscious patient. Commonly cited in the literature are the Glascow Coma Scale (Teasdale and Jennett, 1974), the Reaction Level Scale (Starmark, 1988), the Edinburgh-2 Coma Scale (Sugiura and others, 1983), and the Grady Coma Scale. While such scales help quantify data and facilitate comparison of patients by severity of symptoms, they are fraught with problems that make their use for stroke patients unacceptable. For example, the Glascow Coma Scale was developed to measure consciousness in patients with severe head injuries. Because of this, the scale does not account for speech deficits or unilateral symptoms frequently seen in stroke patients. Also, more detailed neurologic assessment parameters so important to determine in stroke patients (such as degree of weakness, abnormal extraocular eye movements, tone, and reflexes) are not part of the scale. For the most accurate assessment of baseline clinical status and for ongoing neurologic monitoring, the following guidelines for use with stroke patients are recommended.

Besides the history and general physical examination, the first area of evaluation should be verbal responses. A lesion in the region of the speech centers may render the patient unable to participate in this portion of the evaluation. However, if the patient can communicate, the determination should be made as to whether the patient is oriented or confused or has inappropriate or incomprehensible speech. For a detailed outline of speech assessment refer to Chapter 11.

The next area of asssessment involves the eyes. Do the eyes open spontaneously, or must there be verbal or noxious stimulation applied to get the patient to open her eyes? Some patients may not open their eyes at all. While assessing eye opening, the pupillary light reflex can be tested. It should be noted whether the pupil responds normally, briskly, sluggishly, or not at all. Testing of the corneal reflex can also be done at this time. Further testing of the eyes includes spontaneous eye movements and oculovestibular and oculocephalic reflexes. The last two should be performed by a person knowledgeable about the procedure and only after it is certain there is no cervical injury.

Respiratory pattern must be documented. Both the rate and rhythm and any periods of apnea should be assessed. If severe alterations in respirations are present, blood gas determinations should be carried out to assess respiratory status. Any state that could produce hypercapnia should be avoided, because the increase in $Paco_2$ results in cerebral vessel dilation. Such dilation can produce further increased intracranial pressure.

Detailed assessment of movement patterns is imperative for the stroke patient with a depressed level of consciousness. Because strokes can produce both unilateral and bilateral weakness or paralysis, assessment of both sides of the body should be performed. The highest level of movement is the ability to obey commands. Asking the patient to lift his arms and legs can determine his ability to move. If the patient has an impairment in speech or language interpretation, he may not be able to understand what you are asking him to do. In this case, stimulating the extremity can produce movement.

The next level of movement is localization of a stimulus. While a patient may be unable to move an extremity because of weakness, noxious stimulation on the impaired side can elicit movement of the unaffected side in an attempt to remove the stimulus. Several varieties of progressively noxious stimulation can be tried, including pinprick, pinch, sternal rub, and pressure on the supraorbital ridge. Plum and Posner (1985) suggest that placing a pencil across the nailbed and applying pressure is an excellent method of producing noxious stimulation, with little tissue damage. This assessment in stroke patients is especially important because it can help differentiate between paralysis on one side of the body and a decreased level of consciousness as the reason for lack of movement. In the latter case, patients show generalized response to the stimulus by poor attempts at stimulus localization.

More indicative of severe motor impairment is abnormal flexion or extension of an extremity. With stimulation, patients who have lost cortical control over movement will have internal rotation and flexion of the arms and internal rotation and extension of the legs. Termed *decorticate posturing* because of the lack of cortical input, the reflex movement can be present on one or both sides of the body. If an individual has lost cerebral hemispheric control over movement, stimulation will produce internal rotation and extension of both upper and lower extremities. This type of decerebrate posturing indicates severe hemispheric dysfunction. Use of the terms *decorticate* and *decerebrate* to describe motor patterns has been found extensively in the literature, but their use with stroke patients is less accurate. Such terminology encompasses many other clinical features found more typically in neurologic trauma. Thus it is preferable to describe exactly what movement occurs with stimulation in each limb. Finally, the lack of any motor movement is an ominous sign. Such a clinical picture indicates dysfunction in central motor areas adjacent to the RAS in the medulla and pons.

The last assessment parameter is that of muscle tone and deep tendon reflexes. Tone should be determined in each extremity and graded as normal, hypertonic with increases in flexor or extensor tone, or hypotonic. Complete guidelines for assessing muscle tone can be found in Chapter 7. Increased flexor tone or spasticity is frequently seen after stroke, expecially if there is severe weakness or paralysis of an extremity. Rigidity, or increased extensor tone, is found more commonly in massive cerebral hemispheric lesions (such as an intracerebral hemorrhage) in patients with supratentorial herniation, and in cerebellar hemorrhage in which there is compression of the midbrain and pons. Hypotonia is indicative of damage to the medulla and pons.

For the comatose patient, assessment of deep tendon reflexes is important. (Deep tendon reflex physiology is discussed in detail in Chapter 7.) Increased deep tendon reflexes indicate central nervous system damage. They are generally hyperactive in patients who have had a stroke. In addition, several abnormal reflexes can be elicited, such as grasping reflexes of the hand and primitive sucking reflexes with frontal lobe lesions. The Babinski sign, or dorsiflexion of the great toe and fanning of the other toes when the bottom of the foot is stroked, is another abnormal reflex. These are all indicative of cerebral hemisphere damage or diffuse central nervous system damage.

INTERVENTIONS

The goals in caring for the stroke patient with a depressed level of consciousness are to maintain normal functioning of body systems; to prevent complications from occurring; and to stimulate the patient's neurologic system to facilitate a return to normal functioning. As neurologic dysfunction on such a grand scale affects numerous body processes, other chapters describe in detail issues such as safety, immobility, and nutrition.

Unique to the comatose patient is the need for neurologic stimulation. The concept of coma stimulation arises from three areas of theory. The first theory is based on normal child development. Children develop with environmental stimulation, and those who have not had the typical stimulation most children receive may suffer developmental abnormalities. The second theory arises from studies of sensory deprivation in humans. People who experience little sensory stimulation have diminished responsiveness to internal and external stimuli. The third theory comes from studies of comatose patients. Tosch (1988) interviewed 15 patients who had recovered from coma. Six of the patients recalled sensory experiences during coma while five had death-like experiences and three had feelings of imprisonment or being held against their will. Recent research has demonstrated that comatose patients show changes in heart rate, respiratory rate, blood pressure, and skin temperature. While no direct link has been made between stimulation and changes in bodily functions, there has been increased interest in determining if the brains of comatose patients have "idling" neurons, which, with appropriate stimulation, can begin to function normally.

All types of coma stimulation programs have three general principles: structured stimulation, combined stimuli, and repetition. The idea is to apply sensory stimulation to the body to arouse the patient via the reticular activating system, which receives sensory input and transmits it to the cerebral hemispheres. Key to all programs is the stimulation of individual sensory modalities, but the frequency and duration of stimulation may vary. The senses to be stimulated include visual, vestibular, taste, olfactory, temperature, proprioception, auditory, and touch.

Exactly what to use for stimulation and when to do the stimulation can vary. For example, DeYoung and Grass (1987) describe shining very bright lights (650 watts) into the patient's eyes for 1 second and then turning them off for 1 second. This is repeated while the patient is assessed for responses, such as blinking. Other types of visual stimulation include having the patient follow the movement of bright lights, or using pictures of objects or familiar photographs of family members. In general, in the areas of visual stimulation and other sensory areas, patients at the lower end of the coma spectrum need more intense or noxious stimuli to facilitate a response than do those who are at the higher end.

Olfactory stimulation can be accomplished by a variety of techniques. Noxious stimuli include ammonia or smelling salts, while more pleasant stimuli include perfume, flowers, mint, and coffee. When using noxious stimuli, care should be taken to not overly stimulate because both the olfactory nerve and the nose itself can become irritated. Taste usually follows application of olfactory stimulation. Sweet items, such as sugar, can be applied to the tongue with cotton applicators. Other stimuli are salt and peppermint. Noxious stimuli for taste include lemon and hot (Tobasco) sauce.

Daily caring for patients in coma involves many opportunities for touch and skin stimulation. In stimulation programs, however, specific stimuli are applied repetitively and observation for a response is made. Different tactile stimuli to use include rough fabrics, such as terry cloth, or wool, and soft objects, such as cotton balls. Stimulation of the temperature receptors can be accomplished by using water bottles filled with warm and cold water.

Auditory stimulation also has a wide spectrum of treatments. The most primitive is loud noise. Slamming a door, blowing a whistle, or tooting a horn can be used to stimulate the low-level patient. At higher levels of coma, music and reading to the patient can be tried.

Finally, vestibular stimulation can be accomplished by turning the patient in bed, swiveling him in a chair that turns, rolling him on large balls or log mats in physical therapy, and standing him upright. When doing vestibular stimulation it is hard to keep the stimulation pure. For example, putting the patient in a swimming pool stimulates the vestibular system but also stimulates touch and temperature.

Assessing patients' responses to coma stimulation techniques involves both the monitoring of vital functions and the observation of specific responses to the stimuli. Because vital functions are controlled in the brainstem, adjacent to the reticular activating system, stimulation techniques can stimulate not only the RAS but also affect heart rate, respiratory rate, and blood pressure. For this reason, all coma patients should have their vital signs monitored during stimulation sessions. This is especially true for low level coma patients who may already have difficulty stabilizing their vital signs. The duration and variety of response to any of the sensory stimulation techniques should also be recorded. Various responses that are often overlooked include turning the head toward or away from the stimulus; facial movement, such as smiling or grimacing; eye movements; and changes in muscle tone. If responses are noted, future stimulation sessions should focus on increasing the magnitude and duration of response.

Sometimes patients will respond to combined sensory modalities better than single modalities presented individually. For example, when using auditory stimulation to get eye movement responses, the person doing the assessment can combine calling the patient's name with a command and a loud noise. The dialogue would go as follows: "John, John look, John look now," (accompanied by a clap of the hands).

As people gradually awake from coma, they move into a higher level of awareness. During this stage, arousal increases and the cerebral hemispheres attempt to respond to the incoming sensory stimulation. Sometimes responses are appropriate, but frequently there is too much sensory stimulation and the patient is unable to manage the overwhelming input and responds with agitation and confusion. At this level, stimulation programs are continued, but the environment is controlled to reduce the incidence of agitation and confusion. Stimulation sessions are given in one-on-one patient-nurse interactions in a neutral room where there are few visual distractions or loud noises. As stimulation proceeds, the goal is to focus the patient's attention on performing simple tasks and reducing the increased muscle tone that often accompanies improvement in level of consciousness. Soothing touch by the nurse who is in charge of the sessions facilitates familiarity on the patient's part. Keeping a daily routine and limiting the sessions to a specific period of time assists the patient in controlling his actions.

Patient assessments made during coma stimulation sessions can often be grouped according to responses on the Rancho Los Amigos Scale. Following are summaries of the eight levels of response:

1. No response—absence of any observable response to stimulation.
2. Generalized response—reflex responses to stimulation. May have physiologic changes, such as increases in heart rate, respirations, or blood pressure.
3. Localized response—withdraws or turns away from stimuli but is unable to respond consistently to simple commands.
4. Confused-agitated—increased activity level but with reduced processing; nonpurposeful behavior.
5. Confused-inappropriate, non-agitated—alert, but exhibits difficulty paying attention. May become agitated with stimulation and have inap-

propriate behavior. Severe memory impairment.

6. Confused-appropriate—inconsistently oriented to time and place. Impaired recent memory. Can follow simple directions. Actively participates in therapy.
7. Automatic-appropriate—appropriate response and oriented. Carryover for new learning and still needs minimal supervision. Demonstrates some insight into disabilities.
8. Purposeful-appropriate—alert and oriented. Functions independently, within physical capabilities. Sets realistic goals and applies judgement to daily living.

While the interest in coma stimulation programs has grown over the past several years, several issues regarding the structure of the stimulation sessions and their frequency have not been resolved. At the International Coma Recovery Institute, the coma stimulation program starts in the acute care facility and continues in the patient's home. Intensive stimulation occurs every hour for 11 hours. Other programs stimulate the patient every 4 hours during the day and evening. Determining the best way to provide coma stimulation has not been subjected to any rigorous research, and outcomes have been based on case reports and overall institutional outcomes. While some reports claim up to 92% recovery from coma (DeYoung and Grass, 1987), the level of recovery varies from complete functional independence to only minor improvement or changes in low level responses. Such reports are even more difficult to evaluate because there are individual differences in each coma case, such as site of injury, age of the patient, complicating medical illnesses, and the natural course of recovery from coma.

Complicating the situation even more is the economical impact on the patient and society. Intensive stimulation programs are expensive because of the number of personnel needed and the amount of time devoted to each patient. Insurance programs may not cover such a rehabilitation program, and the only alternatives to this are a nursing home or skilled care within the patient's home. Added to this is the question of how long must the patient participate in a coma stimulation program when there has been only minimal improvement over a long period of time? Only further research will help answer many of these questions.

Any time a stroke patient has an impaired level of consciousness there is a decreased chance of recovery. Recovery depends on the site of the lesion and whether it is the primary cause of coma. With large lesions, such as massive cerebral hemorrhage, the degree of brain swelling impairs consciousness in the initial stage and often leads to death within a few days. Brainstem hemorrhages and infarcts can present with a similar scenario. However, if the patient can survive the initial stage, then recovery may gradually occur. Bates and others (1977) reviewed 310 cases of nontraumatic coma, 102 of which had focal cerebral vascular disease. Of these patients, 71 had no recovery, 9 remained in a vegetative state, 12 had severe disability, 6 had moderate disability, and only 4 had a good recovery. Generally, cerebral hemorrhage has a better prognosis than ischemic strokes, possibly because the blood is gradually reabsorbed over time and neurons that have been idling can function again.

Certainly, with more aggressive stroke management and better care in the initial stroke period, the statistics on stroke-coma recovery will improve.

NURSING CARE PLAN

Nursing Diagnosis	Interventions	Expected Outcomes
Decreased Arousal related to impaired central nervous system processing **Defining Characteristics** ■ Change in alertness, orientation, eye movements, motor responses, and verbalization ■ Pupillary, respiratory, or cardiac abnormalities ■ Increased deep tendon reflexes and posturing	**Ongoing Assessment** ■ Assess level of consciousness at regular intervals as indicated by patient condition (every 15 minutes to hourly) ■ Assess motor, respiratory, and cardiac function ■ Assess patient for protective responses and ability to prevent injury **Therapeutic Interventions** ■ Record assessments and notify physician of any changes ■ Orient to person, place, and time as needed ■ Prevent injury by keeping bed in low position with rails up at all times ■ Protect eyes and airway if the patient has decreased corneal, blink, or gag response ■ Institute range of motion exercises and turning schedule related to decreased mobility ■ For those patients with sustained depressed consciousness, institute stimulation program based on sensory modalities and patient's ability to respond ■ See Care Plans for chapters related to loss of sensory, communication, etc., for additional interventions	■ Stable or improved level of consciousness ■ Absence of injury to patient ■ Ongoing stimulation program, if decreased level of consciousness continues ■ Family actively involved in care and long-term care planning

Patient Education

- Teach family about patient's inability to respond and ways they can become involved in care, such as bringing photographs and items familiar to the patient.
- Discuss safety requirements of the patient and ways to prevent injury.
- Encourage verbalization of concerns by family and refer to appropriate resources, such as social service agencies and pastoral care.

Continued.

NURSING CARE PLAN — cont'd

Nursing Diagnosis	Interventions	Expected Outcomes

Related Nursing Diagnoses
- Impaired CNS integrative functions
- Potential for injury
- Self-care deficit
- Potential for skin breakdown
- Impaired mobility
- Nutritional deficit

REFERENCES

Amerian Academy of Neurology: Position of the American Academy of Neurology on certain aspects of the care and management of the persistent vegetative state patient, Neurology 39:125, 1989.

Bates D, Caronna JJ, Cartlidge NEF and others: A prospective study of nontraumatic coma: methods and results in 310 patients, Ann Neurol 2:211, 1977.

DeYoung S and Grass RB: Coma recovery program, Rehabilitation Nursing 12:121, 1987.

Hansotia PL: Persistent vegetative state: review and report of electrodiagnostic studies in eight cases, Arch Neurol 42:1048, 1985.

La Puma J, Schiedermayer DL, Gulyas AE and others: Talking to comatose patients, Arch Neurol 45:20, 1988.

Manders KL: The head injury-coma arousal center: a new program for the care of brain-injured patients, Indiana Med 78:1094, 1985.

Norrsell U: Awareness, wakefulness and arousal, Acta Neurochir 36:86, 1986.

Plum F and Posner JB: The diagnosis of stupor and coma, Philadelphia, 1985, FA Davis Co.

Price DJ: Factors restricting the use of coma scales, Acta Neurochir 36:106, 1986.

Stalhammar D and Starmark JE: Assessment of responsiveness in head injury patients, Acta Neurochir 36:91, 1986.

Stalhammar D, Starmark JE, Holmgren E and others: Assessment of responsiveness in acute cerebral disorders, Acta Neurochir 90:73, 1988.

Starmark JE and Lindgren S: Is it possible to define a general "consciousness level?" Acta Neurochir 36:103, 1986.

Starmark JE, Stalhammar D, and Holmgren E: The Reaction Level Scale (RLS85): manual and guidelines, Acta Neurochir 91:12, 1988.

Sugiura K, Muraoka K, Chishiki T and others: The Edinburgh-2 coma scale: a new scale for assessing impaired consciousness, Neurosurgery 12:411, 1983.

Teasdale G and Jennett B: Assessment of coma and impaired consciousness, Lancet 2:81, 1974.

Tosch P: Patients recollections of their posttraumatic coma, J Neurosci Nurs 20:223, 1988.

Chapter 6

Alterations in Integrated Regulation

The nervous system does not function in isolation. Rather, it maintains intimate relationships with other organ systems of the body, exerting an integrated regulatory function. In specific, control is exerted over the heart and lungs, and the nervous system plays an important role in temperature, fluid, and electrolyte balance. Stroke, therefore, has implications for systemic function. Stroke may produce cardiac dysfunction, pulmonary alterations, hyperthermia, fluid and electrolyte abnormalities, and coagulopathy. In this chapter, selected systemic complications resulting from stroke will be discussed and nursing implications reviewed.

CARDIAC ALTERATIONS

Although certain types of cardiac disease are known to cause stroke, there is also strong evidence that stroke may directly contribute to cardiac dysfunction. Specifically, stroke may produce ECG changes, cardiac dysrhythmias, and changes in cardiac enzymes.

Characteristic ECG changes associated with stroke include:

Prolonged QT interval
Shortened PR interval
Peaked P waves
Peaked T waves
Depressed ST segment
Tall U waves

These changes may occur singly or in combination. Interestingly, peaked P waves, in combination with shortened PR intervals and prolonged QT intervals and tall U waves, have been shown to indicate poor prognosis after stroke. In addition, ECG changes may be noted, which are suggestive of cardiac ischemia mimicking myocardial infarction. Such changes include inverted T waves, ST segment elevation, and pathological Q waves, which evolve over time.

Virtually any type of cardiac dysrhythmia may occur following stroke. Dysrhythmias may result from abnormalities in impulse formation or disturbances in conduction (see box on p. 70). Premature ventricular contractions are the most commonly occurring cardiac dysrhythmia following stroke. There are two major consequences related to stroke-induced cardiac dysrhythmias. First, life-threatening dysrhythmias may occur, even without a past history of cardiac disease. Second, cardiac dysrhythmias may decrease cardiac output, contributing to a decrease in cerebral perfusion pressure. Thus the size of the cerebral infarct and the extent of neurologic deficit may be secondarily increased.

Cardiac enzymes have been shown to be elevated after stroke. Creatine kinase, released with tissue destruction, may be seen with cardiac tissue damage but can also be elevated because of damage to brain or muscle tissue or as a nonspecific response to stress. Creatine kinase-methylated bovine (CK-MB) is an isoenzyme specific to cardiac tissue. The extent of CK-MB elevations is directly related to

CARDIAC DYSRHYTHMIAS ASSOCIATED WITH STROKE

Sinus arrhythmia
Sinus bradycardia or tachycardia
Premature atrial contractions
Atrial flutter, fibrillation
Wandering pacemaker
Supraventricular tachycardia
Premature ventricular contractions
Ventricular tachycardia, fibrillation
Atrioventricular blocks
Bundle branch blocks

the extent of cardiac tissue damaged. Dramatic elevations in CK-MB are associated with poor prognosis after stroke.

Given that heart disease also produces ECG abnormalities, cardiac dysrhythmias, and elevated cardiac enzymes, the question arises whether cardiac manifestations are truly complications or causes of stroke. Current research in this area identifies these cardiac changes as a response to stroke. Similar ECG changes have been noted following both ischemic and hemorrhagic stroke, and it is obvious that cardiac changes cannot cause intracranial hemorrhage. Premature ventricular contraction, the most common dysrhythmia following stroke, is a very unlikely cause of stroke. Changes in cardiac enzymes following stroke are characteristically different from those seen with myocardial infarction. With myocardial infarction, CK-MB peaks within 24 hours of injury then gradually declines. However, CK-MB peaks after stroke about the sixth day after brain injury and returns to normal by the tenth day. Each of these observations supports the argument that these cardiac changes occur as a response to stroke.

Cardiac changes are thought to result from a neurogenically mediated autonomic response. Beta-adrenergic hyperactivity is thought to occur, producing a local and systemic release of catecholamines, particularly norepinephrine. Clinically, increases in plasma norepinephrine have been measured after stroke. High levels of catecholamines may produce cardiac myofibrillary exhaustion, leading to subendocardial ischemia and myocardial necrosis. Interestingly, the myocardial necrosis is often evident only at autopsy, and it is quite diffuse rather than focal (as would be seen with myocardial infarction). Changes in the ECG pattern and cardiac dysrhythmias may result from both the microscopic cardiac changes and the catecholamine surge. Cardiac enzyme elevation occurs with underlying cardiac damage. Alpha-adrenergic hyperactivity may also occur. Rarely, parasympathetic dominance may result. The exact etiology of the autonomic response is not known. Initially, cardiac changes were thought to be associated with hemorrhagic stroke, with studies reporting an incidence of poststroke cardiac abnormalities in this population of 70% to 100%. More recent studies have identified cardiac changes following ischemic stroke, although the incidence may not be as high (50% to 68%) and the changes may not be as pronounced. At present, cardiac changes are thought to be a nonspecific response as similar changes are noted in response to a variety of neurogenic stimuli, including head injury, brain tumor, and intracranial surgery. Also, increased intracranial pressure may indirectly produce a sympathetic response by stimulating release of catecholamines.

Because of its interrelationship with the autonomic nervous system, the limbic system and its connections are thought to be implicated in the cardiac response to stroke. Involvement of the cingulate gyrus, orbitofrontal region, thalamus, hypothalamus, amygdala, and/or midbrain is expected to produce autonomic alterations. However, cardiac changes have been noted when stroke has spared these areas, again highlighting the lack of specificity of the cardiac response. Cardiac alterations are more common with hemispheric rather than brainstem involvement.

It was previously thought that coexisting heart disease and age were important factors contributing to poststroke cardiac dysfunction. However, in studies where preexisting cardiac disease was equivalent in both the stroke and nonstroke (control) groups, and groups were equal in age, cardiac alterations in the stroke group were significantly greater. Therefore, preexisting heart disease may not be a contributory factor in poststroke cardiac changes.

The influence of cardiac changes on poststroke outcome is not clearly understood. While it appears that these changes may spontaneously resolve without any residual deficits, some studies have indicated certain changes (e.g., extreme elevations in CK-MB and ventricular fibrillation) may negatively influence outcome. Study results conflict in this area, warranting additional research.

Because the exact influence of cardiac changes on outcome is not known, clinicians disagree about whether these cardiac changes should be treated. Some physicians advocate the use of the beta-blocker, propanolol (Inderal) for its cardioprotective effects. Since stroke may produce both alpha- and beta-adrenergic responses, phentolamine (Regitine) may be used for alpha blockade. Calcium channel blockers have also been recommended for cardiac protection. The limited number of studies that have been performed question the benefit of pharmacologic intervention. Again, additional study is warranted.

Nursing intervention begins with a realization of the connection between stroke and cardiac changes. The most obvious implication is the need to monitor the ECG following acute stroke. Continuous ECG monitoring is preferred and daily 12-lead ECGs are indicated. Changes in ECG configuration and rhythm should be noted.

Related cardiac isoenzymes (in particular, CK-MB) are also monitored as ordered. Emergency drugs and equipment should be available in the event life-threatening dysrhythmias occur. It may be advisable to periodically measure cardiac output via thermodilution, particularly when cardiac compromise is evident.

Nursing intervention should focus upon minimizing myocardial oxygen consumption. Blood pressure should be closely monitored for hypertension and antihypertensive drugs administered as ordered. Physical activity is restricted and gradually resumed as cardiac condition improves. Heart rate should be monitored during physical activity, and the activity stopped if tachycardia occurs. To ensure that adequate oxygen is available to the heart, arterial blood gases are checked periodically and supplemental oxygen provided as necessary.

Factors related to cardiac function should be controlled. Hypokalemia may contribute to myocardial necrosis and should be quickly reversed. Current medications should be reviewed, climinating, if possible, medications that decrease cardiac output or produce electrolyte abnormalities. Attempts should be made to control intracranial pressure. When medications are used to treat the cardiac response, the patient should be closely observed for adverse effects. Beta-blockers may produce bradycardia and subsequently decrease cardiac output. Alpha blockade may produce tachycardia, which ultimately increases the workload of the heart.

PULMONARY ALTERATIONS

Several respiratory changes may occur as a consequence of stroke. Alterations in respiratory rhythmicity and neurogenic pulmonary edema occur directly as a result of neurologic abnormalities. Other respiratory complications result from immobility imposed by stroke (e.g., pulmonary embolus and pneumonia). Since these respiratory complications potentially affect cerebral oxygenation, the effects should be understood and interventions provided accordingly.

Alterations in Respiratory Rhythmicity

Initiation of inspiration and expiration and rhythmicity of the respiratory pattern are controlled by the brainstem to adjust the alveolar ventilatory rate to meet the demands of the body. The medulla contains neurons responsible for initiating inspiration and expiration. The pneumotaxic and apneustic centers in the pons modify respiratory rhythm and provide a smooth respiratory pattern.

Other inhibitory and facilitatory impulses from the lungs, spinal cord, and vasomotor centers also play a role in altering respiratory rhythmicity in response to certain stimuli. In addition, the medulla contains centers that respond to input from systemic chemoreceptors (namely the carotid and aortic arch bodies). This allows the brainstem to adjust respiratory rate, depth, and rhythm in response to arterial oxygen and carbon dioxide levels. Although respiration is largely an involuntary function, higher areas in the cerebral cortex play a role in voluntary control of respiration, allowing a person to increase or decrease respiratory rate and depth as desired.

Stroke may impair respiratory control by affecting voluntary control (via higher cerebral centers) or by affecting the brainstem to produce various respiratory rhythm alterations. Hemorrhagic infarction of the pons or basilar artery occlusion have been cited as the most common causes of respiratory alteration following stroke. Increased intracranial pressure produced as a result of stroke may secondarily compress the brainstem and alter respiratory function. Specific types of respiratory alterations, characteristic patterns, and level of involvement are described in Chapter 5.

Brainstem stroke generally carries a poor prognosis because vital motor and physiologic centers are involved. Appearance of respiratory alterations indicative of brainstem involvement is generally an ominous finding. Because these respiratory alterations may produce changes in arterial oxygen and carbon dioxide levels, intubation, with mechanical ventilation to override brainstem control, is necessary. Early intervention is advocated because blood gas abnormalities have been related to poor return of motor function. While the patient receives mechanical ventilation, abnormal respiratory patterns may be difficult to evaluate. Often the nurse relies on descriptions of spontaneous respiration before intubation or notes the pattern upon removal of the patient from the ventilator for suctioning.

Central sleep apnea (CSA), or Ondine's curse, deserves special mention. Probably the least common of all sleep apneas, CSA results from involvement of the medulla. The most common cause of CSA is lateral medullary infarction, although other neurologic diseases may produce a similar response. Characteristically, the person with CSA is able to fall asleep quickly, but awakens frequently, usually because of snoring or a feeling that he cannot breathe, and complains of not feeling rested. More commonly, the ventilated patient may initiate spontaneous respirations while awake yet require assisted ventilation while asleep. Automatic breathing ceases during sleep in CSA, resulting in a decrease in arterial oxygen saturation. This produces arousal and resumption of breathing. The patient is able to breathe normally while awake but has prolonged periods of apnea or even respiratory arrest during sleep.

Treatment of CSA is essential but can be quite complex. Pharmacologic interventions have been used with varying degrees of success in an attempt to increase output of respiratory neurons. Drugs most commonly used include protriptyline, acetazolamide, pemoline, and methoxyprogesterone; however, these drugs seem to be more effective in obstructive rather than central types of sleep apnea. Ventilatory support during sleep, in the form of continuous positive airway pressure (CPAP), is helpful. Ventilation may also be assisted during sleep by other mechanical means, such as the rocking bed or cuirass (tank) respirator. Surgical intervention in the form of placement of an electrophrenic pacer has been recently studied with somewhat promising results. In addition, current medications should be reviewed, eliminating, if possible, those with respiratory-depressant effects. Since obstructive sleep apnea may coexist with CSA, the airway should be completely evaluated and measures instituted to relieve any obstructive problems.

Neurogenic Pulmonary Edema

The pulmonary response to severe neurologic insult was described over 100 years ago. Increased survival from the initial neurologic insult in recent years has afforded a greater understanding of the "brain-lung" connection. Neurogenic pulmonary edema (NPE), also known as an adult respiratory distress syndrome, is an acute respiratory failure, occurring in response to a neurologic insult. Although respiratory failure may occur following stroke, it is not as common a response as that seen with other types of neurologic involvement (such as head injury or subarachnoid hemorrhage). In general, NPE is associated with severe rather than mild to moderate stroke.

It appears that stroke (or other neurologic insult) stimulates sympathetic pathways, which produce vasoconstriction of the pulmonary vasculature. The resultant pulmonary hypoperfusion leads to obstruction of the pulmonary vasculature because of platelet aggregation. Damaged platelets release vasoactive substances that also contribute to vasoconstriction. Blood stagnates in pulmonary vessels and capillary permeability is altered, allowing fluid to leak into the extravascular (extracellular) space. Secondarily, decreased surfactant is produced and lungs become stiff (noncompliant). Thus a neurogenic stimulus produces edematous, noncompliant lungs with impairment of gas exchange. A variety of neurologic (and other) insults produce the same response, the severity of which is thought to be related to the severity of the insult.

Clinical findings vary based upon individual patient response. Minor NPE may produce nonspecific signs, such as a slightly increased respiratory rate and decreased arterial Po_2. More severe states of NPE produce dyspnea, tachypnea, rales and rhonchi, profuse secretions, and a decline in level of consciousness. Diagnosis is based upon the presence of characteristic infiltrates on chest x-ray and accompanying changes in arterial blood gases.

Because mortality rates are high with NPE, early identification of clinical symptomatology and supportive treatment is essential. Intensive pulmonary hygiene is vital to prevent retention of secretions and closure of small airways. Since mortality increases with infection, infection control measures should also be incorporated. Most importantly, measures to promote optimum pulmonary ventilation and tissue perfusion should be considered. This usually requires administration of supplemental oxygen, positioning to facilitate the work of breathing, and usually, provision of mechanical ventilation. Although difficult, the underlying cause or pathophysiologic response should be eliminated. There is some evidence to indicate administration of a hypothalamic depressant medication, such as chlorpromazine, may decrease the sympathetic response. Some clinicians have advocated the use of corticosteroids to provide pulmonary protection. Because use of these medications is generally controversial, treatment focuses on providing supportive pulmonary care. The nurse's role is vital in early recognition and provision of supportive care.

Pulmonary Embolus

Pulmonary embolization (PE) is unfortunately a common occurrence in stroke patients. The third highest incidence overall of PE has been reported in the stroke patient, with the paralyzed leg serving as the source for embolization. Although not all stroke patients develop venous thrombosis, evidence indicates that the incidence of venous thrombosis in the stroke patient is higher than previously thought. In a recent study, almost 33% of stroke patients admitted to a rehabilitation hospital without evidence of venous thrombosis demonstrated in impedance plethysmography abnormalities indicative of thrombosis. Another author reports incidence of venous thrombosis in the stroke patient at 45% to 75%, with only about half of the patients being symptomatic. The high incidence of venous thrombosis in this population is thought to result not only from immobility but also from platelet abnormalities known to exist after stroke. An estimated 10% to 50% of patients with venous thrombosis will develop PE. Considering that PE may be preventable, mortality rates from PE may be quite high; reports range from 18% to 30%. As a result, preventive measures, early identification, and aggressive intervention are vital.

Increasing age and dense hemiplegia contribute to venous thrombosis and PE. Venous thrombosis and PE tend to be slightly more common in males and edema in the extremities may be a contributing factor. Most often, venous thrombosis occurs within 10 to 14 days of the onset of stroke but may occur up to months later. PE most often occurs (if it does) within 3 to 7 days of thrombosis.

Clinical findings reported to be associated with venous thrombosis in the stroke patient include swelling, warmth, and tenderness in the affected leg. Leg hyperpigmentation, an indication of venous disease, may be another important clinical finding. Clinical findings associated with PE in the stroke patient include chest pain, dyspnea, fever, hypotension, hemoptysis, and transient neurologic deficit. Interestingly, symptom clarification was regarded as most difficult in the aphasic patient.

Preventive treatment remains controversial. The incidence of venous thrombosis in the stroke patient is an argument for prophylactic anticoagulation, using low-dose, subcutaneous heparin. However, studies to date have been contradictory. In addition, prophylactic anticoagulation is contraindicated in the patient with hemorrhagic stroke. Once venous thrombosis and/or PE occur, aggressive anticoagulation using intravenous heparin remains the treatment of choice. Supportive pulmonary care may also be necessary. Because of the incidence of occult venous thrombosis, it is recommended that all stroke patients be screened, using noninvasive studies (such as impedance plethysmography).

Pneumonia

A preventable and unfortunately common complication of stroke is pneumonia. Incidence is estimated at about 40%. Pneumonia is a major cause of death (34% of stroke-related deaths) following stroke. A number of factors in the stroke patient may contribute to pneumonia. Imposed bedrest or immobility induced by motor deficits may contribute to pooling of secretions. Respiratory movements may also be decreased on the hemiplegic side. Aspiration, resulting from dysphagia, impaired cough, and an impaired gag reflex, may occur with brainstem stroke. Overall, immune function may be depressed because of the stress of stroke.

To complicate the stroke patient's situation, diagnosis of pneumonia may be difficult. Expected pulmonary findings may not be readily apparent. Confusion or behavioral changes are common presenting symptoms. Fever is a relatively unreliable indicator. Therefore, close observation of the stroke patient for subtle changes in respiratory function, behavior, and temperature is essential.

Because of the high incidence of pneumonia among stroke patients, preventive measures are advocated. Preventive measures recommended in the literature include head elevation to facilitate breathing and frequent positioning and deep breathing to prevent pooling of secretions. Chest physiotherapy and prophylactic antibiotics may also be used. Once pneumonia occurs, these measures are also indicated. Aggressive antibiotic therapy is vital, and supportive pulmonary care is important. Tracheostomy with cuff inflation may be indicated to minimize risk of aspiration. Unfortunately, there is little conclusive evidence to date to support efficacy of any of these measures.

Nursing Implications

Nursing care begins with the realization that every stroke patient is at risk for pulmonary compromise, thus warranting a detailed pulmonary assessment. Respiratory rate and rhythm should be monitored every 2 to 4 hours for the first 3 days following stroke and as necessary after that. Increased or decreased rate or alteration in rhythm should be reported and noted in the patient's chart. The patient may offer subjective complaints of respiratory difficulty or the nurse may question the patient directly. Peripheral evidence of respiratory distress may be noted in the physical examination, such as nailbed or circumoral cyanosis, nasal flaring, or restlessness. The lungs should be auscultated for clarity of breath sounds. Rales or rhonchi are to be reported and noted in the patient's chart. The patient's ability to handle secretions should be noted, and presence of the gag reflex determined, particularly in the patient with brainstem stroke.

Clinical indicators of respiratory function should be monitored. Baseline arterial blood gas (ABG) assays should be obtained and repeated as necessary, particularly with any evidence of change in respiratory status or when changes in ventilatory support are instituted. The patient's white blood count should be monitored, observing for elevation that might indicate infection. This is particularly important since fever indicative of pneumonia may not occur in the older stroke patient. However, temperature should still be determined every 4 to 8 hours. Chest radiographs should be ordered by the physician as a baseline and rechecked as necessary or when evidence of pulmonary dysfunction exists.

Patients with brainstem stroke who maintain spontaneous respirations and are alert, should be monitored for hypoventilation and apnea during sleep. Application of an apnea monitor may provide additional information. Patients with hemiparesis, hemiplegia, or prescribed prolonged bedrest should be assessed twice a day for evidence of venous thrombosis, including edema, warmth, and tenderness in one or both legs.

Obtaining adequate information on the patient's past history is also important. The patient should be questioned about smoking, past history of pulmonary disease (such as, asthma or chronic obstructive lung disease), and congestive heart failure. Ongoing assessment of respiratory status through discharge is essential because pulmonary complications may arise at any time.

Nursing interventions focus on prevention of respiratory complications and provision of respiratory support. If possible, the patient could be positioned upright, but blood pressure should be monitored closely because the upright position may lead to hypotension, contributing to additional ischemia and neurologic deficit. Early mobilization is generally advocated to minimize the risk of pneumonia and other hazards of immobility. The patient's blood pressure must be stable before mobilization and activity increased gradually. Changing positions frequently may prevent pooling of secretions. If alert and cooperative, the stroke patient may be encouraged to deep breathe every 4 hours. Incentive spirometry may also be incorporated. Humidity may be added to the environment to decrease tenacity of secretions; adequate hydration should be provided for the same reason. If prophylactic antibiotics are ordered, the patient should be observed for adverse effects.

The nurse is involved in providing respiratory support as ordered by the physician. Evidence indicates that even subtle respiratory changes occur acutely after stroke. Therefore, supplemental oxygen, 2 to 4 liters per minute per nasal cannula may be ordered. More obvious respiratory changes require intubation and mechanical ventilatory support to preserve neurologic function. Intubation may be accomplished using a high-volume, low-pressure cuffed tube. Ventilator settings are adjusted to maintain arterial PCO_2 at 25 to 30 torr and arterial PO_2 at 85 to 100 torr or within age-adjusted normal limits. (Normal arterial PO_2 in the older population may be decreased to 70 to 80 torr as a result of age-related changes of the respiratory system.) Care is taken to avoid respiratory measures that may increase intracranial pressure (such as positive end expiratory pressure). The patient should be monitored for adverse effects of intubation, mechanical ventilatory support, and oxygen toxicity.

BODY TEMPERATURE ALTERATIONS

Body temperature is adjusted to a predetermined level by the preoptic area of the hypothalamus. This area, known as the hypothalamic thermostat, serves to balance heat production and heat loss in the body. Body temperature elevation above the predetermined level (set-point) is known as *fever.** In contrast, when the hypothalamic set-point is increased above the normal level, and body temperature increases to achieve that level, *hyperthermia** (or central fever) results.

Central fever may occur as a result of stroke involving the hypothalamus or brainstem, usually hemorrhagic in origin. Characteristically, the fever is quite high, usually greater than 103° F (39.44° C).

*These two terms, *fever* and *hyperthermia,* are often used interchangeably.

FACTORS AFFECTING ADH RELEASE

Stimulating Factors

- Anxiety
- Hyperosmolality
- Hypertension
- Hyperthermia
- Hyponatremia
- Hypovolemia
- Myocardial failure
- Pain
- Physiologic stress response

Suppressant Factors

- Alcohol
- Drugs-
  - Acetaminophen
  - alpha-adrenergic drugs
  - Anticholinergic drugs
  - Barbiturates
  - beta-adrenergic drugs
  - Carbamazepine
  - Chlorothiazide
  - Chlorpromazine
  - Chlorpropamide
  - Cholinergic drugs
  - Clofibrate
  - Corticosteroids
  - Cyclophosphamide
  - Demeclocycline
  - Lithium
  - Meperidine
  - Morphine
  - Nicotine
  - Phenytoin
  - Vincristine
- Hypernatremia
- Hypervolemia
- Hypoosmolality
- Hypotension
- Hypothermia

Heat loss mechanisms appear impaired. Flushing is absent, respirations may be slow, and sweating is absent. As a result, central fever generally responds poorly to conventional heat reduction mechanisms, such as topical cooling, bathing, or administration of antipyretic agents. The fever may respond to medications that depress hypothalamic activity, such as chlorpromazine, meperidine, or promethazine. Other autonomic dysfunctions may accompany central fever (such as labile heart rate and blood pressure).

It is important to note that central fever is quite uncommon in the stroke patient. Rather, fever is usually attributable to a pulmonary source, most often pneumonia. However, because treatment differs radically, and since fever may increase cerebral metabolic demand, it is essential that the source of fever be identified and appropriately treated. Fever in the stroke patient is considered to be an unfavorable prognostic sign, contributing not only to a higher mortality but also to increased morbidity and prolonged recovery.

FLUID BALANCE ALTERATIONS

Three major mechanisms control the body's fluid balance: the antidiuretic hormone (ADH) system, the thirst mechanism, and the renin-angiotensin-aldosterone system. These three mechanisms work jointly to promote normovolemia. Only the first two mechanisms, mediated primarily by the central nervous system, will be addressed here.

The neurohypophyseal system of the hypothalamus is responsible for production, storage, and release of ADH. This hormone increases permeability of the distal tubules of the kidney to water, allowing water to be reabsorbed. Without ADH, water is not reabsorbed and, subsequently, is lost in the urine. Production and release of ADH are trolled by volume status and blood pressure. Hypovolemia or hypotension trigger ADH release, while hypervolemia or hypertension inhibit ADH release. These factors are intended to be normal physiologic control mechanisms. Factors affecting ADH release are listed in the box at right. Abnormal release of ADH may occur because of a neurologic insult involving the hypothalamus. ADH abnormalities are not common, but may occur following hemorrhagic or ischemic stroke. Abnormalities of ADH are the syndrome of inappropriate ADH secretion and diabetes insipidus.

Syndrome of Inappropriate ADH Secretion (SIADH)

With SIADH, the amount of ADH released is greater than that required by the body, resulting in water retention and intoxication. Clinical characteristics associated with SIADH are listed in the box on p.78. The therapy provided for SIADH depends on severity of water retention. Mild SIADH is usually treated by restricting overall fluid intake to 1000 ml or less in 24 hours. More severe cases of SIADH may require more stringent fluid restriction (500 ml/24 hours) and cautious sodium replacement using a 3% sodium chloride solution. Medications may be ordered to facilitate the body's removal of excess fluid; drugs such as furosemide (Lasix) or mannitol have been helpful. Drugs that inhibit ADH release have been used more recently. Examples include demeclocycline (Declomycin), butorphanol (Stadol), lithium, and oxilorphan. Resolution of SIADH may occur over days to weeks; rarely is the problem permanent.

Diabetes Insipidus (DI)

In classic DI, ADH production and release is impaired, resulting in decreased reabsorption of water in the renal tubules, leading to dehydration. Clinical characteristics associated with DI are listed in the box on p.78. Treatment of DI focuses on fluid replacement and administration of replacement ADH. Since severe polyuria may occur, fluid replacement may be difficult to achieve. Replacement of ADH may be accomplished by administering the medications listed in Table 6-1. Replacement of ADH is usually considered when fluid loss is severe or when DI symptoms persist for more than 12 hours. Additional medications may be used to enhance the kidney response to ADH or to stimulate ADH production and release. Examples of such drugs include chlorpropamide (Diabinese), carbamazepine (Tegretol), and clofibrate (Atromid-S). Stroke-related DI is usually temporary; however, permanent DI may occur, requiring lifelong ADH replacement. Patients with permanent DI require detailed teaching about the pathophysiology and effects of DI and the necessity for lifelong medication.

Nursing Implications

Fluid and electrolyte abnormalities following stroke require skilled nursing assessment and intervention. The patient's intake and output must be closely monitored, especially over a 24-hour period. Specific gravity is assessed a minimum of once each shift but preferably every 2 to 4 hours (if catheterized) or with each void. Daily weights are important indicators of fluid loss or gain. One kilogram of weight gained (or lost) is roughly equal to 1000 ml of fluid retained (or lost). Central measures of volume status, such as central venous pressures or pulmonary capillary wedge pressure, may be necessary with more severe or difficult to control volume alterations. Laboratory indicators, including urine and serum osmolarity and electrolytes, must be closely monitored. With acute ADH abnormalities, testing may be ordered as frequently as every 6 hours. The patient should also be monitored for evidence of fluid and electrolyte abnormalities. Most important, the patient with SIADH should be observed for signs related to hyponatremia, including decreased level of consciousness, confusion, weakness, muscle cramping, headache, and seizures. If possible, factors should be eliminated that affect ADH production and release (see the box on p.76). Since fluid and electrolyte abnormalities may predispose the patient to skin breakdown, a skin care program and frequent repositioning are warranted.

Patient education is essential in chronic or long-term stroke-induced fluid and electrolyte abnormalities. Patients and families should be informed about the pathogenesis underlying the abnormality and the need for medication. A Medic-alert bracelet is usually indicated. The need for fluid restriction

CLINICAL CHARACTERISTICS OF STATES OF ALTERED ADH RELEASE

Syndrome of Inappropriate ADH Release

Decreased urinary output (<500 ml/24 hr)
Increased urine specific gravity (>1.020)
Decreased serum osmolality (<275 mOsm)
Increased urine osmolality
Decreased serum sodium (<130 mEq/l)
Increased urine sodium
Weight gain
Signs of hyponatremia
- mild—lethargy, fatigue, headache, muscle cramping
- severe—nausea, vomiting, seizures, coma, fasciculations

Diabetes Insipidus

Increased urinary output (>4000 ml/24 hr)
Decreased urine specific gravity (<1.005)
Increased serum osmolality (>290 mOsm)
Decreased urine osmolality
Increased serum sodium (>150 mEq/l)
Decreased urine sodium
Weight loss
Thirst
Signs of dehydration

Table 6-1 Drugs used in the treatment of diabetes insipidus (DI)

Name	Usual adult dose	Duration	Comments
Aqueous vasopressin	5 to 10 units SC	3 to 6 hours	Short duration; used for patients who have immediate postoperative DI or who cannot be monitored frequently
Vasopressin tannate in oil	5 units IM	24 to 72 hours	Painful injection; must be warmed and shaken to mix properly; need to rotate injection site; used if diabetes insipidus expected to last for a period of time
Lypressin nasal spray	Spray intranasally 3 to 4 times a day	4 to 6 hours	Nasal mucosa must be intact; useful for mild DI; patient may develop nasal congestion which will interfere with absorption
Desmopressin acetate (DDAVP)	0.1 ml to 0.4 ml intranasally	12 to 24 hours	Causes minimal nasoconstriction; administered once or twice a day; used for severe permanent or transient complete central DI
In milder forms of DI (when ADH is secreted in small amounts), the following drugs may be used to enhance the secretion of ADH or to increase the response of the kidney to ADH:			
Chlorpropamide (Diabinese)	250 mg to 500 mg/qd/PO	24 hours	Stimulates release of ADH from the posterior pituitary and enhances its action on renal tubules
Clofibrate (Atromid S)	500 mg/qid/PO	24 hours	Same as above
Carbamazepine (Tegretol)	400 mg to 600 mg/qd/PO	24 hours	Same as above
Hydrochlorothiazide (HydroDiuril)	50 mg/qd or bid/PO	12 to 24 hours	Used for nephrogenic DI

From Hickey JV: The clinical practice of neurological and neurosurgical nursing, ed 2, Philadelphia, 1986, JB Lippincott.

or replacement should be explained and reinforced as should the need for accurate monitoring of intake, output, and specific gravity. The patient and family must also be taught the importance of controlling factors that affect ADH release.

Changes in serum osmolarity affect the thirst center located in the hypothalamus. As osmolarity increases, the thirst center is stimulated and the person becomes thirsty. This response may be directly altered by stroke by either inhibiting or accentuating the response. The thirst response may also be indirectly affected by dysphagia or a decreased level of consciousness, impairing the person's ability to drink. Changes in the thirst response are uncommon and often superimposed on other fluid alterations.

COAGULOPATHY

Massive cerebral infarction produces extensive brain tissue damage, which can lead to disseminated intravascular coagulation (DIC). This clinical syndrome occurs only as a complication of a primary disease and results from numerous neurologic and nonneurologic disorders. DIC is characterized by simultaneous clotting and hemorrhage.

With extensive stroke, thromboplastic substances are released from damaged tissue. The thromboplastic substances activate the extrinsic clotting system to produce both the hemorrhage and clotting characteristic of DIC. As the clotting cascade is initiated, diffuse intravascular clotting occurs, occluding microcirculation to produce further tissue damage and release of thromboplastic substances. The fibrinolytic process begins as a normal part of the clotting cascade, and plasmin is activated to break down the clotted cells into fibrin-split products (FSPs). FSPs combine with fibrinogen to produce a paracoagulable product that hemolyzes red blood cells, releasing additional thromboplastin. This process can be self-perpetuating.

Simultaneously, as clotting occurs, the supply of coagulation factors may be depleted, leading to hemorrhage. Circulating FSPs released in the fibrinolytic process act as anticoagulants, also contributing to hemorrhage. Hence, the seemingly contradictory picture of hemorrhage and clotting occurs. In most patients, evidence of both processes usually exists but one process dominates.

Clinical characteristics of DIC include manifestations of hemorrhage and/or clotting. Hemorrhagic signs include:

- Slow bleeding or oozing of blood—may exude into body fluids (i.e., urine and nasogastric aspirate) or around sites of altered skin integrity
- Bruising
- Major hemorrhage—usually evident from a gastrointestinal site but may be intracranial or exude into the urine

As a result of consumption of coagulation factors, clotting profiles will be prolonged and platelet count decreased. Clotting signs are related to occlusion of the microcirculation and include:

- Acral cyanosis
- Organ failure—particularly pulmonary and nal
- Seizures

Treatment for DIC consists of replacement of clotting factors. Heparinization has been used in situations in which the clotting process dominates; however, its use remains controversial. This is because a precise dose of heparin cannot be determined because the partial thromboplastin time will be prolonged. Nursing care focuses on assessment for hemorrhagic and clotting effects as described; clotting profiles should be closely monitored and compared with the patient's baseline. Bleeding precautions are also indicated. If alert and mobile, the patient may be prescribed bedrest to minimize the risk of hemorrhagic injury.

NURSING CARE PLAN

Nursing Diagnosis	Interventions	Expected Outcomes
Alteration in Integrated Regulation* related to consequences of stroke **Defining Characteristics** ■ Electrocardiogram (ECG) abnormalities ■ Cardiac dysrhythmias ■ Elevated cardiac enzymes ■ Abnormalities in respiratory rhythm ■ Neurogenic pulmonary edema ■ Pulmonary embolism ■ Pneumonia ■ Hyperthermia (central fever) ■ Alteration in fluid balance, excess or deficit ■ Clotting abnormalities	**Ongoing Assessment** ■ Assess past history of systemic problems: A. Previous cardiac disease, hypertension, smoking, previous pulmonary disease ■ Monitor vital signs every 2 to 4 hrs as needed ■ Monitor baseline ECG and observe for changes ■ Monitor cardiac enzymes as ordered ■ Monitor hemodynamic status if at risk for compromise (requires pulmonary arterial catheter) ■ Monitor electrolytes, arterial blood gases, white blood count, osmolality, PT, PPT, platelet count ■ Observe for adverse effects of medications ■ Monitor respiratory rate, rhythm, breath sounds, and ability to handle secretions every 2 to 4 hours ■ Check presence of gag reflex ■ Observe for evidence of respiratory distress: patient complaints, cyanosis, restlessness, shortness of breath, nasal flaring ■ Monitor body temperature every 4 hours, more frequently if elevated ■ Monitor for evidence of deep venous thrombosis: edema, warmth, tenderness in legs ■ Monitor for adverse effects of respiratory support ■ Monitor intake and output, urine specific gravity every 2 hours ■ Monitor volume status ■ Observe for subtle or overt bleeding ■ Monitor daily weights	■ ECG pattern and rhythm will be stable without changes in cardiac enzymes ■ Respiratory status will be stable ■ Patient will achieve a stable body temperature (normothermic) ■ Patient will be normovolemic with electrolyte balance ■ Patient will not show evidence of coagulopathy

*This is proposed as a working diagnosis and is not a NANDA-approved nursing diagnosis. At present, no such diagnosis exists to address the many systemic problems that occur as a consequence of stroke.

NURSING CARE PLAN — cont'd

Nursing Diagnosis	Interventions	Expected Outcomes
	Therapeutic Interventions ■ Notify physician of any abnormalities in assessment parameters ■ Minimize myocardial oxygen consumption: A. Restrict physical activity initially; gradually resume physical activity as tolerated B. Provide supplemental oxygen ■ Control cardiac related factors: A. Administer medications to reverse hypokalemia B. Review medications for potential cardiac effects or electrolyte abnormalities; discuss changes in medications with physician C. Institute measures to control intracranial pressure ■ Position upright to facilitate work of breathing: A. Monitor blood pressure closely during any position change ■ Prevent pooling of secretions: A. Change position every 2 to 4 hours B. Encourage deep breathing C. Add humidity to the environment D. Assure adequate hydration ■ Provide respiratory support: A. Administer supplemental oxygen as ordered B. Provide endotracheal or tracheal care if warranted C. Oversee ventilatory support if used D. Avoid respiratory measures that increase intracranial pressure ■ Control body temperature: A. Administer antipyretics as ordered B. Initiate topical cooling methods as ordered	

Continued.

NURSING CARE PLAN — cont'd

Nursing Diagnosis	Interventions	Expected Outcomes
	C. Administer hypothalamic depressants as ordered ■ Review medications for effects on fluid and electrolyte balance; discuss changes with physician ■ Maintain volume status by replacing or restricting fluids as ordered ■ Administer vasopressin as ordered	

Patient Education

- Explain need for close monitoring of physiologic parameters
- Instruct in deep breathing techniques
- Instruct patient in incentive spirometry
- Instruct patient in bleeding precautions
- Explain pathophysiology underlying abnormalities in production of antidiuretic hormone and need for patient cooperation in treatment:
  A. Fluid restriction or replacement, need for monitoring intake and output, need for medication
- Inform patient and family about factors influencing release of antidiuretic hormone

REFERENCES

Askenasy JJ and Goldhammer I: Sleep apnea as a feature of bulbar stroke, Stroke 19:637, 1988.

Brott T and Reed RL: Intensive care for acute stroke in the community hospital setting, Stroke 20:694, 1989.

Brouwers PJ, Wijdicks EF, Hansan D and others: Serial electrocardiographic recording in aneurysmal subarachnoid hemorrhage, Stroke 20:1162, 1989.

Chokroverty S: Sleep and breathing in neurologic disorders. In Edelman NH and Santiago TV, editors: Breathing disorders of sleep, New York, 1986, Churchill Livingstone.

Dexter JR, Banasiak GA, Corcoran LJ and others: Sleep apnea syndromes. In Burton GC and Hodgkin JE, editors: Respiratory care, Philadelphia, 1984, JB Lippincott.

Guyton AC: Textbook of medical physiology, ed 7, Philadelphia, 1986, WB Saunders Co.

Horner J and Massey EW: Silent aspiration following stroke, Neurology 38:317, 1988.

Kaplan PE and Cerullo LJ: Stroke rehabilitation, Stoneham, Ma, 1986, Butterworth Publishers.

Lloyd T: Effect of stroke on lung function. In Price TP and Nelson E, editors: Cerebrovascular diseases, New York, 1979, Raven Press.

Mulley GP: Avoidable complications of stroke, J R Coll Physicians Lond, 16:94, 1982.

Myers MG, Norris JW, Hachinski VC and others: Cardiac sequelae of acute stroke, Stroke 13:838, 1982.

Norris JW: Effects of cerebrovascular lesions on the heart, Neurologic Clinics 1:87, 1983.

Plum F and Posner JB: The diagnosis of stupor and coma, Philadelphia, 1986, FA Davis.

Przelomski MM, Roth RM, Gleckman RA and others: Fever in the wake of a stroke. Neurol 36:427, 1986.

Randall WC: Autonomic nervous system effect on cardiac arrythmias and conduction. In Price TR and Nelson E, editors: Cerebrovascular diseases, New York, 1979, Raven Press.

Sioson ER, Crowe WE and Dawson NV: Occult proximal deep vein thrombosis: its prevalence among patients admitted to a rehabilitation hospital, Arch Phys Med Rehabil 69:183, 1988.

Subbarao J and Smith J: Pulmonary embolism during stroke rehabilitation, Illinois Med J 165:328, 1984.

Vincent GM: Cardiac electrophysiologic abnormalities in the stroke syndrome. In Price TR and Nelson E, editors: Cerebrovascular diseases, New York, 1979, Raven Press.

Chapter 7

Alterations in Mobility

The ability to move different parts of our body depends on many systems interacting with one another. The motor system is easily understood if it is thought of as a feedback loop within an open system that can be influenced by outside components. As such there is input, throughput, and output specifically within the motor system, and there are regulatory mechanisms that assist in controlling the quantity, quality, and smoothness of the action. Movement—with the proper amount of speed, coordination, and strength—results from a delicate balance between the central nervous system (brain and spinal cord) and the peripheral nerve input.

A stroke can interrupt the central nervous system component of mobility. The resulting degree of impaired movement depends on many factors, including size and location of the stroke, causative mechanism, and potential for recovery. This chapter discusses the anatomy and physiology of normal movement, specifics of how a stroke can impair mobility, assessment parameters, and nursing interventions related to alterations in mobility.

ANATOMY AND PHYSIOLOGY OF MOBILITY (see Fig. 7-1)

Input

Sensory nerve (afferent) fibers originate in the dorsal root ganglia of the spinal cord and possess one nerve process that eventually divides into a peripheral nerve component and a central nervous system, or spinal cord, component. Humans have two types of afferent fibers: somatic and visceral. Somatic afferent fibers transmit input sensory information from the muscles, tendons, and joints and information from the skin, such as pain, touch, and temperature. The visceral fibers transmit sensory information from the internal body organs. In movement, the somatic afferent fibers are the primary input mechanism.

Output

Efferent, or motor, fibers have divisions similar to afferent fibers. The somatic division, originating in the spinal cord, consists of skeletal motor fibers, while the visceral division regulates smooth and cardiac muscles and is referred to as autonomic. Further classification is based on the size of the fibers and the speed by which information can be transmitted. Large fibers, which are myelin covered, or insulated, are divided into alpha, beta, gamma, and delta categories according to the speed of transmission. Of the four, alpha and gamma fibers are key in motor movement because they are responsible for extrafusal and intrafusal muscle contraction. These fibers are found in the long skeletal muscles of the body. Alpha neurons receive input from many sources, including afferent nerves and the descending tracts of the spinal cord, which include corticospinal, lateral vestibulospinal, and reticulospinal fibers. They in turn innervate the muscle end plate, specifically, the extrafusal fibers

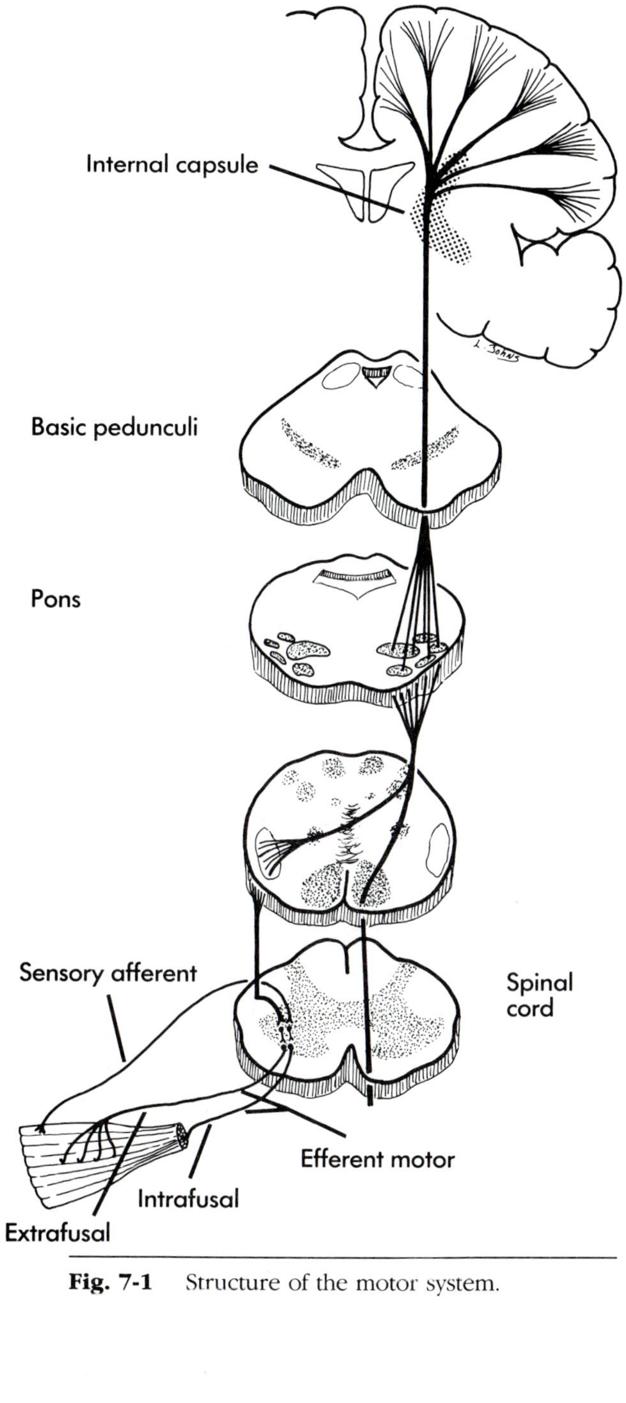

Fig. 7-1 Structure of the motor system.

responsible for muscle contraction. The smaller muscle spindle fibers (intrafusal), which control muscle length, are innervated by gamma neurons. In addition to receiving input from the same sources as alpha neurons, gamma neurons are mediated by the reticular system, basal ganglia, and cerebellum. For normal muscle movement and tone, the alpha and gamma neurons work as a negative feedback loop.

Throughput

At the simplest level, movement is generated by two nerves, one afferent and one efferent. Deep tendon reflexes are best recognized for this monosynaptic system. For example, input or stimulation from a reflex hammer striking the biceps tendon is transmitted via an afferent nerve that meets, or synapses, with an efferent motor nerve in the spinal cord. This nerve then transmits the message to contract to the biceps muscle. More complex throughput exists in which the afferent fibers transmit their message to interneurons located in the spinal cord before the message is given to efferent nerves.

Higher Level Throughput

Several components of the central nervous system affect the throughput of motor movement. For voluntary movement to occur there must be integration of the various components. The three major components are the motor areas of the cerebral cortex, which are assisted by the descending tracts from the cortex and the brainstem; the basal ganglia; and the cerebellum. Once this higher level throughput is initiated, the spinal cord (specifically, the anterior aspect) transmits the message to the peripheral nerves.

Cerebral Cortex

Located in the precentral gyrus of the frontal lobe is the primary motor area or the motor strip (Fig. 7-2). Toward the top of the strip reside controls for the lower part of the body—the leg, foot, and perineum. Located at the bottom of the strip

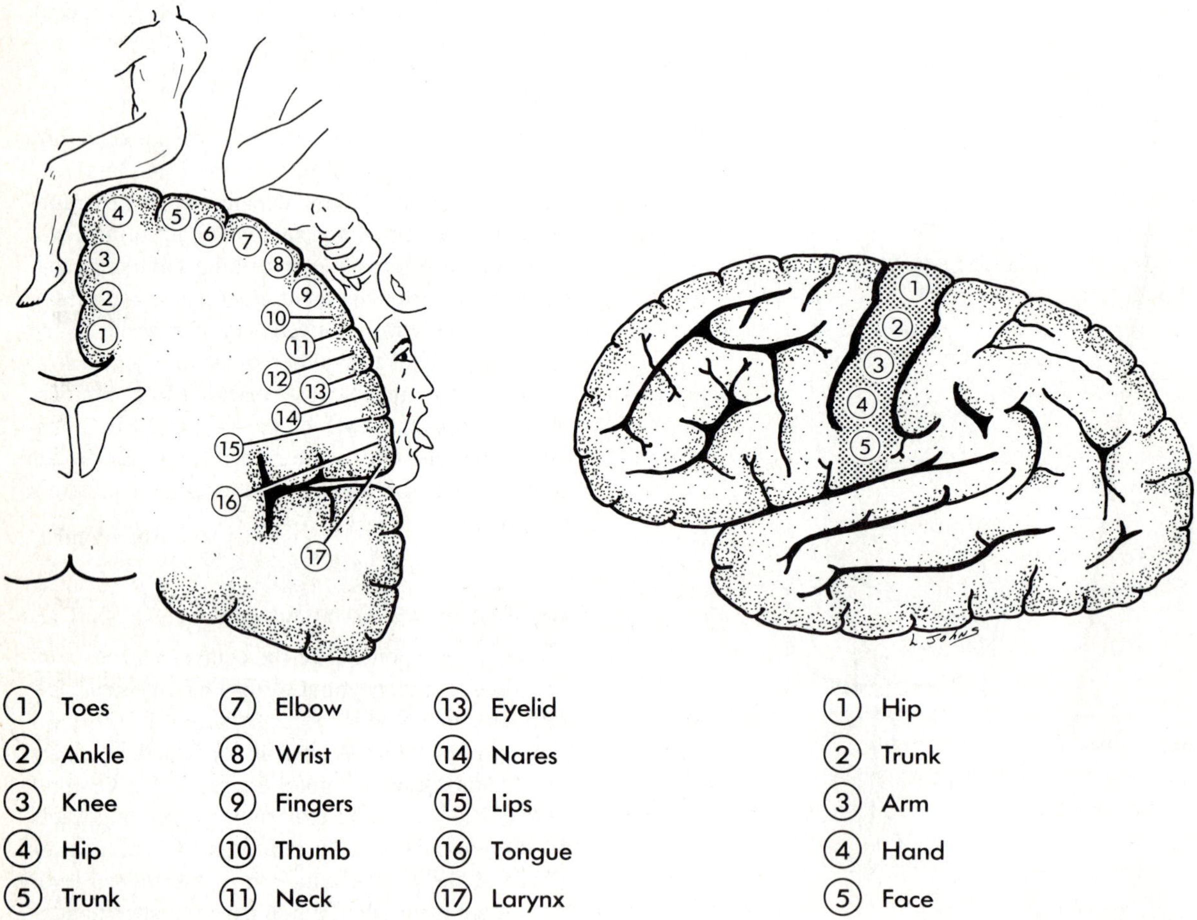

1 Toes
2 Ankle
3 Knee
4 Hip
5 Trunk
6 Shoulder
7 Elbow
8 Wrist
9 Fingers
10 Thumb
11 Neck
12 Brow
13 Eyelid
14 Nares
15 Lips
16 Tongue
17 Larynx

1 Hip
2 Trunk
3 Arm
4 Hand
5 Face

Fig. 7-2 Motor strip of the cerebral cortex.

are portions which control the upper part of the body, including the arm, hand, face, and tongue. The mapping of the body on the motor strip is easily remembered if one thinks of a person standing upsidedown on the side of the brain.

Nerve fibers that originate in this area travel downward through the brain, cross over (decussate) to the other side of the body in the brainstem, and eventually innervate muscles on the opposite side of the body from which they originated. Thus the left motor strip controls muscles on the right side of the body and the right motor strip controls muscles on the left side of the body.

From the motor strip, motor neurons travel down through the spinal cord and connect with more motor neurons that have their cell bodies within the central nervous system and their axons connecting with muscles. The nerves that run through the brain, brainstem, and spinal cord are called upper motor neurons (UMN) and are divided into several different tracts based on the area of origin and termination. The primary tracts that are involved with movement follow.

Corticospinal tract (pyramidal) — arises from motor areas of the cerebral cortex, passes through the posterior portion of the internal capsule, crosses over to the other side of the body in the medulla, and continues downward through the spinal cord. While this tract has many functions, its main role is in voluntary movement of limb muscles, specifically, the flexor muscles innervated by alpha and gamma neurons.

Corticobulbar tract — arises from motor areas of the cerebral cortex and travels through the brain to the brainstem. At various levels within the brainstem, the fibers exert control over several cranial nerve nuclei, including CN III through CN VII and CN IX through CN XII. Most cranial nerves are innervated by fibers from both sides of the brain, except for the upper division of the facial nerve, which is only innervated from one side. This exception is important to note, however, because it can help distinguish facial weakness of central nervous system origin (stroke) vs facial weakness of peripheral origin (Bell's palsy).

Corticotectal tract — arises from the occipital lobe and terminates in the brainstem, eventually influencing eye movements.

Corticorubral tract — arises from the motor areas of the cortex and terminates in the red nucleus of the midbrain. It then forms the rubrospinal tract, which travels down through the spinal cord. Its primary function is flexor movement, especially in the arms.

Corticoreticular tract — travels from the cortex to the reticular formation within the brainstem. From the brainstem, these fibers give rise to the reticulospinal tracts that run through the spinal cord. The nerves in this tract promote extension in the legs and also influence gamma neurons.

Regulatory Components of Throughput

Basal ganglia. The basal ganglia influences motor function by feedback loops that interconnect with the cerebral cortex and cerebellum (Fig. 7-3). The basal ganglia has three components: the caudate nucleus, the putamen, and the globus pallidus. The three are closely connected and can be considered as a whole when discussing movement. The primary role of the basal ganglia is to integrate input information from visual, vestibular, and other sensory modalities into movement. Interruptions in this system can cause unusual movements, such as tremor, choreiform movements (sudden involuntary movements in groups of muscles), athetosis characterized by slow, irregular twisting movements mainly in the arms, and hemiballismus or twitching of muscles.

Cerebellum. The cerebellum plays a key part in any type of motor movement (Fig. 7-4). It regulates the maintenance of posture and balance, the ability to perform repetitive tasks, and sequential motor movements. Disease or injury of the cerebellum produces striking changes in movement, such as difficulty in walking, staggering gait, in-

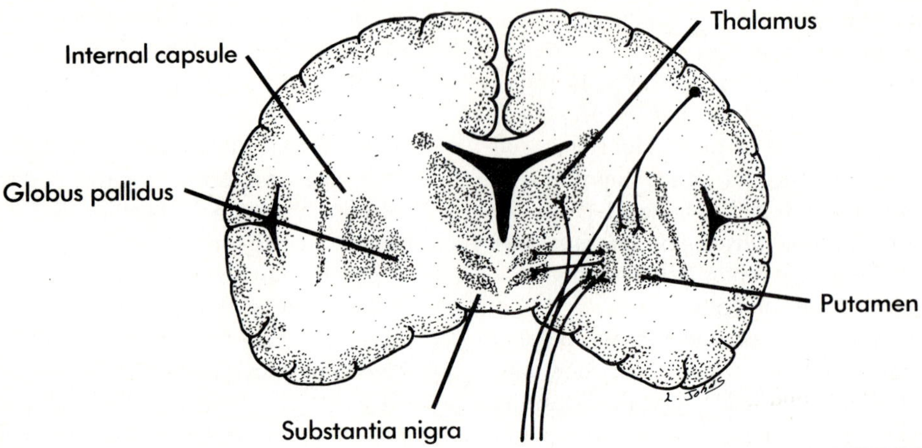

Fig. 7-3 Basal ganglia.

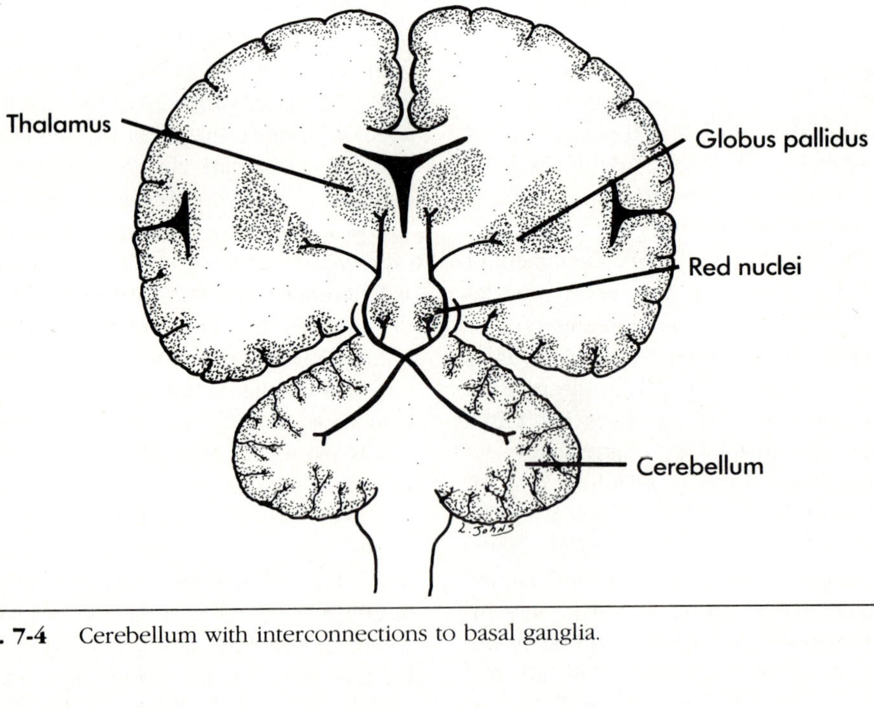

Fig. 7-4 Cerebellum with interconnections to basal ganglia.

ability to perform coordinated movements with both the upper and lower limbs, and hypotonia.

EFFECTS OF STROKE ON MOBILITY

A stroke can produce varying levels of decreased mobility, from mild weakness that impairs a person's ability to carry out the activities of daily living, to hemiplegia or quadriplegia that severely limits any type of movement. Besides such striking changes in quantity of movement, some patients experience a change in the quality of movement. Cerebellar strokes produce ataxia in movements, and a stroke in the basal ganglia results in extrapyramidal signs, such as tremor.

Besides weakness and tremor, the most striking feature of most strokes is spasticity. Stroke impairs the normal balance that results in both alpha and gamma neurons being stimulated to initiate voluntary movement. Both types of neurons are normally stimulated by excitatory and inhibitory input from areas in the cerebral cortex and brainstem. It is easiest to think of the cerebral cortex as producing the inhibitory stimulus and the brainstem structures as generating the excitatory input. The excitatory input from the brainstem to the motor neurons is constant. To moderate the brainstem stimulus, the cerebral cortex sends inhibitory transmissions, especially to the gamma neurons, to balance the system. Thus an interruption of the inhibitory stimulus from the cortex, as in stroke, produces unregulated excitatory stimulation of the motor neurons. Gamma neurons are constantly being excited, resulting in shortening of the muscle. This pattern of uncontrolled stimulation is clinically demonstrated as spasticity.

Complications of Immobility

In 1967, Olson described the complications of bedrest on the different body systems, and in 1988, Rubin detailed the physiology of changes in the organs, muscles, and bones when a person is confined to bed. These two articles outline the various effects and complications arising from immobility that can lead to major life-threatening situations. Whenever anyone is confined to bed several changes occur that are directly related to the mere reduction in activity, such as orthostatic hypotension, increased thrombus formation, changes in cardiac output, and changes in the respiratory system. Decreased gas exchange and pooling of secretions impairs lung functioning. Decreased activity increases catabolic metabolism and leads to negative nitrogen balance. The increased nitrogen in the system decreases appetite so the patient does not consume sufficient nutrients for healing. Immobility also increases the release of calcium from bones and contributes to the development of osteoporosis. The combination of increased catabolism, caloric needs, breakdown of skeletal muscle, and decreased mobility leads to skin breakdown, unless measures are taken to prevent pressure and ulceration of the skin.

ASSESSMENT

Based on the many components of the motor system, assessment proceeds through various phases so that each component is evaluated individually and then combined with the others to complete the clinical picture. The major assessment parameters include muscle, reflex, and cerebellar function.

The Muscles

Four muscle characteristics should be assessed when examining the patient: size, strength, tone, and involuntary movements.

Size. The patient's overall muscle size should be assessed, with comparisons made between the right and left halves of the body. If differences are noted, measuring the muscles and recording the data for a baseline reading are important. Muscle size can be recorded on a scale of 0 to 5 as follows:

5 to 4 = Hypertrophy
3 = Normal
2 to 1 = Atrophy
0 = Muscle is absent

Strength. Both flexion and extension movements are assessed in the major muscle areas of the arms and legs. In each individual muscle group, the examiner applies resistance to the muscle action being tested. For example, to test flexion of the arm, the examiner exerts gentle resistance in the opposite direction. Strength is recorded on a 0 to 5 scale as follows:

5 = Normal, 100%
4 = Mild weakness or paresis, 75% of normal
3 = Moderate weakness or paresis, 50% of normal
2 = Marked weakness or paresis, 25% of normal
1 = Severe weakness, 10% of normal
0 = Complete paralysis

Tone. Muscle tone is assessed while the patient is at rest. The proximal and distal joints are slowly moved throughout their normal range of motion. Hypotonicity is evidenced by joints that move with increased ease and have an increased range of movement. It is most often found in patients who have peripheral nerve disorders or lesions that interrupt the facilitatory UMN pathways. Hypertonicity is divided into three categories: paratonia, spasticity, and rigidity. Resistance to movement in all directions, or *paratonia*, can be produced by lesions in the frontal lobe. Increased resistance to stretching of the extremities is referred to as *spasticity*. As the examiner stretches the extremity farther, the resistance grows. Most lesions that produce spasticity are located in the descending motor tracts. Increased resistance that is uniform throughout the stretching of the extremity is called *rigidity*. It can be found in persons with lesions of the basal ganglia. Once the type of tone is identified, it can be graded as mild, moderate, or severe. Contractures of the muscle are often seen in persons with hypertonia who have not had adequate mobilization. In these patients, the muscles actually become physiologically shorter and incapable of being stretched.

Involuntary movements. While the patient is at rest, the major muscle groups should be inspected for any abnormal movements, such as tics, rapid twitches of muscles (fasciculations), jerking, or tremors. Most often these signs are produced by disturbances in the basal ganglia and their connections.

Reflexes

Deep tendon or muscle stretch reflexes assess the integrity of the monosynaptic reflex. Reflexes are tested by delivering a quick, direct blow to the tendon with a reflex hammer. This produces stretching of some muscles and contraction of others. The chart on p. 91 represents the major deep tendon reflexes and the muscles that are assessed for contraction.

Grading of reflexes

5 = Hyperreflexia with clonus
4 = Moderate hyperreflexia
3 = Normal
2 = Moderate hyporeflexia
1 = Marked hyporeflexia
0 = Areflexia

Hyperreflexia is seen most commonly with lesions involving the UMNs, such as with a stroke. Hyporeflexia reflects lesions within the monosynaptic reflex arch.

Cerebellar Assessment

The cerebellum is responsible for balance and coordination; thus assessment involves tests of these two functions. For the upper extremities, the patient is asked to keep his eyes open and then touch his finger to his nose with one hand and then the other. Next, the patient is asked to touch his nose with his finger and to then touch the examiner's upheld finger. This is repeated several times while the examiner moves her finger to various points in front of the patient. Another test for the upper extremity is for the patient to make rapid alternating movements by pronating and supinating his hands.

Assessment of the lower extremity is similar. The patient is asked to slide the heel of one foot down the shin of the other leg and then repeat the action with the other heel. Testing cerebellar function also involves having the patient walk heel-to-toe in a straight line with his eyes open and then

CHART OF DEEP TENDON REFLEXES

Muscle Group	Segment Stimulated	How to Elicit	Reflex Produced
Biceps	C 5 and 6	Strike biceps tendon	Biceps contracts
Brachio-radialis	C 5 and 6	Strike radius	Flexion of arm
Triceps	C 6, 7, and 8	Strike triceps tendon	Elbow extends
Patellar	L 2, 3, and 4	Strike patellar tendon	Leg extends
Achilles	S 1 and 2	Strike achilles tendon	Flexion of foot

with his eyes closed. All of these actions should be carried out smoothly and accurately. Any impairment noted, such as tremor or ataxia, can be due to lesions within the cerebellum.

INTERVENTIONS

Planning care for stroke patients with impaired mobility is multi-faceted. It includes preventing skin breakdown, loss of functional mobility, and complications. The focus of rehabilitation is to improve the patient's functional ability and promote independence. While the nurse is the person who has the most contact and can most easily incorporate these goals into patient care delivery in the actue stages of stroke, the goals of rehabilitation become a team effort as the patient becomes medically stable and can actively participate in the recovery process. Care conferences that include nurses, physical, occupational, and speech therapists, physiatrists, and other specialists in stroke rehabilitation, facilitate coordination of the many goals in the postacute phase.

After careful baseline assessment of muscle tone and strength is complete, a plan of care must be developed that prevents complications that can develop from immobility and at the same time promotes improved function. By focusing on the motor system and functional abilities in the early phase after stroke, the patient may have less long-term functional loss and may have a shorter rehabilitation period. During the acute phase it is the primary responsibility of members of the health care team to ensure maintenance of functional ability, along with help from the patient and her family. Teaching significant family members and the patient how to participate in the recovery process, and also the reasons behind carrying out needed exercises, facilitates successful outcomes in the plan of care.

General Principles

A major focus of nursing care is to increase the functional ability of the person with decreased mobility. Getting the patient with hemiparesis to use his weak arm and leg in daily activities increases strength and facilitates rehabiliation. For the hemiplegic patient, getting her to incorporate the affected extremities into daily care activities, such as washing, grooming and dressing, decreases the risk of contractures and maintains functional mobility. Often the completely hemiplegic patient has accompanying loss of spatial orientation, hemineglect, and hemiagnosia. The lack of awareness of the involved side of the body and neglect of the environment necessitates a more complex approach to increasing mobility.

Traditionally, nurses have been taught to position patients so that their unaffected side faces areas of activity and to place needed objects in the room in

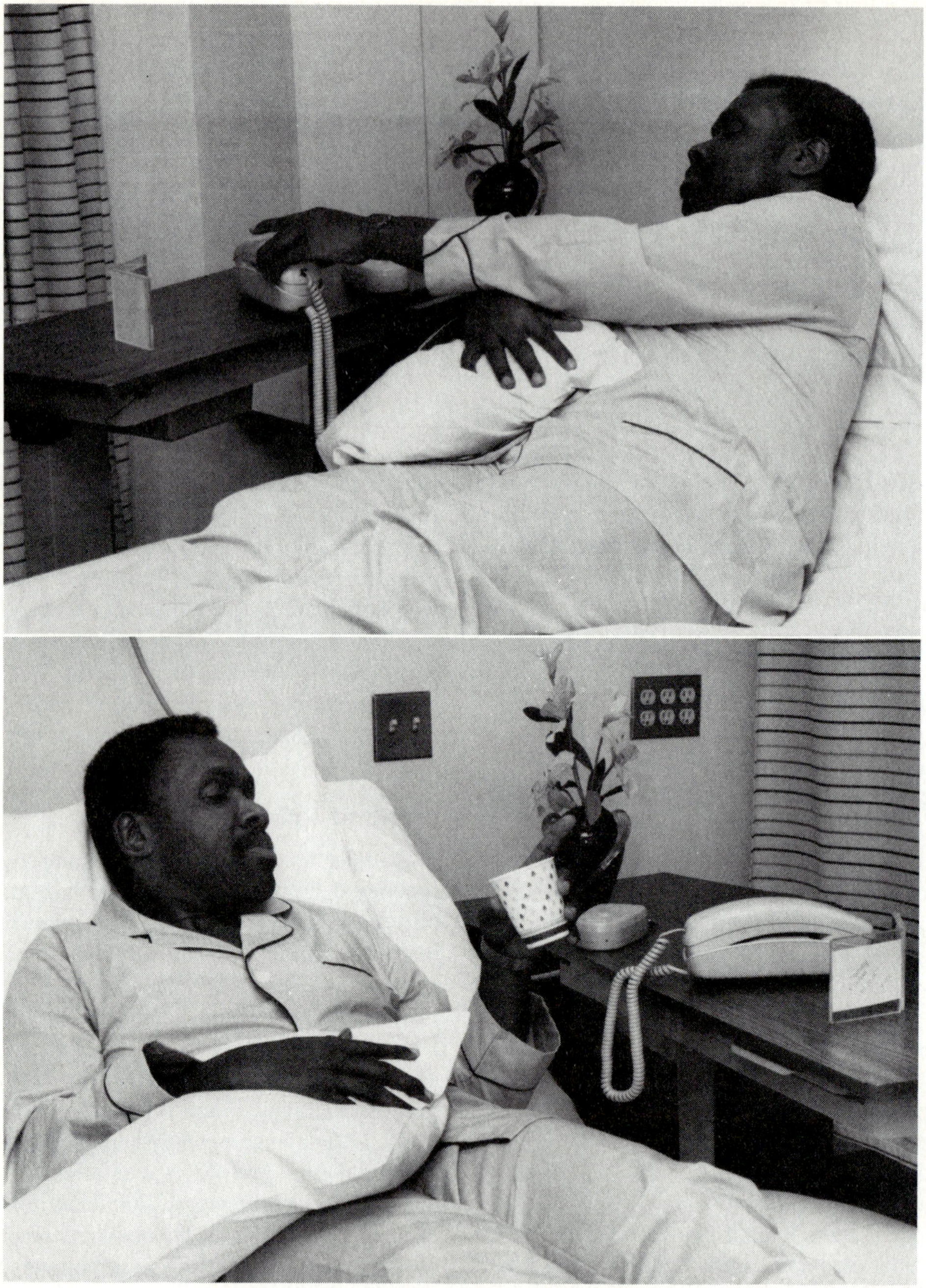

A

B

Fig. 7-5 Arrangement of needed items for the patient with stroke. **A,** Placement of objects on affected side promotes the goals of rehabilitation. **B,** Placement of objects on the unaffected side allows independence when patient is alone.

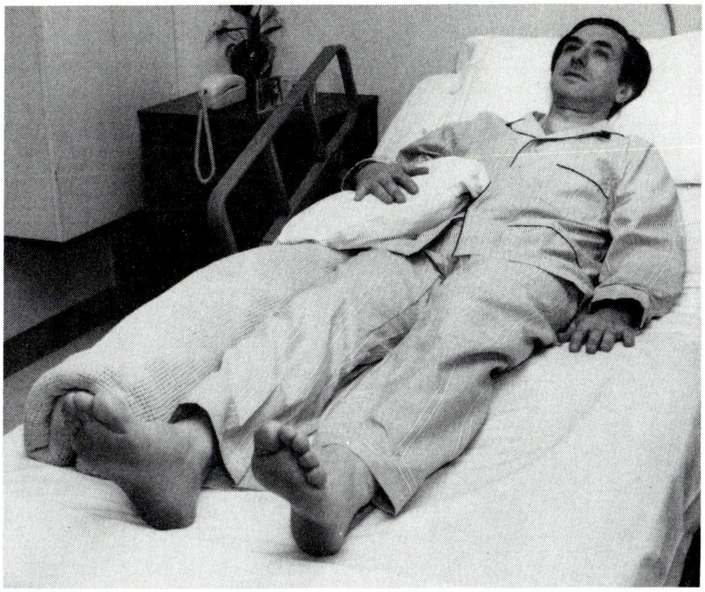

Fig. 7-6 Lying supine, the patient should be in midline with head and spine aligned.

a manner that enables the patient to see and use objects with his unaffected side. While this theory is excellent for the times when the patient is alone in his room, it does not encourage the goal of rehabilitation, which is to increase his awareness and use of the affected side. To balance these concepts, it is best to evaluate the patient's needs individually and combine approaches (Fig. 7-5). An example of such a combined approach is to have the patient positioned so that his unaffected side faces areas of activities and his environment is arranged on his unaffected side, but so that nursing care and activities are planned to be delivered from his affected side to encourage his awareness and use of that side of space. This plan gives stimulation and independence to the patient when care and activities are not being delivered while incorporating the goals of rehabilitation.

Impaired Physical Mobility Related to Paresis or Paralysis

Whenever the patient has weakness or paralysis, his ability to move about in the enviroment is decreased. The severely impaired patient must rely on the nurse for basic positioning, turning, and maintenance of joint mobility, which would normally be done on a voluntary basis. The overall goals for the patient with decreased mobility are to maintain normal alignment and function; to prevent edema from forming in the extremities, which can contribute to decreased movement; to reduce spasticity; and to prevent complications of immobility.

Positioning while in bed

Lying supine. The patient should be in midline with his head aligned with his spine (Fig. 7-6). The affected arm should be raised slightly on pillows with the hand and fingers extended. The tendency of the affected leg to externally rotate can be minimized by placing a pillow along the lateral aspect of the leg below the level of the knee.

Lying on the side. If the patient is to be placed on his unaffected side, his entire body should be rotated more than 90° to achieve alignment (Fig. 7-7). The affected arm and leg should be beyond

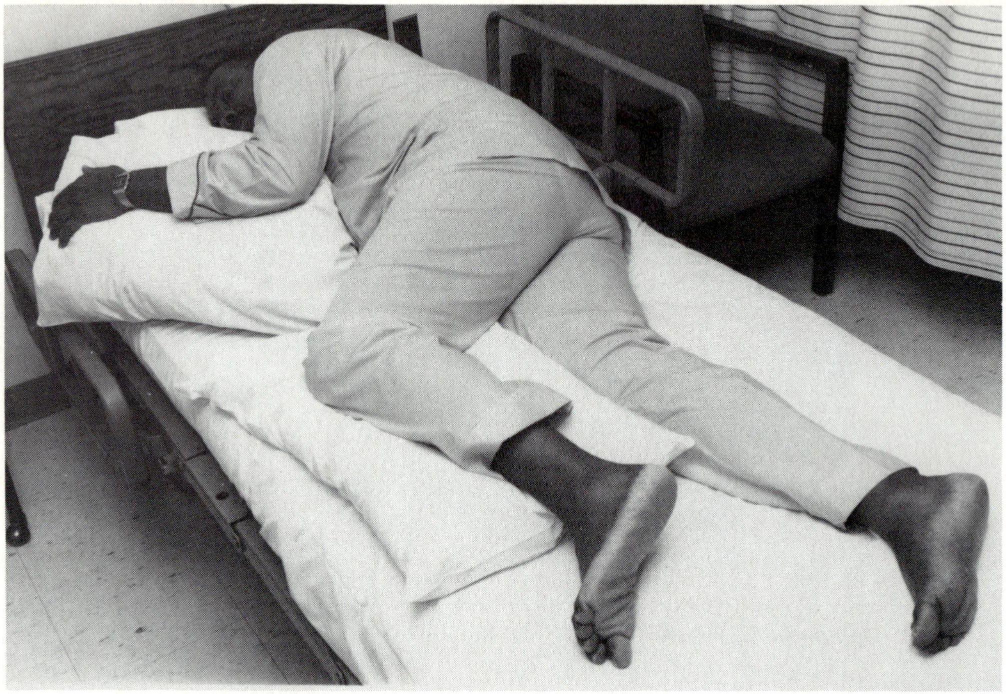

Fig. 7-7 Patient positioned on unaffected side.

midline, with both extremities elevated on pillows. The arm is maintained in an extended position while the leg is flexed. Pillows behind the upper and lower back can aid in maintaining the correct position.

When placing the patient on his affected side, the body should be rotated slightly less than 90º so that the weight of the body is not on the paralyzed arm and leg (Fig. 7-8). The arm should be extended perpendicular to the body and the leg flexed. Placing pillows behind the back can facilitate keeping the patient in the proper position.

Lying prone. The patient is turned onto his abdomen with his head rotated to one side (Fig. 7-9). Pillows are placed under the chest, hips, and lower legs. Placing the patient toward the lower end of the bed allows the feet to rest between the mattress and the footboard. The arms are either flexed with the affected arm supported with a pillow or extended along the patient's side. This position may not be medically indicated or comfortable for certain patients. If the patient has any respiratory or cardiac problems, this position is contraindicated. For older patients, decreased ability to rotate the neck may make this position infeasible and uncomfortable.

Several ways of managing the weak or paralyzed side that were used in years past have become controversial. These include the use of footboards and high top tennis shoes to prevent footdrop and placing hand cones in the patient's affected hand to prevent contractures. Researchers report conflicting results using hand splints and cones to reduce spasticity (Dayhoff, 1975; Jamieson and Dayhoff, 1980; and Scherling and Johnson, 1987). Rather than decrease the possibility of contractures, these measures may actually stimulate input to the sensory system and increase tone within the affected extremities. Each patient should be individually assessed for his or her response to splinting or positioning measures.

Sitting in bed. Many patients spend time sitting

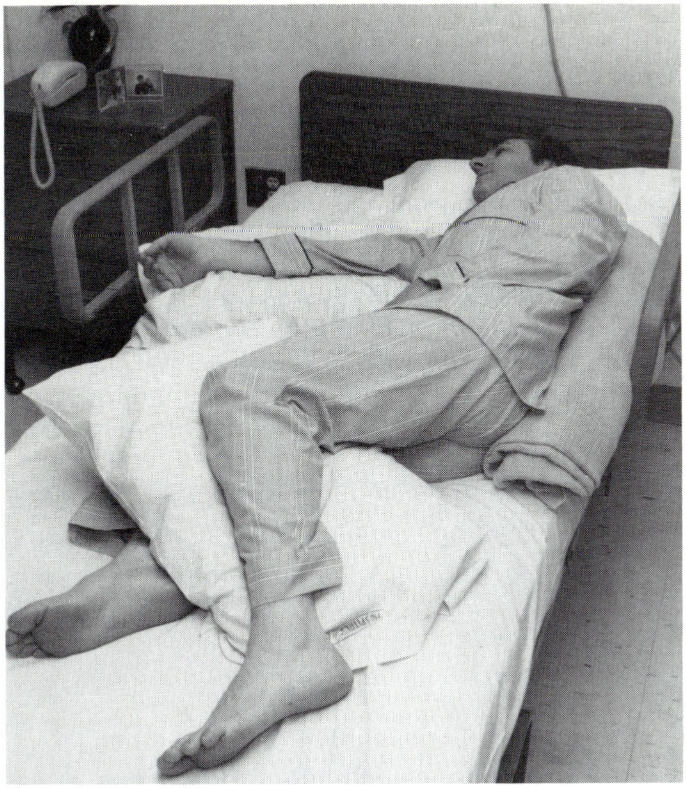

Fig. 7-8 Patient positioned on affected side, rotated to avoid bearing weight on the paralyzed side of body.

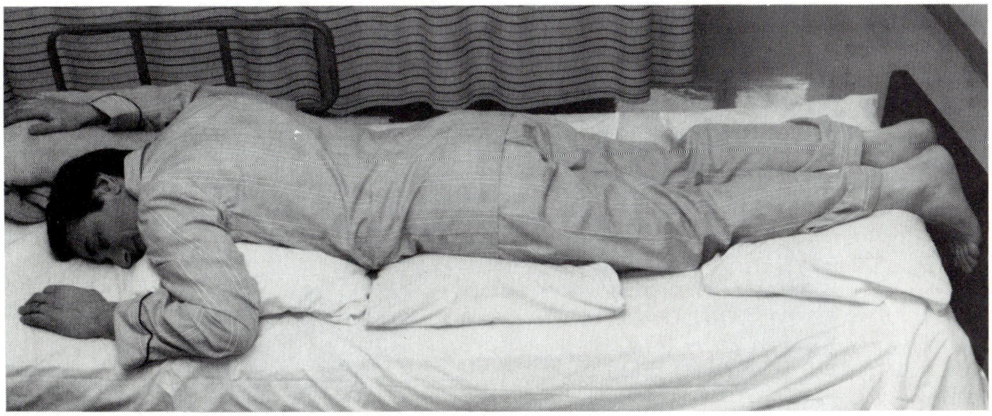

Fig. 7-9 To achieve the prone position the patient is turned onto his abdomen with his head rotated to one side.

in bed. During these periods proper alignment and positioning should be maintained. The patient should have a lap board or overbed stand placed in front of him with the affected arm supported on the table. A pillow can be placed under the arm if needed. If the patient has a tendency to fall to one side, a pillow can be used to maintain an upright position.

Turning in bed. Unless the patient is unusually heavy or uncooperative, most changes in position can be accomplished by one nurse with the aid of the patient. The most frequent position changes (from side to side or back to side) are easily managed if the patient is taught to assist in the movement. To move from lying on the back to either side, the patient should bend his knees and place his feet flat together on the bed. He then clasps his arms together and raises them upward and away from the body. From this position, the patient then pushes with his unaffected leg and uses his arms to guide the body to the right or left side (Fig. 7-10).

Rolling from a side position to the back is accomplished in the reverse order, however, more assistance may be needed from the nurse. The nurse should never pull or push the patient but facilitate the motion the patient is trying to make.

Moving the patient up in bed. One of the most

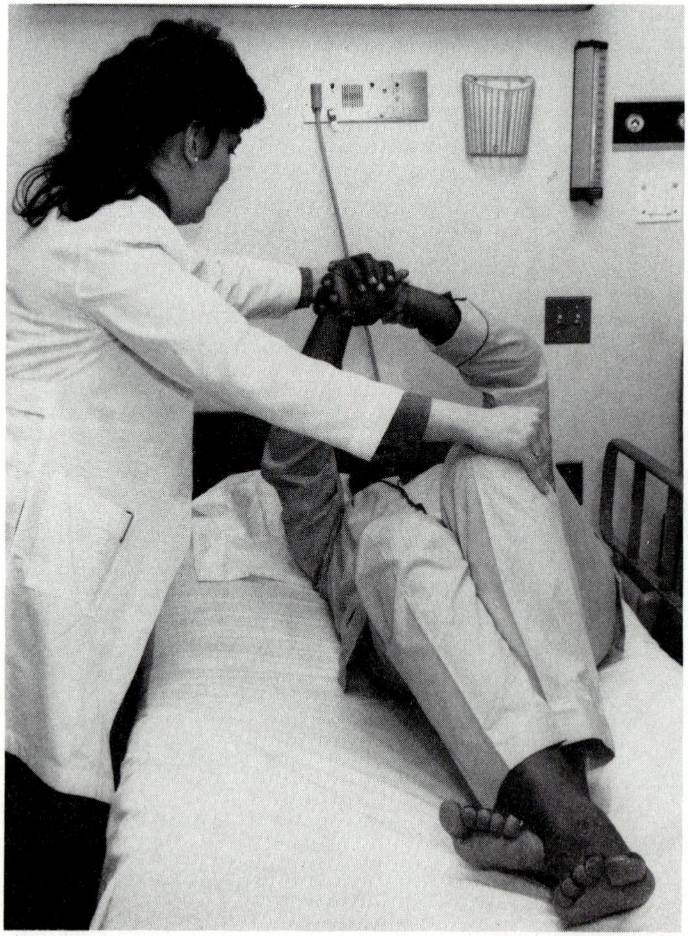

Fig. 7-10 Turning in bed is accomplished by nurse with the aid of the patient.

difficult tasks for the patient to perform is to move himself from the foot of the bed toward the head of the bed. To assist the patient in this activity, the head of the bed is lowered to a flat position. The patient then bends both legs at the knee and places his feet flat on the bed. The nurse uses her arms to encircle the patient's upper body and clasps her hands behind his back. The patient pushes with his feet while the nurse lifts and moves the upper part of the body toward the head of the bed. Sometimes this activity is easier with two nurses; however, the same approach should be used. When additional persons are assisting, there is a tendency for poor technique to be used because some persons think it may be easier to lift or slide the patient upward in bed. In these instances, the patient is lifted under the arms and dragged across the linens. Lifting the patient in such a manner increases the chance of subluxation of the shoulder, and dragging the patient causes shearing of the skin and increases the chance of skin breakdown.

Preventing pressure sores. Decreased movement by the patient, combined with other factors known to increase risk of skin breakdown, make the stroke patient particularly susceptible to the development of pressure sores. Factors include: under or over weight, incontinence, changes in cognitive function, advanced age, decreased nutritional status, and decreased sensation. When any of these factors are present in the patient who has been confined to bedrest or who has decreased capabilities to adjust her body to relieve pressure, then preventative measures must be instituted to maintain skin integrity.

The primary way to prevent skin breakdown is to alleviate pressure on the prominent body areas that are particularly prone to high pressures when the patient is lying or sitting. This can be accomplished by regularly changing the position of the body so that pressure is on these areas only briefly. Turning schedules, according to which the patient's position is adjusted every 2 hours from side to side and back to prone, can facilitate a plan for relieving pressure. This combined with skin care techniques to prevent skin breakdown is what most stroke patients need to maintain skin integrity.

Despite efforts at prevention, some patients have a propensity to develop skin breakdown. For these patients, pressure-relieving equipment can be placed on the bed or chairs to assist in reducing pressure on the key body parts. Jester and Weaver (1990) compared various pressure relieving devices for their ability to relieve pressure on bony prominences, specifically the sacrum and trochanter. Decreased tissue perfusion and tissue damage occur when the pressure on the bony prominences is greater than 32 mm Hg. In evaluating pressure-relieving capabilities of the various devices, the equipment was categorized as devices that are laid on top of the normal hospital mattress, air mattresses, water mattresses, and special beds. Consistently, the special bed was the only device that reduced pressure to a level below 32 mm Hg. Few of the air or foam overlays or special mattresses reduced the pressure below 32 mm Hg, although many significantly reduced the pressure from the levels found with the regular hospital mattress. Some of the speciality overlays were able to reduce the pressure to below 32 mm Hg. Many of these devices can be expensive for clinical use and are not appropriate for all patients. Assessing the patient for risk factors and degree of impaired movement can assist the nurse in determining the best method for preventing skin breakdown.

Range of motion exercises. All patients must perform range of motion (ROM) exercises several times each day. For the patient who does not have an altered level of consciousness or a severe lack of comprehension, active participation in the exercises is encouraged. The purposes of these exercises are to maintain strength in the muscles, reduce spasticity, and maintain joint mobility.

Arm mobility. Three joints must be exercised when performing range of motion on the arm — the shoulder, the elbow, and the wrist. The patient can easily assist in these exercises by using the unaffected arm to grasp and move his affected arm.

For the shoulder, with hands clasped, the patient should raise his arms from in front of him to above his head. The elbow is exercised in a similar fashion except that elbows are rested on a table or bedside stand and the arm is flexed and extended.

Exercising the hand is accomplished by clasping the hands and having the strong hand move the affected hand right and left, then up and down. A circular motion then completes the exercises for the upper extremity.

One of the major concerns with upper extremity immobility is shoulder subluxation on the affected side. Paralysis of the arm impairs not only the upper and lower arm muscles but also the muscles of the shoulder. Often the weight of a person's affected arm is unable to be supported by the shoulder muscles, and the shoulder joint separates. Two positions promote subluxation: moving the arm sideways away from the body (abduction) and allowing the arm to hang unsupported from the shoulder. Previously it was believed that use of an arm sling would prevent shoulder subluxation; however, current practice has demonstrated that slings not only do not prevent shoulder subluxation but also can actually do more harm by keeping the arm flexed and increasing the likelihood of contracture formation. The best method for maintaining shoulder mobility is to support the affected arm with pillows whenever it is placed in a dependent position.

Leg mobility. As with the arm, three major joints require exercise: the hip, the knee, and the ankle. The knee and hip can be exercised at the same time with the following technique. The nurse should lift the affected leg at the knee and heel. The leg is then gently flexed at the knee and the hip is flexed so that the leg moves toward the abdomen. The leg is then gently extended to the original position. The ankle can be exercised by flexing and extending the foot toward and away from the patient's face, similar to pressing and releasing the gas pedal on a car.

Grooming and dressing. Whenever possible patients should groom and dress themselves with the nurse acting only as an assistant. This not only promotes functional ability but also increases feelings of independence. Nurses who think they are helping the patient or saving time by doing these activities for the patient are actually doing a disservice to the patient and may ultimately lengthen

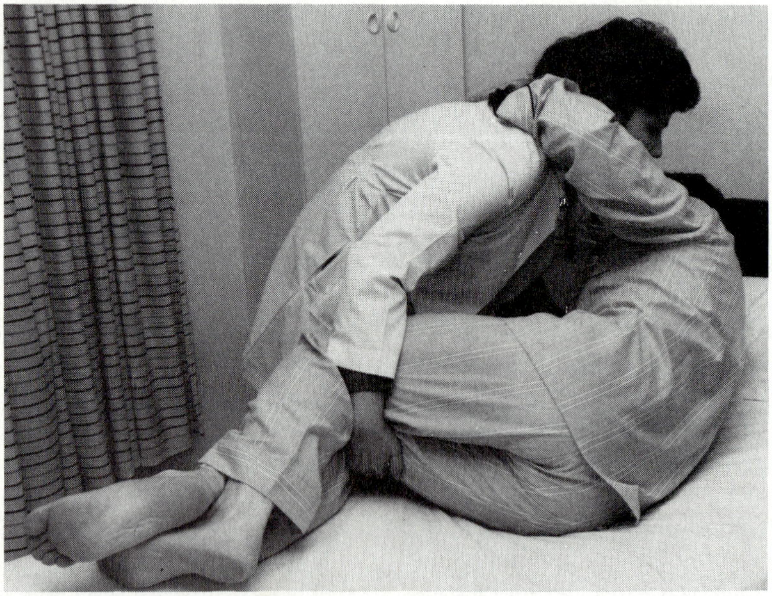

A

Fig. 7-11 Transferring patient from bed to a chair. **A,** Transfer begins with patient lying on affected side, knees bent. Patient encircles nurse's neck with unaffected arm.

the rehabilitation period. The patient can use his unaffected side to do activities such as brushing his teeth, combing his hair, and washing. Whenever possible, the affected arm is included in the motions of these activities. Handles on the various utensils needed for grooming can be adapted for easier use by attaching Velcro hand straps or wrapping the handle in large foam for easier grasping with a weak hand.

The patient can dress himself by using the unaffected side to dress the affected limb first and then dress the unaffected limb. This may be cumbersome with certain styles of clothing, such as those that pull over the head or fit tightly. The patient should experiment with various types of clothing to determine those which can be mastered.

Transferring the patient from bed to chair. This complex activity should be broken down into two steps: (1) getting the patient to a sitting position on the side of the bed and (2) transferring from the bed to a chair (Fig. 7-11). To start, the patient should be lying on the affected side with the knees bent. The nurse slides one arm underneath the affected arm and shoulder and grabs the patient's unaffected leg behind the knees with the other arm. The patient uses his unaffected arm to reach up and encircle the nurse's neck. While pivoting, the nurse lifts the patient's trunk and slides his legs over the edge of the bed. Next, transfers can be made to either the unaffected or

B

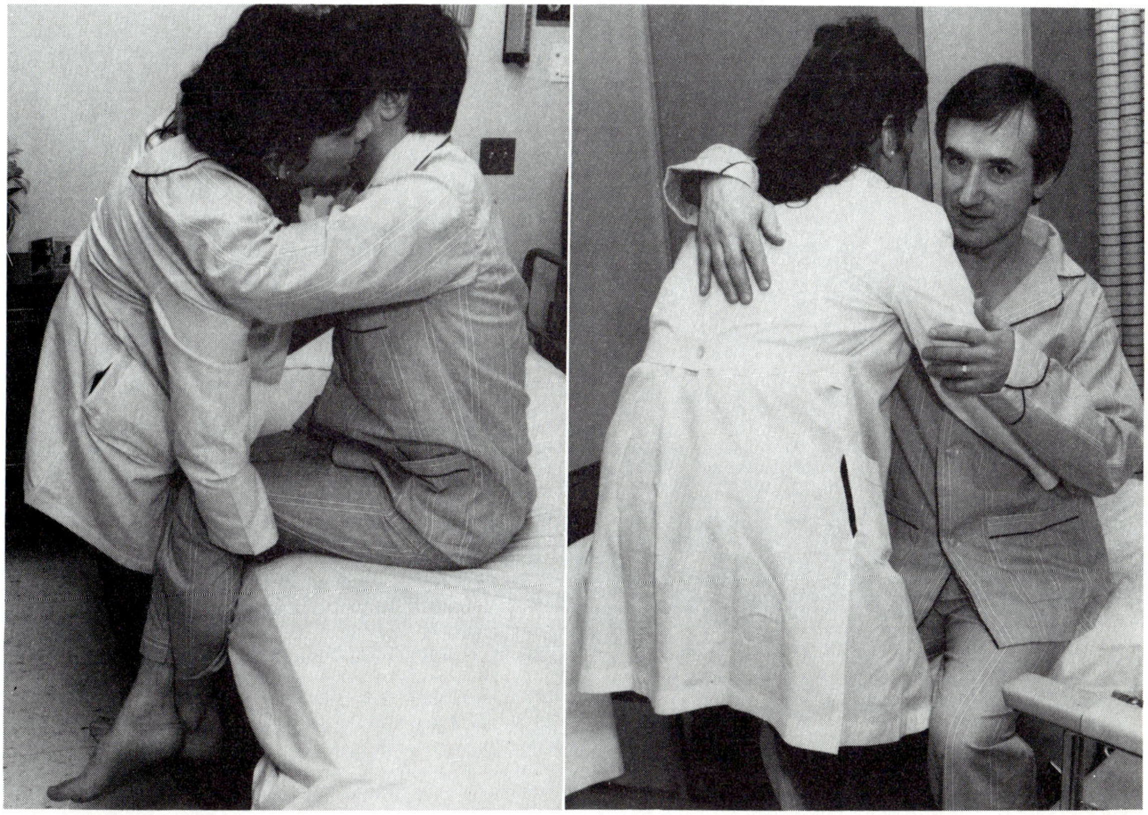

C

Fig. 7-11, cont'd **B,** Nurse lifts patient and slides his legs over the edge of the bed. **C,** With nurse bracing the affected leg, the patient moves to the edge of the bed.

Continued.

D

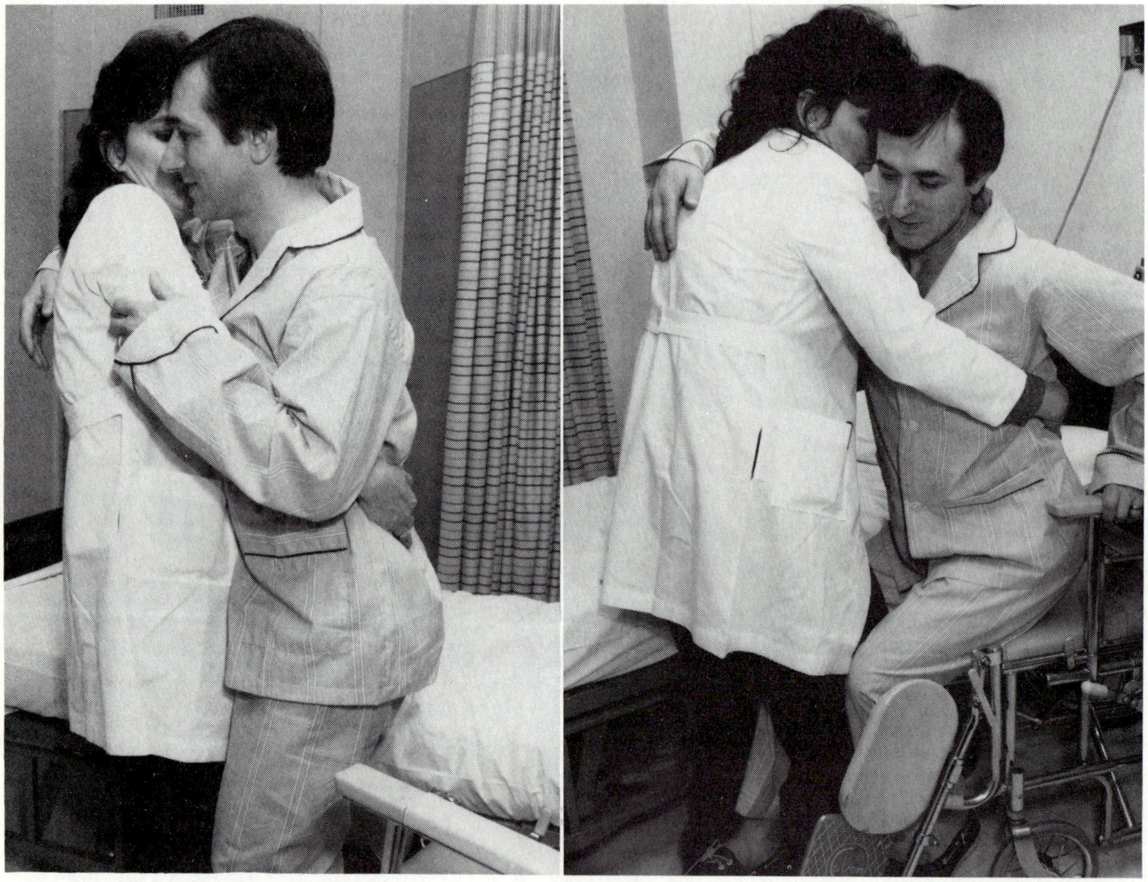

E

Fig. 7-11, cont'd **D,** Patient leans forward and stands up. **E,** Patient is pivoted and uses strong arm to reach for chair on unaffected side.

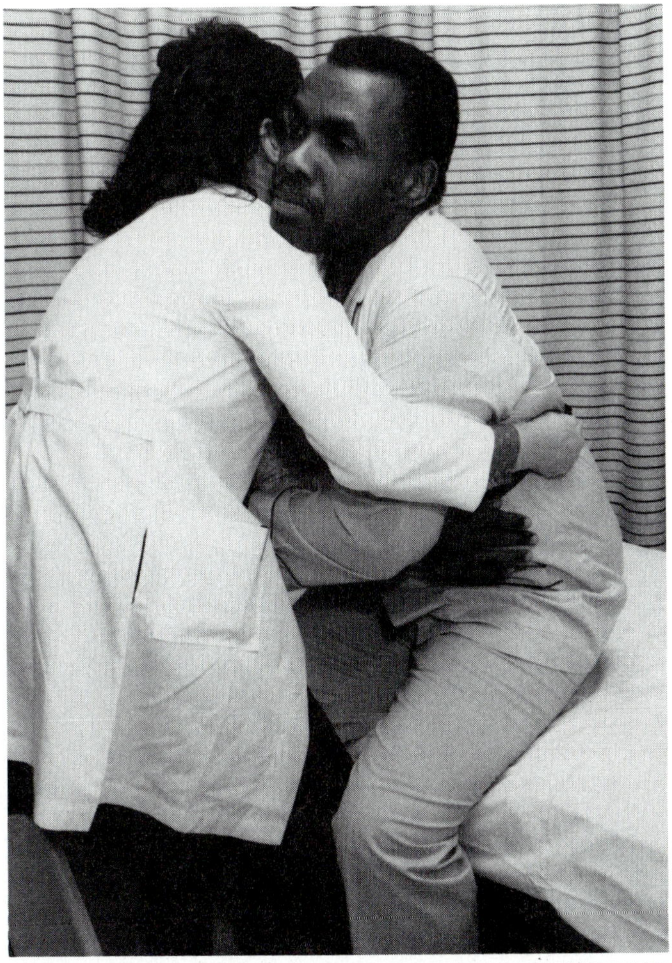

A

Fig. 7-12 **A,** A lifting belt facilitates transfer to chair on affected side.

Continued.

affected side. To transfer to the unaffected side, a wheelchair is placed at a 90° angle to the bed on the unaffected side. The nurse braces the affected leg between her two legs, slides the patient's hips to the edge of the bed, and the patient leans forward and stands up. The patient is pivoted and with his strong arm reaches for the arm of the chair. He can then be eased into a sitting position.

To transfer to the affected side, the chair is placed at a 90° angle on the affected side of the body. The patient folds the affected arm across his chest and holds it with his strong arm. Again the same method is used for standing and pivoting the patient into the chair. For transfers a lifting belt can facilitate helping the patient to stand and lowering him into the chair (Fig. 7-12).

Ambulation. The patient may initially require two persons to assist with ambulation, but as strength increases and the patient becomes more comfortable with the process, only one person may

B

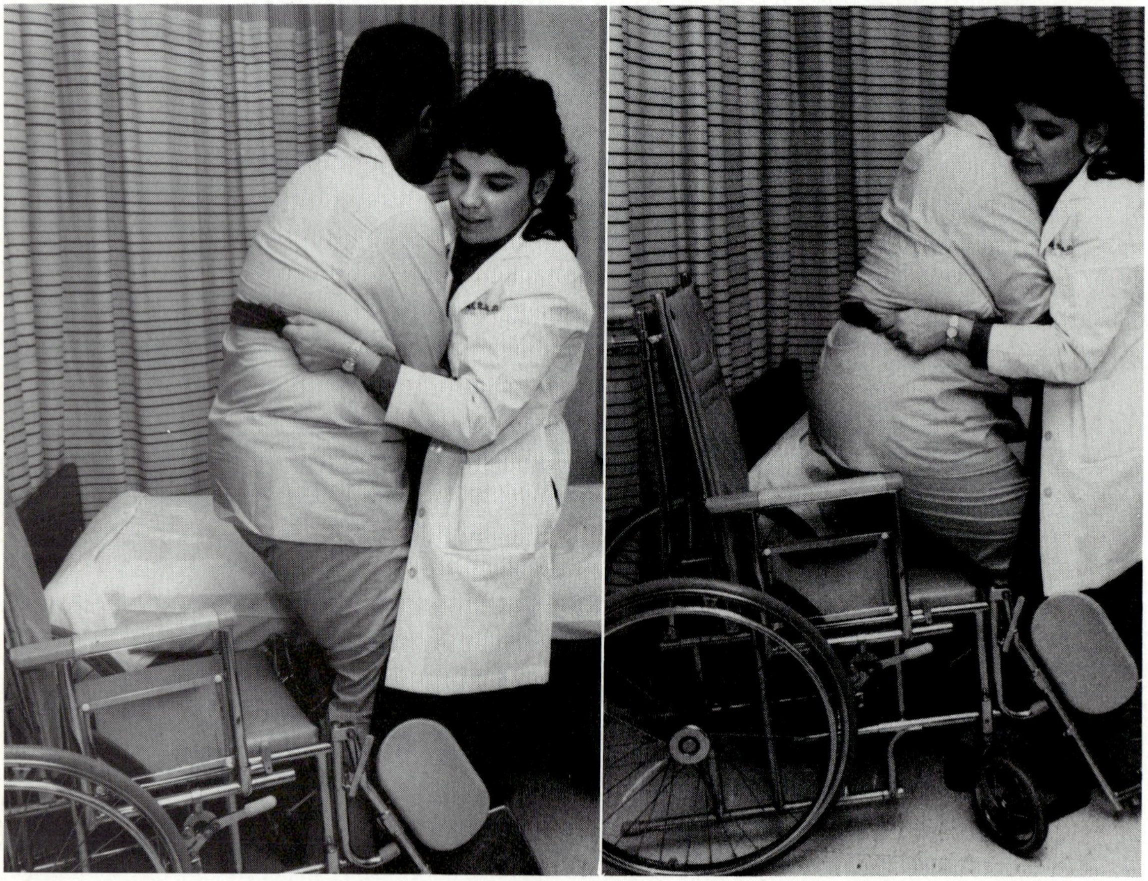

C

Fig. 7-12, cont'd **B,** With nurse providing support, patient stands and is pivoted into chair. **C,** Patient is lowered into sitting position.

be needed or the patient may use an assistive device to aid in walking. Before starting to walk, the patient should be standing, with good posture and his weight evenly distributed. A lifting belt can be useful for the assisting person(s) to grasp. The assisting person(s) supports the patient by holding underneath the axilla or grasping the belt and placing the other hand in the palm of the patient's hand. To begin walking, the patient places his weight on the strong leg (Fig. 7-13). The weak leg is then swung forward to a point in front of the strong leg. Weight is then distributed between the weak leg and cane and the strong leg brought forward. The patient continues to make steps in this pattern. For some patients the affected leg may be unstable when they first begin to walk. Assisting persons can help the patient stabilize the leg by standing in front or to the side and bracing the affected leg with their own legs(s).

Assistive devices enable the patient to walk independently. Patients who can walk with the as-

A

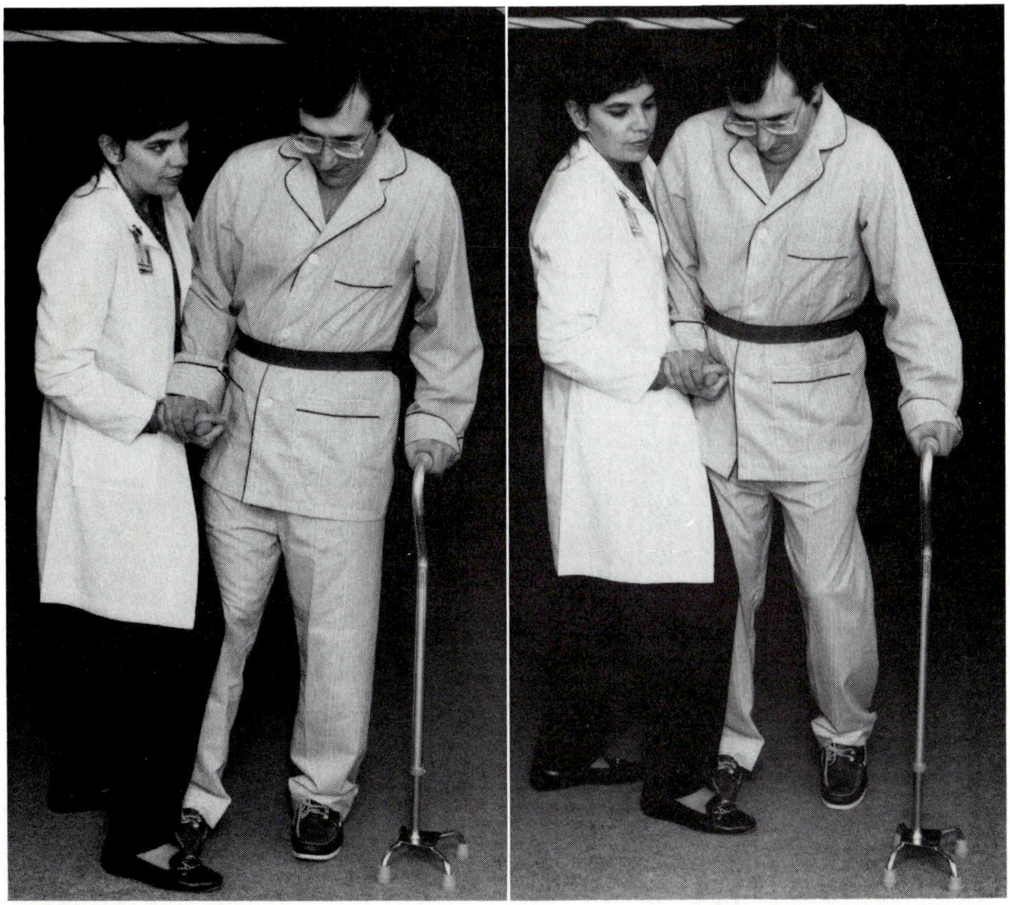

B

Fig. 7-13 **A,** Patient begins ambulation by placing weight on strong leg and swinging the weak or paralyzed foot forward. **B,** With nurse providing support, patient moves affected leg in front of strong leg.

sistance of one person may benefit from using a hemiwalker or quad cane for independent ambulation. The patient holds these devices in his strong hand as a substitute for the assisting person. When walking with the hemiwalker or quad cane, the patient moves the affected leg forward, transfers weight to the cane and affected leg, and then moves the strong leg forward (Fig. 7-14).

Some patients may have difficulty bringing the affected leg forward while trying to walk because of foot drop and outward turning of the weakened ankle. These patients can benefit from an ankle-foot orthosis that is fitted to the shoe and braces the upper calf muscle (Lehmann and others, 1987). This maintains the foot in a functional position and facilitates walking. These orthoses can be extended above the knee for patients who have instability in the knee and who need support to permit weight transfer.

For the patient who will spend a significant amount of time in a wheelchair, assessment must be made for the type and dimensions of the wheel-

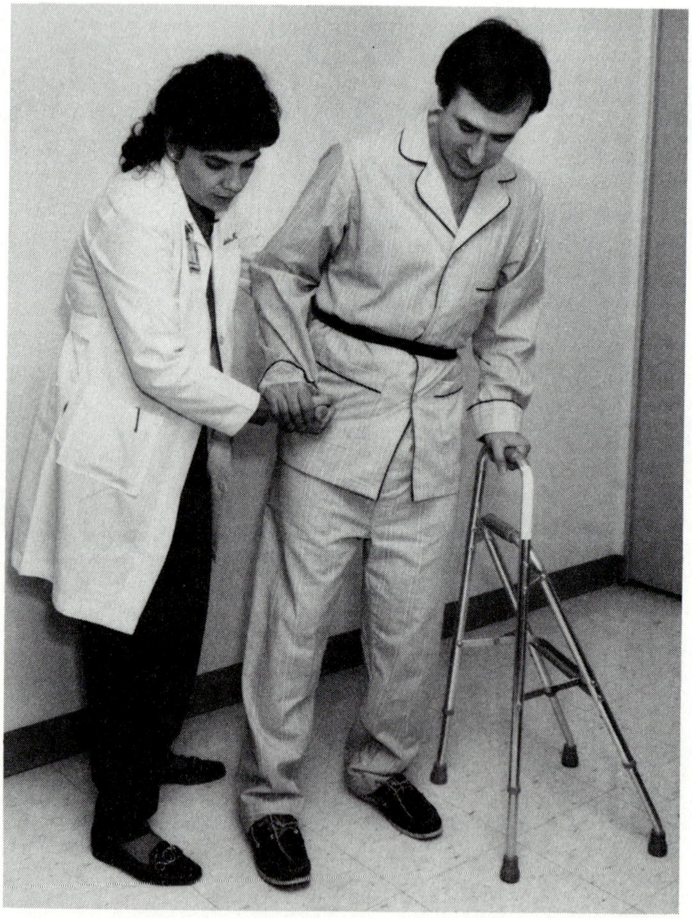

A

Fig. 7-14 **A,** Patient moves hemiwalker and affected leg forward.

chair. Typically, stroke patients fare better in a lower than standard wheelchair so that the strong leg can assist in propelling the chair (Fig. 7-15). Additionally, special brake handles are needed so that the unaffected arm can reach both brake handles for locking the wheelchair and permitting stable transfers. If edema is a problem in the affected leg, the leg rests should be adjustable to elevate the extremity. These chairs can also be fitted with support boards for the patient or molded arm rests to maintain the arm in a functional position.

Impaired Physical Mobility Due to Change in Muscle Tone

Spastic extremities complicate the process of rehabilitation and decrease the functional level many

B

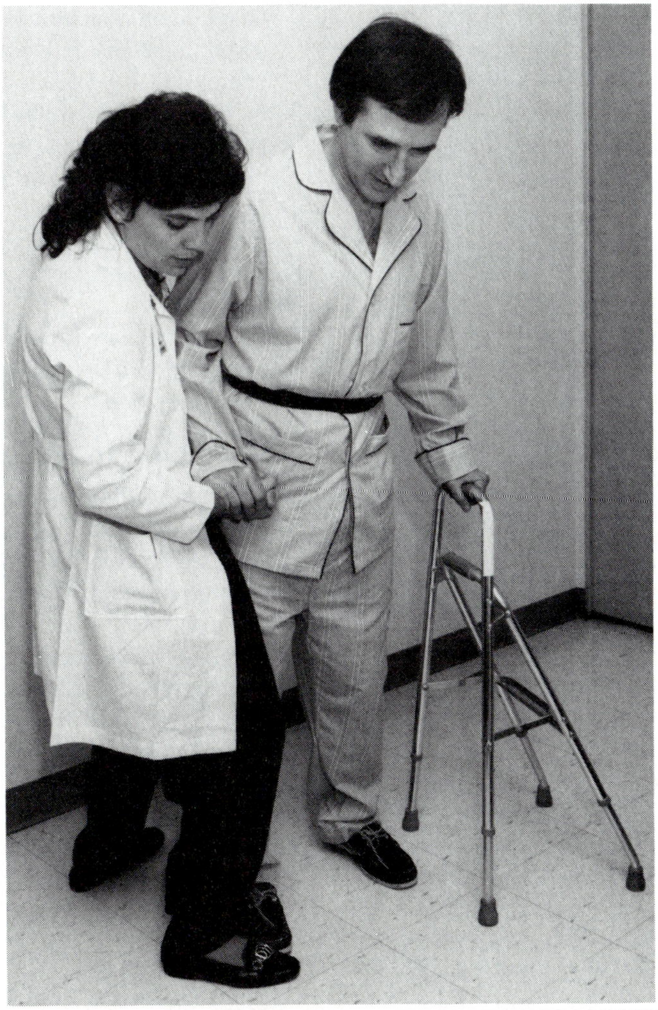

Fig. 7-14, cont'd **B,** Then patient moves strong leg forward.

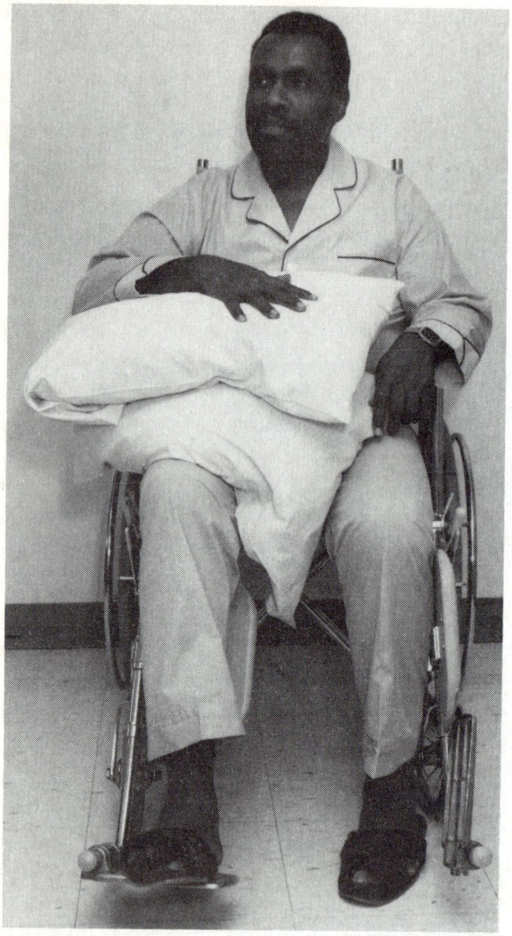

Fig. 7-15 Stronger leg assists in propelling the wheelchair.

stroke survivors can achieve. For these reasons it is important to minimize spasticity and the resultant contractures that can form in the extremities. Several nursing measures can benefit the patient and assist in reducing spasticity. Range of motion exercises have already been discussed as important in maintaining functional capacity. Typically, the stroke patient initially has decreased tone in the extremity and can easily carry out ROM exercises. Tone in the extremities gradually increases in stroke patients several weeks after the initial insult and impedes the ability to perform the exercises. As part of the care plan for patients with increases in tone, physical measures can be instituted to reduce tone so that greater ROM exercises can be carried out. The following techniques can be tried with the patient to reduce tone:

1. Application of wet cold towels or soaking the affected extremity in cold water to decrease the excitability of the muscle spindle.
2. Application of warm towels. Heat can produce an inhibitory stimulus to the reticular activating system, thereby reducing input to the gamma neurons.
3. Stimulation of vestibular and proprioceptive pathways by rolling the patient in bed or on a physical therapy log or ball to reduce excitatory stimuli.
4. Stroking the patient along the spinous processes to reduce sympathetic input and relax the patient.
5. Gradual, repeated stretching of the muscle with extension and rotation combined followed by gradual flexion.

Medications to reduce spasticity

Dantrolene sodium—relaxes skeletal muscles. Doses start at 25 mg tid and can be gradually increased according to response. Side effects include nausea and vomiting, drowsiness, and GI disturbances.

Baclofen—is a synthetic neurotransmitter that has a suppressant effect at nerve synapses. Total daily doses range from 15 mg to 80 mg. Side effects include GI distress, drowsiness, and headache.

Diazepam—decreases central nervous system excitability and relaxes muscles. Dosage ranges from 6 mg to 40 mg per day. Side effects include dependency, drowsiness, and weakness.

Impaired Physical Mobility Related to Loss of Balance and Coordination

Stroke patients who have interruption in the cerebellar component of movement or those who have infarction in the basal ganglia have difficulty controlling the quantity and quality of movement. These problems are often manifested when the person tries to perform a voluntary action with her arms or legs. Examples of dysfunction include ataxic gait because of the inability to coordinate leg movements and tremors that occur with initiation of arm movement.

Nursing interventions focus on assisting the patient to gain control over the movements and on preventing falls or injuries. To improve muscle control the patient must learn first how to control the proximal muscles (e.g., shoulder, upper arm, hip and upper leg). Subsequently, distal muscles can be incorporated into movement. Using weights on the distal muscles can help improve stability.

Instability while sitting and walking is a potential safety hazard. Patients should practice aligning their center of gravity when in both positions. Arms should be at both sides and weight evenly distributed when attempting to walk.

FUNCTIONAL OUTCOME AFTER STROKE

Adaptation to stroke, particularly functional outcome, has been the focus of many research endeavors. Studies have focused on stroke type, neurologic deficits, complications, and predictors of long-term outcome. As early as 1966, persons in the health care field were interested in developing methods to evaluate and predict outcome from stroke. Initial efforts focused on short-term outcome and survival. Ford and Katz (1966) identified high mortality in the early poststroke phase that was associated with variables such as type of stroke, age, damage to vital centers of the brain, and the presence of other major diseases. During this time, Katz and others (1966) focused on long-term survival and examined the influence of chronic illness, aging, and the natural history of the disease. Rehabilitation outcomes related to walking and the ability to carry out the activities of daily living (ADL) were measured as part of the overall recovery process. While only a handful of participants were alive 2 years after having a stroke, survivors showed the greatest functional recovery in the first 6 months.

The trend in attempting to assess outcome in terms of the neurologic examination and functional return grew during the next 20 years. In attempting to predict functional outcome following stroke, Prescott and others (1982) used the standard neurologic examination along with memory recall, problem solving ability, sensory and motor function, speech comprehension, and ADL capabilities. Upper limb function was the only area found to be predictive of outcome at 4 weeks after stroke. A similar study conducted by Dove and others (1984) compared neurologic examinations and functional recovery. While patients with transient ischemic attacks were included in the population, half of the patients with stroke had a successful outcome—they were ambulatory and independent at discharge.

Developing from the preceding studies was the awareness that functional ability was an important outcome variable to be used when assessing recovery. A standard scale or set of measurements was not available, making comparison of study results impossible. For example, while some investigators defined a patient's ADL as dependent or independent, others tried to assign various weights to different levels of ADL ability. Resulting from these early attempts at quantifying functional recovery was the development and refinement of several scales that could be used for assessing a patient's functional capacity. Currently, these scales are used for assessing patient's progress in rehabilitation and overall outcome (see box on p. 108). Perhaps the most widely used scale is the Barthel Index (Mahoney and Barthel, 1965). It includes categories for feeding, transferring, grooming, toileting, bathing, walking, stair climbing, and bowel and bladder control. Numerous studies have used this instrument to evaluate patients and to measure its predictive value in determining long-term functional gains (Granger, Albrecht, and Hamilton, 1979; Granger and others, 1979; Granger and others, 1988; and Wade, 1983).

FUNCTIONAL ASSESSMENT SCALES

INDEX OF ACTIVITIES OF DAILY LIVING (ADL)	**A.** Six categories: bed activities, transfers, hygiene, dressing, feeding, and locomotion. **B.** 0 to 4 point scale, with 0 being complete dependence.
BARTHEL INDEX	**A.** Nine categories: feeding, transfers, grooming, toileting, bathing, walking, climbing stairs, bowel and bladder control. **B.** Weighted scores with partial credit given for functions performed with assistance.
PULSES	**A.** Six categories: medical conditions, upper extremity (self-care), lower extremity (walking), sensory, bowel and bladder control, socialization. **B.** Four point Likert scale for each item, grading from dependent to independent.
MOTOR ASSESSMENT SCALE	**A.** Nine categories: one for general tone and eight for motor activity. **B.** Ratings are on a 0 to 6 scale, with 6 indicating the patient's ability to perform more complex tasks.
FUGL-MEYER ASSESSMENT	**A.** Three categories: balance and motor activities, sensation, and joint motion. **B.** Scoring on a 0 to 2 point scale, with 0 being inability to perform a task.

High reliability and validity have been established for most scales when used by persons familiar with assessing and scoring function in stroke patients. These scales can also be used in following the patient after discharge to assess ongoing rehabilitation progress. Shinar and others (1987) reported a high correlation between information gathered by telephone on level of functioning and assessment made on the same patients when evaluated in person. This means that in certain instances when patients are unable to return for follow-up, assessment may be reliably carried out over the phone.

As such scales have been incorporated in assessing stroke patients, quantitative measurements have been made in terms of functional recovery. For upper limb function, it has been estimated that 24% of patients will persist in having a moderate or severe paralysis 3 months after stroke (Parker and others, 1986). Recovery of lower limb function has higher percentages, with one half to two thirds of patients being able to eventually walk independently (Wade and others, 1987). Several techniques and programs increase the chances of such recovery, including stroke units that focus on the unique needs of these patients (Strand and others, 1985); biofeedback (Basmajian, 1983); and intensive rehabilitation efforts (Dombovy, 1986).

NURSING CARE PLAN

Nursing Diagnosis	Interventions	Expected Outcomes
Mobility, Impaired Physical related to paresis or paralysis **Defining Characteristics** ■ Inability to move within the environment ■ Decreased muscle strength ■ Central nervous system insult	**Ongoing Assessment** ■ Assess patient's degree of weakness in both upper and lower extremities ■ Assess ability to move and change position in bed ■ Assess ability to transfer and walk **Therapeutic Interventions** ■ Change position of patient at least every 2 hrs, keeping track of position changes with a turning schedule ■ Monitor skin integrity for areas of blanching or redness as signs of potential skin breakdown ■ If patient is at high risk for pressure ulcer development, then use pressure-relieving devices on the bed and chair. ■ Perform active and passive range of motion exercises in all extremities several times daily ■ Increase functional activities as strength improves and patient is medically stable.	■ Patient's level of function is maximized ■ Complications of immobility are avoided

Continued.

NURSING CARE PLAN — cont'd

Nursing Diagnosis	Interventions	Expected Outcomes
Mobility, Impaired Physical related to loss of balance and coordination **Defining Characteristics** ■ Tremor ■ Ataxia ■ Impaired righting reflexes ■ Wide base stance in walking	**Ongoing Assessment** ■ Assess ability for fine muscle movements ■ Assess ability for gross muscle movements **Therapeutic Interventions** ■ When assisting or having the patient independently perform a movement or task, begin with small range of movements and encourage control ■ Patients should be encouraged to focus on proximal muscle control initially, and then distal muscle control ■ For sitting and standing activities, ensure center of gravity is over pelvis or equally distributed over stance	■ Patient's sitting and walking capabilities are improved ■ Patient's ability to perform fine and gross motor activities is increased ■ Patient learns how to identify where his extremities and center of balance are located in relationship to the environment

Continued.

NURSING CARE PLAN — cont'd

Nursing Diagnosis	Interventions	Expected Outcomes
Mobility, Impaired Physical related to increased muscle tone **Defining Characteristics** ■ Increased tone in extremities ■ Hyperreflexia ■ Possible clonus ■ Decreased range of motion	**Ongoing Assessment** ■ Determine active and passive range of motion capabilities ■ Assess for activities or situations that increase or decrease tone **Therapeutic Interventions** ■ Perform activities in a quiet environment with few distractions ■ Apply heat or cold to the extremities in an effort to reduce tone before initiating movement ■ Perform muscle stretching activities in gentle, rhythmical motions to provide input into the central nervous system ■ Integrate inhibiting patterns for reducing spasticity as instructed by physical therapy ■ Give medications to reduce spasticity as ordered by physician ■ Apply splinting devices to spastic extremities as ordered, with ongoing assessment for increasing tone	■ Muscle tone will be reduced ■ Range of motion in spastic extremities will be increased ■ Patient's functional abilities will improve

Patient Education
- Teach patient and family exercises and transferring techniques
- Discuss potential complications of bedrest and preventive techniques
- Reinforce safety precautions with patient and family
- Teach patient and family exercises and techniques to improve balance and coordination
- If increased tone is present, teach patient and family about concepts of spasticity and ways to reduce tone
- Discuss medications, dosage, and side effects

REFERENCES

Basmajian JV: Biofeedback: principles and practice for clinicians, ed 2, Baltimore, 1983, Williams and Wilkins.

Dayhoff N: Rethinking stroke: soft or hard devices to position hands?, Am J Nurs 75:1142, 1975.

Dombovy ML, Sandok BA, and Basford JR: Rehabilitation for stroke: review, Stroke 17:363, 1986.

Dove HG, Schneider KC, and Wallace JD: Evaluating and predicting outcome of acute cerebral vascular accident, Stroke 15:858, 1984.

Ford AB and Katz S: Prognosis after strokes part I: a critical review, Medicine 45:223, 1966.

Granger CV, Dewis LS, Peters NC, and others: Stroke rehabilitation: analysis of repeated Barthel Index measures, Arch Phys Med Rehabil 60:14, 1979.

Granger CV, Albrecht GL, Hamilton BB: Outcome of comprehensive medical rehabilitation: measurement by PULSES profile and Barthel Index, Arch Phys Med Rehabil 60:145, 1979.

Granger CV, Hamilton BB, and Gresham GE: The stroke rehabilitation outcome study—part I: general description, Arch Phys Med Rehabil 69:506, 1988.

Jamieson S and Dayhoff N: A hard hand-positioning device to decrease wrist and finger hypertonicity: a sensorimotor approach for the patient with nonprogressive brain damage, Nurs Res 29:285, 1980.

Jester J and Weaver V: A report of clinical investigation of various tissue support surfaces, Ostomy/Wound Management 26:39, 1990.

Katz S, Ford AB, Chinn AB, and others: Prognosis after strokes. Part II: long-term course of 159 stroke patients, Medicine 45:233, 1966.

Lehmann JF, Condon SM, Price R, and others: Gait abnormalities in hemiplegia: their correction by ankle-foot orthoses, Arch Phys Med Rehabil 68:763, 1987.

Mahoney FI and Barthel DW: Functional evaluation: Barthel Index, Maryland Med J 14:61, 1965.

Olson EV: The hazzards of immobility, Am J Nurs 4:781, 1967.

Parker VM, Wade DT, and Langton HR: Loss of arm function after stroke: measurement, frequency, and recovery, Int Rehabil Med 8:69, 1986.

Poole JL and Whitney SL: Motor assessment scale for stroke patients: concurrent validity and interrater reliability, Arch Phys Med Rehabil 69:195, 1988.

Prescott RJ, Garraway WM, and Akhtar AJ: Predicting functional outcome following acute stroke using a standard clinical examination, Stroke 13:641, 1982.

Rubin M: The physiology of bedrest, Am J Nurs 88:50, 1988.

Scherling E and Johnson H: Dorsal dynamic wrist/hand splint in achieving improved control of spasticity in the upper extremity, Arch Phys Med Rehabil 68:594, 1987.

Shinar D, Gross CR, Bronstein KS, and others: Reliability of the activities of daily living scale and its use in telephone interview, Arch Phys Med Rehabil 68:723, 1987.

Strand T, Asplund K, Eriksson S, and others: Nonintensive stroke unit reduces functional disability and need for long-term hospitalization, Stroke 16:29, 1985.

Wade DT, Skilbeck CE, and Hewer RL: Predicting Barthel ADL score at 6 months after an acute stroke, Arch Phys Med Rehabil 64:24, 1983.

Wade DT, Wood VA, Heller A, and others: Walking after stroke: measurement and recovery after first three months, Scand J Rehabil 19:25, 1987.

Chapter 8

Alterations in Nutrition

Metabolic needs of the body are met primarily by oral intake of nutrients. Oral intake is influenced by a number of factors, including appetite and thirst, the ability to obtain food and feed oneself, and the ability to chew and swallow. A person's ability to meet his own nutritional needs is also influenced by his metabolic state. With metabolic homeostasis, nutritional needs are adequately met through oral intake. In contrast, with a hypermetabolic state, as is often seen with disease, increased nutrients are required and the person may not be able to increase oral intake sufficiently to meet the nutritional demands. The stroke patient may be at risk for developing an altered nutritional status (less than body requirements) because of decreased oral intake, a hypermetabolic state, or a combination of both. In this chapter, physiologic changes underlying altered nutritional status are discussed, along with an approach to nutritional assessment. Interventions for providing adequate nutrition are also presented.

ANATOMY OF NUTRITIONAL INTAKE AND STROKE EFFECTS

A person's interest in or craving for food is commonly known as hunger. Although the terms *hunger* and *appetite* are often used interchangeably, appetite actually refers to the desire for a specific type of food. In contrast, *satiety* is the feeling of fulfillment that follows eating. Hunger and satiety are functions mediated by the hypothalamus. The lateral nuclei of the hypothalamus produce the drive to seek out food and eat. Satiety is a function of the ventromedial nuclei. Evidence indicates that the hypothalamus contains feedback mechanisms that regulate the desire for intake of specific nutrients in relation to body requirements. For example, with a deficiency in protein, an individual may develop an appetite for a food that is high in protein.

Although it is not common, stroke may affect either area in the hypothalamus. Stroke involvement of the lateral nuclei produces lack of interest in food, or anorexia, resulting in extreme weight loss. Excessive eating may result from involvement of the ventromedial nuclei, leading to extreme obesity. Other areas appear to be involved in hunger and appetite. The amygdala, closely allied with the olfactory nerve, plays a role in taste likes and dislikes and food preference. Bilateral destruction of the amygdala results in the inability to control food selection. As a result, nonnutritive objects may be ingested, resulting in malnutrition. The hippocampal and cingulate gyri play a role in the drive to seek food when hungry. Involvement of these areas may produce inactivity in food searching behaviors in spite of hunger.

Thirst may be described as the conscious desire for water. Guyton, 1986. The thirst center is located in the lateral hypothalamus. Closely related to the thirst center is the antidiuretic hormone (ADH) secretion system. Both mechanisms work together to control osmolality, volume status, and serum sodium concentration. ADH is secreted by the posterior pituitary. Although not common, stroke may involve the hypothalamus and affect one or both of these mechanisms. The thirst response may be blocked or severe thirst may occur, causing the patient to drink excessively, leading to water intoxication. Abnormalities in ADH secretion may also result. More common is the inappropriate ADH syndrome (SIADH) in which ADH secretion is excessive and leads to water retention and intoxication. The opposite, or diabetes insipidus, in which ADH secretion is decreased, may occur. As a result, volume is depleted and dehydration results.

The ability to obtain and prepare food and feed oneself is obviously important to oral intake. Neurologic deficits resulting from stroke influence this ability. Deficits, such as hemiplegia, incoordination, and hemisensory loss, make the mechanical act of feeding difficult. This leaves the previously independent person to rely on others to feed her. Feelings of inadequacy or dependency may also decrease food interest. Hemianopia may also influence the ability to feed oneself. The stroke patient with this deficit may not see food in the affected field of vision and subsequently may leave that food untouched. Cognitive and perceptual deficits, such as decreased attention span or impulsiveness (common in right hemispheric stroke), may also impair oral intake. Patients with such deficits may find it difficult to complete mealtime activities, even when hungry.

Perhaps the most important factor influencing oral intake is the ability to chew and swallow. Chewing is essential for digestion of food because only the food surfaces may be affected by digestive enzymes. Chewing is under both voluntary and reflex control. Voluntary control of chewing is mediated by the frontal lobe, with the trigeminal (fifth) nerve innervating muscles used for chewing. Reflex chewing is controlled by the reticular formation in the brainstem with the same muscular innervation. However, other areas of the brain, such as the limbic system, sensory cortex (areas responsible for interpreting taste and smell), or lateral hypothalamus (hunger center) may stimulate reflex chewing. Stroke affecting any of these areas may result in less automatic chewing and require greater concentration than normal. Patients with brainstem stroke and coma may have reflex chewing movements and may even swallow when food is placed in their mouths. Unfortunately, swallowing mechanisms may be impaired and the risk of aspiration is high. More commonly, the chewing reflex is lost along with the decrease in arousal because of the closeness of the respective centers.

Swallowing is a more complex phenomenon, primarily because the multifunctional pharynx must be converted to a passageway for food. Swallowing occurs in three phases. In the first, or voluntary, phase, the tongue pushes food up and back against the palate toward the pharynx. Tongue movement is a function of the hypoglossal (twelfth) nerve. Once reaching the pharynx, swallowing becomes involuntary. As the food reaches the pharynx, sensory impulses are transmitted through the trigeminal (fifth) and glossopharyngeal (ninth) nerves and tractus solitaris into the lower pons and medulla. Here the swallowing center is stimulated to produce the reflex act of swallowing. Motor impulses via cranial nerves V, IX, X, and XII play a role in this response. The pharyngeal phase of swallowing consists of:

1. Closure of the posterior nares to prevent nasal reflux of food
2. Approximation of palatopharyngeal folds to facilitate passage of chewed food while preventing passage of too large a bolus
3. Closure of the larynx by epiglottal movement and vocal cord approximation to prevent aspiration of food into the lungs
4. Upward/forward laryngeal movement, which enlarges the esophageal opening with simultaneous relaxation of the upper esophageal sphincter
5. Contraction of the pharynx with initiation of a peristaltic wave to propel food into the esophagus

This activity occurs in the very short time span of 1 to 2 seconds.

The third, or esophageal, phase consists of primary and secondary peristaltic movement occurring over 5 to 10 seconds. Primary peristalsis is the esophageal continuation of the pharyngeal movement. If food is retained in the esophagus after the peristaltic wave reaches the stomach, a reflex stimulation of additional peristaltic waves occurs *(secondary peristalsis)* until the food is passed. Vagal afferent and efferent fibers mediate activity in this phase, with additional input from the myenteric nerve plexus. Therefore, some reflex peristaltic movement in the esophagus can occur even when vagal input is absent.

Each of these swallowing phases may be affected by stroke, resulting in dysphagia (swallowing disorder). Weakness or incoordination of the mouth or tongue may improperly propel food toward the pharynx or out of the mouth, leading to choking or drooling. Attention deficits, perceptual disorders, lethargy, or confusion may also impair this phase. During the pharyngeal phase, the swallow reflex may be impaired or absent, resulting in choking, aspiration, or nasal regurgitation. Although not common, the esophageal phase may be affected, resulting in regurgitation.

Numerous other factors may influence oral intake of nutrients. These should be considered, particularly when chewing and swallowing mechanisms are preserved. Depression, cognitive or perceptual deficits, and concomitant diseases may decrease appetite. Since eating is a social and often ritualistic endeavor, the social isolation imposed by stroke and hospitalization may also contribute to decreased interest in food. Cultural food preferences may be strong and, if the preferred food is not offered in the hospital setting, may also contribute to decreased interest in food. Taste and salivation, mediated by the facial (seventh) and glossopharyngeal (ninth) nerves, may also be impaired by stroke, contributing to decreased interest in food. A decreased level of consciousness presents serious concerns for oral intake. The ability to obtain food and feed oneself is obviously impaired. Reflex chewing and swallowing may be present, but it is more likely they will be absent. This is due to the closeness of chewing and swallowing reflex centers to arousal mechanisms in the brainstem. A decreased level of consciousness may also contribute to altered integrity of the mucous membranes, leading to anorexia, oral infection, and decreased ability to chew and swallow after returning to consciousness. Other, yet unknown, factors may play a role in oral intake; hence the need for additional research in this area.

METABOLIC RESPONSE

Metabolism is the process by which cells in the body use nutrients to produce energy for cellular function and growth. Metabolic homeostasis represents a fine balance among anabolism (tissue building or growth), catabolism (tissue breakdown), and oral intake of nutrients, which fuels both processes. In response to injury or disease, metabolic needs of the body often increase; this is an important defense mechanism for the body. It is important to understand this *metabolic response* because it ultimately influences the patient's outcome.

Nutrients are generally provided in the forms of carbohydrate, protein, and fat. The body has precise daily requirements for each and will utilize the necessary nutrients provided while storing the remainder. Stored nutrients, known as endogenous fuel substrates, are in the form of glycogen (in liver and muscle) and adipose tissue. Muscle and other body tissues, composed primarily of protein, represent another, though inefficient, source of energy. When metabolic needs exceed that which is supplied by oral intake or when oral intake is restricted, endogenous fuel substrates may be mobilized and converted to a usable source of energy.

A physiologic stressor, such as stroke, stimulates the body's utilization of endogenous fuel substrates. Metabolism and metabolic needs increase and oral intake is often acutely restricted. In response to the stressor, catecholamines are released because of sympathetic hyperactivity that occurs for approximately 72 hours after an insult. Catecholamines convert muscle and liver glycogen to glucose and suppress insulin to increase available glucose. Thus catecholamines produce hyperglycemia while secondarily increasing the body's basal metabolic rate. Glycogen stores may be quickly depleted, forcing the body to resort to gluconeogenesis, catabolizing muscle protein for glucose production. Muscle protein breakdown results in increased urinary excretion of nitrogen (known as nitrogen loss or negative nitrogen balance). Ketones (byproducts of protein metabolisms) accumulate, leading to ketosis and ketonuria. The brain may use ketones, although inefficiently, as a source for energy. Increased heat production and elevated body temperature also result. Clinically, the patient may manifest weight loss, muscle weakness, and wasting. Protein synthesis is decreased, resulting in decreased formation of enzymes and compromise of the immune system, rendering the person prone to infection.

The catabolic phase of the metabolic response may last indefinitely, depending on whether nutritional demands are met and the severity of the response. As the catabolic phase begins to resolve, anabolism dominates. This phase is characterized by weight gain, positive nitrogen balance, and improvements in immune function.

A number of factors influence the extent and duration of the metabolic response. As mentioned previously, the greater the severity of the initial stressor, the more severe and prolonged the response. Other factors that may adversely affect the response include advanced age, decreased level of consciousness, extensor or flexor posturing, fever, infection, concomitant stressors (such as diabetes, heart or liver disease), and poor premorbid nutritional status.

Although studies have not yet been reported that examine the extent and duration of the metabolic response specifically in the stroke population, there is general agreement among clinicians that nutritional requirements are increased during the acute phase following stroke. While the problem may not be as severe as in the patient with major thermal injuries, severe infection, or multiple trauma, it nonetheless does exist in the stroke patient. Therefore, nutritional status must be carefully assessed and nutritional needs determined.

ASSESSMENT

A detailed nutritional assessment is essential to properly identify all factors that contribute to altered nutritional status. Information obtained from the assessment is used in planning a comprehensive approach to the stroke patient's nutritional needs. Assessment data are obtained by the nurse, but a speech pathologist, occupational therapist, and dietitian are likely to be involved. In settings where a nutritional support team is available, a multidisciplinary approach to assessment is incorporated. Nutritional status is assessed on admission and on an ongoing basis as necessary, particularly as mobility or level of consciousness change. Because of the multifaceted nature of alterations in nutritional status, every stroke patient should be assessed for deficiencies.

Nutritional assessment covers aspects directly and indirectly related to nutrition. Multidimensional components of a detailed nutritional assessment follows.

Medical History

Pertinent aspects of medical history include any previous surgery or disease that may impair nutritional status. Examples to consider include vomiting, diarrhea, gastrointestinal ulceration, diabetes, liver or kidney disease, malabsorption syndrome, and bowel resection. Medications should also be reviewed to determine any food–medication interaction.

Nutritional History

A review of prestroke nutritional habits may identify preexisting deficiencies and areas in need of improvement. The patient should be questioned about food attitudes, mealtime rituals, and number of meals consumed per day. The patient or a family member may be asked to describe a typical day's meals or to keep a diary of food consumed in a 24 to 48 hour period. Recent history of weight loss or gain of greater than 10% of body weight should also be noted. The patient should be questioned about any difficulty in chewing or swallowing. A nutritional history should encompass food preferences, dislikes, and allergies. Any religious requirements or cultural preferences should also be identified. In planning for discharge, it may also be necessary to incorporate information, such as who prepares the food, food budget, preparation and storage, and social setting in which meals are consumed.

Physical Examination

Neurologic assessment is important in determining the presence of factors that influence oral intake. Specific aspects to note include hemiplegia, neglect, confusion, attention deficits, or incoordination, all of which influence a person's ability to obtain food and feed oneself. Since visual field deficits may limit oral intake, hemianopia should be identified. The ability to chew and swallow is directly observed. Asking the patient to clamp his jaws together and palpating the masseter muscle may demonstrate trigeminal nerve weakness. At the same time, mobility of the temporal-mandibular joint should be assessed because dislocation or decreased mobility may contribute to difficulty chewing. Hypoglossal weakness is determined by asking the patient to extrude his tongue, noting any deviation from the middle. Presence and condition of teeth or presence and fit of dentures should be determined because this affects chewing ability. Throat strength (function of the vagus and glossopharyngeal nerves) is tested by noting symmetry of the uvula at rest and symmetric movement on vocalization. Asymmetry is noted. Presence of the gag reflex is also noted. In addition, physical examination is conducted to determine changes indicative of poor nutritional status. Indicators to observe for include dryness and bleeding of gums, tongue, and oral mucosa, pale or sunken eyeballs, and muscle wasting or atrophy. Decreased skin turgor, edema, or bruising may also be noted.

Anthropometric Measurements

Anthropometric measurements of nutritional status provide additional information on body composition and nutritional storage. Height and weight are determined and compared with standard height-weight tables. A bedscale may be used to weigh the bedridden patient. Height may be determined from history, actual measurement, or measurement of total arm length. Skinfold thickness (SFT), a measure of subcutaneous fat, is obtained by applying a skin caliper at a point halfway between the elbow and shoulder, overlying the triceps muscle (Fig. 8-1). The ambulatory patient is measured with the arm hanging down, and the bedridden patient is measured with the arm extended vertical to the body. The subscapular skin fold may also be measured. Mid upper arm circumference (MUAC) is determined with a tape measure at the same point as for the SFT. Using the SFT and MUAC values, mid upper arm muscle circumference (MAMC), may be derived, providing an approximation of skeletal muscle mass. The following formula is used:

$$\text{MAMC} = \text{MUAC} - (\text{SFT} \times 3.14)$$

The MAMC value is then compared with a standard. Decreases in any of these values may indicate depletion of protein stores. Extreme obesity or edema may also influence results.

Laboratory Evaluation

Blood and urine analyses may provide additional information to validate other data obtained. Specifically, biochemical state, plasma protein, immunocompetence, and protein metabolism are measured. Specific laboratory testing related to nutritional status, normal values, and purpose of testing is listed in Table 8-1. In the malnourished patient, immunoincompetence occurs as protein stores are depleted. Therefore, anergy (cellular immunity) testing may be useful as an indicator of protein status. Purified protein derivative, mumps, or other immune challenges may be injected. The normal response within 24 hours is inflammation. In the malnourished patient with decreased antibody response (anergy) there is little or delayed response.

Interestingly, several studies have compared results by using objective and subjective measures of nutritional status. Results indicate that history and physical examination are reliable measures of nutritional status when performed by a trained nurse. (Wirth and Ralcheson, 1987).

Abbreviated versions of these measures may be used to initially identify those patients at high risk for nutritional deficiencies and to provide for on-

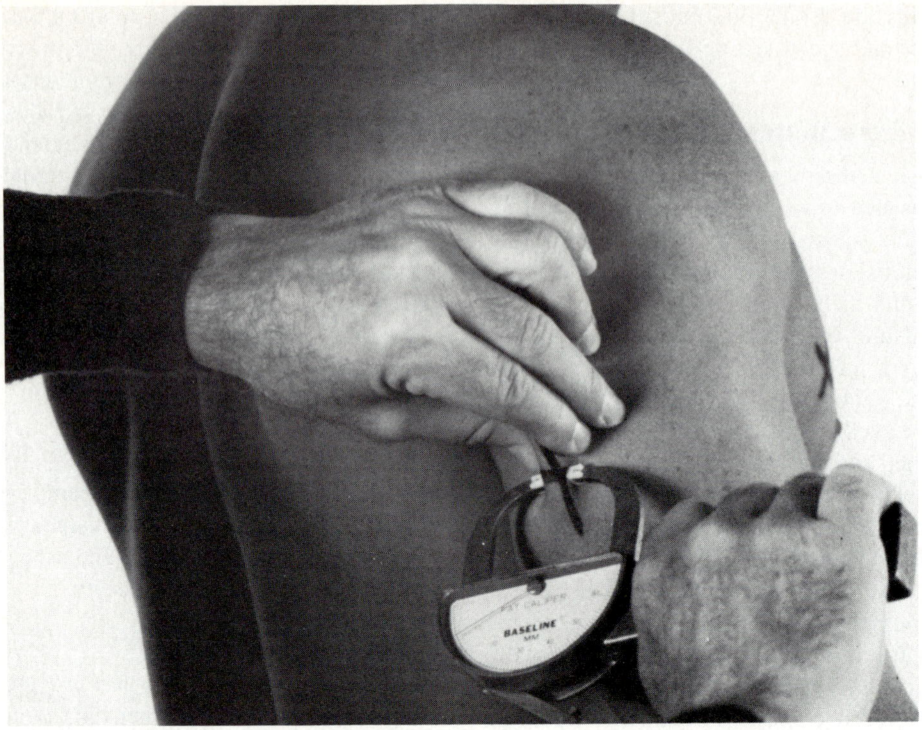

Fig. 8.1 Triceps skinfold measure as part of patient's nutritional assessment.

going assessment. A patient's height and weight, serum transferrin and albumin, and total lymphocyte counts are usually incorporated into such an assessment. Daily observation of energy level, intake and output, skin turgor and muscle bulk may be helpful in ongoing analysis. In addition, the patient should be weighed 1 to 2 times per week.

MANAGEMENT OF ALTERED NUTRITIONAL STATUS

Following an in-depth assessment, a comprehensive nutritional plan is developed. Optimum nutritional support of the stroke patient focuses on facilitating adequate oral intake and/or providing adequate nutrition to promote metabolic homeostasis, replenish nutritional deficiencies, minimize tissue breakdown, and promote tissue growth.

Daily nutritional requirements may be calculated by using a variation of the expression for basal energy expenditure (BEE). The formula used to calculate BEE incorporates height (in centimeters), weight (in kilograms), and age (in years) as follows:

$$\text{Males: BEE} = 66 + (13.7 \times W) + (5 \times H) - (6.8 \times A)$$

$$\text{Females: BEE} = 665 + (9.6 \times W) + (1.9 \times H) - (4.7 \times A)$$

To accommodate for a hypermetabolic state, the BEE is multiplied by 1.2 for bedridden patients and by 1.3 for those who are out of bed. The formula may be applied in the following manner: A 65-year-old male who weighs 70 kg and is 180 cm tall is confined to complete bedrest following his stroke.

Table 8-1 Laboratory testing of nutritional status

Test	Normal adult range of values	Purpose of testing
Serum albumin	3.3-4.5 g/dl	Estimates protein stores
Serum total protein	6.6-7.9 g/dl	Estimates protein stores
Serum total iron binding capacity	Males: 300-400 μg/dl Females: 300-450 μg/dl	Estimates protein stores
Serum creatinine	0.6-1.2 mg/dl	Indicates depletion of muscle mass (protein wasting)
24 hr urine assay for creatinine height index	84-90 ml/min	Indicates degree of protein wasting
Blood urea nitrogen	8-20 mg/dl	Indicates rate of protein metabolism
Serum transferrin	250-390 μg/dl	Indicates rate of protein metabolism and iron-binding capacity
24 hr urine assay for urea nitrogen	64-99 ml/min	Measures nitrogen balance
Blood glucose	70-100 mg/dl	Indicates availability of primary energy source
Serum electrolytes		Provides rough measure of fluid and electrolyte balance and overall nutritional status
Sodium	135-150 mEq/l	
Potassium	3.5-5.5 mEq/l	
Chloride	95-105 mEq/l	
Calcium	8.6-10.5 mg/dl	
Phosphorus	3-4.5 mg/dl	
Magnesium	1.5-2.4 mEq/l	
Serum osmolality	286-305 mOsm/l	Estimates fluid balance
Total white blood count	4500-11,000 mm^3	Indicates immune function
Total lymphocyte count	800-4500 mm^3	Indicates immune function
Hemoglobin	Males: 14-17 g/dl Females: 12-16 g/dl	Provides rough measure of iron-binding capacity, fluid balance, and absence of anemia
Hematocrit	Males: 40%-54% Females: 34%-51%	Provides rough measure of iron-binding capacity, fluid balance, and absence of anemia

Additional studies may be ordered as indicated. Examples include: serum liver and kidney function studies, free fatty acids, and vitamin and mineral levels.

$$BEE = 66 + (13.7 \times 70) + (5 \times 180) - (6.8 \times 65)$$

$$BEE = 1483\text{: then multiplied by } 1.2 = 1779 \text{ kcal}$$

This man should receive 1800 k calories per day. Exact amounts of carbohydrates, proteins, and fat are planned around this caloric figure. Nutritional supplements of vitamins, minerals, or trace elements are added to provide minimum recommended daily requirements.

INTERVENTIONS

Once nutritional needs are determined, the appropriate route for delivery is planned. Oral feedings are preferred as the most natural form of nutrition. Oral feedings are preferred even for the patient who is unable to feed himself, providing oral feedings are otherwise tolerated. Soft or pureed foods may be used for the patient who has difficulty chewing or swallowing. For these patients, solids are generally tolerated better than liquids. Small, frequent meals in a pleasant, nondistracting environment may improve appetite. Oral supplements may be useful to augment oral food intake. Such supplements are not intended to replace oral intake but rather to provide an additional nutrient source. Most oral supplements provide a mixture of nutrients, but modular supplements that are limited to only one type of nutrient (e.g., only carbohydrate or protein) may be used.

Before initiating any oral feeding, certain precautions must be taken. The nurse should evaluate gag and swallow reflexes, bowel sounds, and facial strength. If reflexes or bowel sounds are absent, oral feeding should not be attempted. In the presence of facial weakness, oral feedings are begun with caution. The patient's head is elevated to 90° for meals, and suction equipment should be readily available. The patient should not be left alone while eating. If a tracheostomy is present, the cuff should be inflated before feedings and kept inflated for 1 hour after. (The same precautions apply to the tube-fed patient.)

In situations in which oral intake is inadvisable, or when a patient is otherwise unable to meet nutritional needs through oral intake (for example, the confused or dysphagic patient), tube feedings (TFs) may be provided. To benefit from TFs, the patient's digestive and absorptive processes must be intact. TFs are contraindicated in persons with malabsorption.

Four types of feeding tubes are utilized: nasogastric (NG), nasoduodenal (ND), gastrostomy (GT), and jejunostomy (JT) tubes. Because of nasal irritation, NG and ND tubes are utilized only for short-term feedings of 6 weeks or less. In the patient with dysphagia and an absent gag reflex, a JT is indicated because this minimizes the risk of regurgitation and aspiration. In long-term situations, GT or JT feedings are more beneficial. However, insertion of either of these tubes requires surgical intervention and carries associated risks.

Nutrients provided via TFs may be from blenderized food or nutritional or elemental formulas. Blenderized food is the least expensive and most natural. However, water or other liquid must be added to produce a consistency suitable for feeding. As a result, a large volume may be necessary to provide adequate calories. In addition, blenderized food may block the tube. Because of the consistency of the feedings and the small diameter of the JT, blenderized feedings are usually not given through this type of tube.

Commercially prepared nutrient formulas are ideal for TFs. These formulas are completely balanced nutritional sources and may also be used as oral supplements. Formulas usually comprise complex carbohydrates and proteins, so digestive processes must be intact to tolerate these types of feedings. The formulas are generally palatable but can be quite expensive.

Elemental formulas are specially developed and nutritionally complete. Carbohydrates and proteins are provided in their simplest forms (usually glucose and amino acids) so little digestion is required and little residue remains. Most of these formulas are lactose-free and have been fortified with vitamins and minerals. These formulas are not at all palatable and are recommended only for TFs. They

Table 8-2 Commercially available tube feeding formulas

Product	Calories	Protein (gm)	Carbohydrates (gm)	Fat (gm)	mOsm/ kg*	Comment
Ensure	1060	37	143	37	450	Lactose free May be used as a full liquid diet, liquid supplement, or tube feeding
Ensure Plus	1500	54	197	52.5	600	High-calorie liquid diet For tube or supplemental oral feeding
Citrotein	533	32	97	1.4	496	For tube or supplemental oral feedings; lactose free
Flexical	1000	22.5	152	0.34	805	For tube or oral feeding; lactose free
Isocal (regular)	1000	33	125	43	350	Lactose free
Isocal (high calorie and nitrogen)	2000	73.5	221.6	89.6	690	Lactose free For tube feeding only
Magnacal	2000	70	250	80	590	High caloric density Nutritionally complete for oral or tube feeding
Osmolite	1006	37	143	38	300	Tube or oral feeding; lactose free
Sustacal	1000	65	148	24	625	Tube or oral feeding
Vivonex	1000	20.4	225	13	550	Lactose free
Vivonex HN (high nitrogen)	1000	43	210	0.9	844	High nitrogen feeding to restore positive nitrogen balance For tube feeding only Requires no digestion Full-strength Vivonex HN is hypertonic and has an osmolarity of 810 mOsm/kg; vomiting, diarrhea, and dumping syndrome can occur

*Formulas of high osmolarity (more than 450 mOsm) are often associated with the dumping syndrome and diarrhea.

From Hickey JV: The clinical practice of neurological and neurosurgical nursing, ed 2, Philadelphia, 1986, JB Lippincott Co.

are also quite expensive. Elemental feedings are most useful via the JT route or when digestive difficulties are present. Table 8-2 lists commonly used formulas for TFs.

Complications may be encountered when using TFs. Nursing measures are important in prevention, and so is early recognition and treatment of the following problems.

Diarrhea. Diarrhea is probably the most common problem related to TFs. Diarrhea usually is due to the hyperosmolarity of the formula or too rapid an infusion rate. Diarrhea may be prevented by giving the formula slowly (usually 30ml/hour) and by diluting it with water. If necessary, metoclopramide or tincture of opium may be given to decrease motility of the gastrointestinal (GI) tract. Lactose intolerance may also cause diarrhea. Patients should be questioned about their tolerance for milk products. Changing to a formula that is lactose-free usually eliminates this problem.

Aspiration. Aspiration is probably the most serious complication because it can lead to pneumonia. Aspiration can be caused by vomiting, regurgitation, or improper tube placement. Risk of aspiration may be minimized by elevating the head of the bed 30° to 40° during feedings and checking position of the tube before feedings. Suction equipment should be readily available. Tube position should be checked every 4 hours. The gag reflexes should be present; if absent, NG and ND tube feedings are contraindicated.

Constipation. Inadequate water content of the feeding is the common cause of constipation; however, immobility may also be a contributing factor. Adequate water should be added and stool softeners or laxatives given as necessary.

Vomiting. Rapid infusion of the feeding or painful stimulation may induce vomiting. Infusion rates should start out slow then gradually increase. If possible, painful procedures could be limited or scheduled around feedings.

Dehydration. Administration of a hyperosmolar formula may lead to hyperglycemia and, ultimately, dehydration. Slow administration of feeding may prevent this problem. Urine sugar and acetone should be checked at least once each shift. Insulin may be necessary to control hyperglycemia. Water may be added to the feedings.

Other problems may occur, including edema, dumping syndrome, intolerance to the formula, and malnutrition. In addition, there are potential problems related to the delivery system. Nasal erosion or ulceration is possible when NG or ND tubes are used. Skin erosion may occur around the GT or JT site, leading to infection. Any tube may become blocked with feeding or GI secretions.

Total parenteral nutrition (TPN) is an alternative means for continuously providing nutrition through an intravenous (IV) route. Nutrients are provided in their simplest and most usable form directly into the bloodstream, bypassing digestion and absorption. TPN may be used when nutrition provided through other sources is inadequate. Oral or tube feedings may not be tolerated, or nutritional needs may be so great it is not possible to provide adequate nutrition through an oral or TF route. TPN represents an important treatment option; studies have shown that TPN contributes to decreased morbidity and mortality (Mitchell, 1989; Wirth and Ratcheson, 1987).

The TPN solution is a complete nutritional source individualized to patient needs. Standard composition of the solution is listed in the box on p. 123. Specific consideration is given to metabolic demands and preexisting or coexisting disease, such as renal, liver, or pancreatic disease. The major source of calories for TPN is 50% dextrose. This is the preferred form of carbohydrate because it is relatively inexpensive, has little risk of metabolic acidosis, and if it causes hyperglycemia, it is relatively easy to treat. The protein (nitrogen) source is usually crystallized amino acids. Vitamins, minerals, and trace elements may be added as needed. In addition, necessary fluids are added to promote hydration. Essential fatty acids are not provided in a TPN solution. Fat emulsions may be administered 1 to 2 times a week as needed.

Because of the hyperosmolarity of the TPN solution, it is poorly tolerated in a peripheral vein. Therefore the TPN solution is usually administered via a subclavian catheter into a central vein. This requires surgical insertion and carries associated

COMPOSITION OF STANDARD TOTAL PARENTERAL NUTRITION (TPN) SOLUTION

Composition of Standard Intravenous Nutrition Solution for Adults

Base solution
- Protein = 10% crystalline amino acid solution, 500 ml
- Calories = 50% dextrose solution, 500 ml

Electrolytes
- Sodium (chloride and/or acetate, lactate, bicarbonate), 50 mEq
- Potassium (chloride/acetate), 20 mEq
- Phosphate (potassium acid salt, 1 mM = 1.5 mEq K^4), 10 mM
- Calcium gluconate, 4.6 mEq
- Magnesium sulphate, 10 mEq
- Zinc sulphate (as Zn ion), 4 mg
- Copper sulphate (as Cu ion), 0.8 mg

Standard formula*—final volume 1060 ml contains:
- 50 gm protein (8.3 gm nitrogen) = 200 kcal
- 250 gm carbohydrate = 850 kcal
- Total calories = 1,050 kcal
- Total calorie:nitrogen ratio = 127:1
- Nonprotein calorie:nitrogen ratio = 102:1

Supplements to daily regimen
- Added to standard formula by pharmacy:
  - Vitamins
    - Multivitamin injection (MVI 12), 10 ml
    - Vitamin K†, folic acid†, and cynacobalamin† (vitamin B_{12})
  - Miscellaneous†
    - Heparin
    - Albumin
    - Human insulin
    - Cimetidine
    - Iron dextran (25 mg Fe/ml)

As separate infusion:
- Fat emulsion 10% or 20% emulsion
- Daily dosage should not exceed 2.5 g/kg
- Proportion of total daily calorie intake 5-50%

From Wirth FP and Ratcheson RA, editors: Neurosurgical critical care, Baltimore, 1987, Williams & Wilkins.

*Standard formula (base solution plus electrolytes) is dispensed in bags containing total daily regimen for infusion over 24 hr.

†As indicated by condition of patient.

COMPLICATIONS OF TOTAL PARENTERAL NUTRITION (TPN) RELATED TO CATHETER INSERTION OR USE

Air embolization
Bacteremia
Brachial plexus injury
Hemothorax
Hydromediastinum
Hydrothorax
Laceration of subclavian artery or vein
Malposition or migration of catheter
Phrenic nerve injury
Pneumothorax
Pulmonary embolization
Subcutaneous emphysema
Thoracic duct injury
Tracheal injury

risks. The above box addresses these risks and those associated with continued usage of a venous access device.

Metabolic complications related to the TPN solution may occur (see box on p. 124). The major concern relates to hyperglycemia. The high glucose concentration of the TPN solution may contribute to hyperglycemia. The excessive glucose causes an osmotic diuresis in which fluids and electrolytes are lost, leading to dehydration and electrolyte abnormalities. To prevent or counteract this problem, and to facilitate use of nutrients provided, insulin may be added to the TPN solution. Close monitoring of blood and urine glucose is essential. In addition, intake, output, and volume status should also be monitored.

Infection is another major concern related to TPN. The access cathether may be a source for sepsis in addition to the solution itself. Disconnection of tubing and administration of other fluids or medications into the TPN line may also contribute to infection. Infections that occur may be bacterial or fungal. Aseptic technique is essential during insertion and any dressing or line changes.

METABOLIC COMPLICATIONS OF TOTAL PARENTERAL NUTRITION

- Glucose metabolism
  - Hyperglycemia, glycosuria, osmotic diuresis, hyperosmolar nonketotic dehydration and coma
  - Ketoacidosis in diabetes mellitus
  - Postinfusion (rebound) hypoglycemia
- Amino acid metabolism
  - Hyperchloremic metabolic acidosis
  - Serum amino acid imbalance
  - Hyperammonemia
  - Prerenal azotemia
- Calcium and phosphorus metabolism
  - Hypophosphatemia, decreased, 2.3-diphosphoglycerate, increased hemoglobin affinity for oxygen, erythrocyte metabolic aberrations
  - Hypocalcemia
  - Hypercalcemia
  - Vitamin D deficiency or excess
- Essential fatty acid metabolism
  - Serum deficiencies of phospholipid linoleic acid and arachidonic acid
  - Serum elevations of 5,8,11-eicosatrienoic acid
- Miscellaneous
  - Hypokalemia
  - Hyperkalemia
  - Hypomagnesemia
  - Hypermagnesemia
  - Biochemical liver dysfunction
  - Bleeding
  - Anemia
  - Hypervitaminosis A
  - Cholestatic hepatitis

From Wirth FP and Ratcheson RA, editors: Neurosurgical critical care, Baltimore, 1987, Williams & Wilkins.

Chance of contamination may be decreased by using the venous access device only for TPN administration. Some institutions have a policy of changing the subclavian catheter every 4 days. Close observation for fever and other signs or symptoms of infection are also important.

Nursing intervention is vital to promoting optimum nutritional status in the stroke patient. It is the nurse who establishes a close relationship with the patient, performs the initial nutritional assessment, and provides nutritional support. However, a multidisciplinary approach is often necessary for stroke-related nutritional deficits. The speech pathologist, occupational therapist, and dietitian are important members of the nutritional support team, each with unique contributions.

Nursing diagnoses may be used to guide intervention. Suggested nursing diagnoses are as follows:

Nutrition, altered: less than body requirements related to decreased appetite. The stroke patient may complain of lack of appetite or the nurse may notice the patient's lack of interest in food. To evaluate the effect of lack of appetite on nutritional status, the nurse may be involved in recording a 24-hour calorie count in which calories of all foods consumed in 24 hours are evaluated to determine nutritional adequacy.

Oral supplements may be offered. In addition, the nurse should question the patient about factors perceived to be related to decreased appetite and intervene accordingly. For example, if meals are scheduled immediately after therapy when the patient is tired, either meals or therapy may be rescheduled. If there are unpleasant odors in the environment, efforts could be made to rid the area of odors, or the patient could be moved to a more esthetic environment for meals. Based on information from the nutritional history, familiar or preferred foods may be offered, and family members may be encouraged to bring in food, if the prescribed diet allows. Small, frequent feedings may also be beneficial. Every effort should be made to allow the patient to eat when hungry, even if it is not mealtime. The family may be encouraged to bring in nutritious snacks that may be kept at the bedside, or snacks may be provided by the dietary service. Nontraditional foods should be allowed if the patient so desires. For example, the patient may prefer a sandwich for breakfast rather than cereal. Efforts should also be made to provide foods that look and smell appetizing to the patient. An appropriate place to eat should be provided for mealtime. If bedridden, the patient should be comfortably positioned upright and an overbed table placed at a convenient height. When the patient is able to be out of bed, a comfortable chair and table should be provided. Every effort should be made to provide an environment conducive to eating by controlling sounds and lighting. Since eating is a social endeavor, providing opportunity for socialization during mealtime may improve appetite. If possible, the nurse may stay with the patient while eating, or family members may be encouraged to visit during that time. Eating in a group setting may also be helpful.

Nutrition, altered: less than body requirements related to inability to feed oneself because of cognitive-behavioral deficits. Distractibility, impulsivity, poor concentration, confusion, and disorientation contribute to feeding difficulties. A quiet, calm environment with minimal distractions may facilitate self-feeding. Distractions such as extra dishes should be removed from the patient's tray or table. The patient may require repeated directions for each step of eating. The nurse may need to redirect the patient's attention to the eating process. Often patients with these problems will not realize they are hungry and must be reminded to eat and supervised during meals.

Nutrition, altered: less than body requirements related to inability to feed oneself because of motor deficits. Stroke may produce hemiparesis, hemiplegia, or incoordination, which decrease patient's ability to feed himself. To facilitate eating, the nurse may help the patient by opening containers or cutting meat. If possible, the patient should attempt to feed himself with his unaffected hand. An occupational therapist may be consulted to provide equipment to help with self-feeding. A handcuff with a palm pocket to hold an eating utensil may be helpful with hand weakness. Foam rubber or plastic grips may be applied to the handles of eating utensils to facilitate holding. A curved "rocker" knife may allow the patient to cut food one-handed. Modified plates or bowls with base grips and end guards may also be helpful. Cups with handles or straws may be used to facilitate drinking. Support to the elbow of a weakened arm is beneficial. Every effort should be made to allow the patient to feed himself. The family should be encouraged to provide verbal rather than physical support. If self-feeding is not possible, the patient is fed, but allowed to choose the order of the food offered.

Nutrition, altered: less than body requirements related to inability to feed oneself because of visual deficits. Hemianopsia, double vision, and decreased visual acuity may contribute to feeding difficulty. For hemianopsia, food should be placed within the patient's visual field. The patient may also be taught to turn her head toward the affected side to scan the tray or table. For double vision, one eye may be patched during meals. For decreased visual acuity, prescribed glasses should be worn and adequate lighting provided. Contents of the patient's tray or plate may be described.

Nutrition, altered: less than body requirements related to difficulty chewing and/or swallowing. Diminished ability to chew or swallow imposed by stroke makes eating a challenge. Before attempting to feed, gag and swallow reflexes should be assessed. If absent, oral feedings are not provided because of the risk of aspiration. Dentures should be cleaned and placed before eating. For the stroke patient with difficulty chewing, soft foods may be provided or food may be cut into small pieces. Food should not be too dry or too liquid because either may cause choking. Small, frequent meals may also be helpful. For the patient with swallowing difficulties, every effort is made to stimulate the swallow reflex to promote normal swallowing. The patient should sit upright, preferably in a chair, with his head positioned slightly forward. A small amount of food is placed in his mouth behind the front teeth on the unaffected side. The patient then tilts his head backward and attempts swallowing. After each swallow, the mouth is checked for remaining food and cleared before the next bite. Because this is a lengthy process, sufficient time for meals must be allotted. Family members may be taught this procedure and assist with feeding the patient. Additional methods may be used to enhance the swallow reflex. Wrapping a collar of ice around the patient's neck or stroking the neck with a soft brush before eating may be helpful. Cold foods may also stimulate a swallow. It is essential that the dysphagic patient have a person in attendance while eating and suction equipment readily available in the event of choking. An occupational therapist may be consulted to provide adaptive equipment to facilitate swallowing. Some dysphagic patients may benefit from a palatal training appliance that maximizes sensory stimulation of the pharynx, thereby facilitating the swallow reflex. The speech pathologist may be consulted to provide this type of device and to assist the patient with swallowing rehabilitation. Evidence indicates swallowing may be relearned even after years of tube feedings. The patient is first taught to suck his own finger until suction strength is increased. Then elevation of the larynx is taught. Using a mirror to view the neck, the patient attempts to imitate upward movement of the thyroid cartilage. Once this is mastered, the two techniques are combined to produce a swallowing movement. Efforts should be made to help the dysphagic stroke patient learn how to swallow rather than rely on TFs. However, TFs may be necessary temporarily to provide adequate nutrition.

Nutrition, altered: less than body requirements related to hypermetabolic state. Stroke may produce a hypermetabolic state with the severity of the response related to severity of the stroke. Since the hypermetabolic state cannot be directly reversed, interventions are geared toward providing sufficient nutrients to meet metabolic demands. Stroke-related deficits may also impair appetite and feeding and swallowing ability. As a result, nutrients provided orally may be inadequate to meet the increased metabolic demands. Therefore tube feedings or TPN may be necessary until the metabolic response resolves. Nursing interventions therefore focus on safe and adequate provision of these nutrient forms. Before initiating tube feedings, bowel sounds and tube placement should be assessed. Dilute feedings (half-strength) are started slowly (usually at 30 ml/hr) and increased as tolerated. The patient is observed for adverse effects as previously discussed. With nasal feeding tubes, the nares should be cleaned daily with soap and water and any sign of erosion reported. Evidence of erosion warrants changing of the feeding tube to the opposite nostril. With the GT or JT, the insertion site should be cleaned daily with sterile saline and hydrogen peroxide and dressed. Any sign of infection or drainage should be reported. The patient's weight and laboratory values indicative of nutritional status are closely monitored. For patients for whom TPN is provided, close physiologic observation is necessary. Continuous infusion of the TPN solution should be closely observed to prevent erratic responses. Daily weights are obtained and intake and output accurately recorded. Urine is checked for the presence of glucose and acetone every 6 hours and laboratory values (mentioned previously) closely monitored. Physiologic parameters, such as blood pressure, heart and respiratory rates, and temperature, should be observed frequently. Care for the TPN access device is provided according to institutional policy, while maintaining aseptic technique.

NURSING CARE PLAN

Nursing Diagnosis	Interventions	Expected Outcomes
Nutrition Altered: Less Than Body Requirements related to decreased appetite **Defining Characteristics** ■ Patient complains of lack of appetite ■ Apparent disinterest in food	**Ongoing Assessment** ■ Record 24 hr calorie count ■ Take a nutritional history with special attention to food preferences ■ Evaluate oral hygiene ■ Question patient about perceived factors related to decreased appetite **Therapeutic Interventions** ■ Offer or perform oral hygiene ■ Reschedule meals as necessary ■ Offer small, frequent meals ■ Provide opportunities for socialization at mealtime ■ Provide aesthetic environment for eating ■ Offer familiar, preferred foods ■ Allow patient to eat when hungry even if it is not mealtime ■ Provide an appropriate place for eating, preferably out of bed	■ Patient's appetite will improve ■ Patient will have adequate oral intake as evidenced by stable weight and physiologic parameters

Continued.

NURSING CARE PLAN — cont'd

Nursing Diagnosis	Interventions	Expected Outcomes
Nutrition, Altered: Less Than Body Requirements related to inability to feed oneself resulting from cognitive-behavioral deficits • **Defining Characteristics** ■ Inability to feed oneself or disinterest in food ■ Distractibility ■ Impulsivity ■ Poor concentration ■ Confusion, disorientation	**Ongoing Assessment** ■ Assess mental status ■ Assess ability to initiate and complete feeding **Therapeutic Interventions** ■ Provide quiet, calm environment for meals to minimize distractions ■ Provide directions for each step of eating ■ Focus patient's attention on eating ■ Supervise during meals, feed if necessary ■ Provide small, frequent feedings	■ Patient will have adequate oral intake as evidenced by stable weight and physiologic parameters
Nutrition, Altered: Less Than Body Requirements related to inability to feed oneself because of visual deficit **Defining Characteristics** ■ Inability to feed oneself ■ Hemianopia ■ Double vision ■ Decreased visual acuity	**Ongoing Assessment** ■ Assess visual acuity ■ Assess visual fields ■ Assess ignored areas of tray ■ Assess patient complaints of visual deficit: A. Blurry or double vision B. Extraocular movements **Therapeutic Interventions** ■ Place food within patient's visual field ■ Patch one eye during meals ■ Assist patient in placement of glasses ■ Provide adequate lighting ■ Review contents of tray with patient at mealtime ■ Feed if necessary	■ Patient will have adequate oral intake as evidenced by stable weight and physiologic parameters

Nursing Diagnosis	Interventions	Expected Outcomes
Nutrition, Altered: Less Than Body Requirements related to inability to feed self due to motor deficits **Defining Characteristics** ■ Inability to feed self accompanied by hemiparesis, hemiplegia, or incoordination	**Ongoing Assessment** ■ Assess extremity strength and equality ■ Assess coordination ■ Assess ability to feed self with unaffected extremity **Therapeutic Interventions** ■ Prepare food for patient to eat as necessary ■ Encourage patient to attempt self-feeding with unaffected extremity ■ Consult with occupational therapy regarding assistive devices ■ Feed patient, but only if necessary, allowing patient to choose food order	■ Patient will achieve adequate oral intake as evidenced by stable weight and physiologic parameters
Nutrition, Altered: Less Than Body Requirements related to difficulty chewing and/or swallowing **Defining Characteristics** ■ Decreased or absent gag reflex ■ Difficulty chewing ■ Difficulty swallowing	**Ongoing Assessment** ■ Assess presence and condition of teeth or dentures ■ Assess ability to chew ■ Assess ability to swallow ■ Determine presence of gag reflex **Therapeutic Interventions** ■ Hold oral feedings if gag reflex is absent ■ Clean teeth or clean and place dentures ■ Provide soft foods or cut food into small pieces ■ Provide small, frequent meals ■ Incorporate methods to stimulate swallow reflex ■ Observe while eating and have suction equipment readily available ■ Collaborate with occupational therapist and the speech-language pathologist to facilitate eating program ■ Provide tube feedings (jejunal) when oral intake is insufficient	■ Patient will have adequate nutritional status as evidenced by stable weight and physiologic parameters

Continued.

Nursing Diagnosis	Interventions	Expected Outcomes
Nutrition, Altered: Less Than Body Requirements related to hypermetabolic state **Defining Characteristics** ■ Weight loss ■ Decline in laboratory values indicative of nutritional status ■ Increased metabolic requirements combined with inability to feed self	**Ongoing Assessment** ■ Assess weight ■ Evaluate laboratory studies indicative of nutritional status ■ Assess nutritional needs for age, previous weight, other factors ■ Assess bowel sounds ■ Check tube placement ■ Monitor intake and output ■ Assess urine for glucose and acetone every 6 hours **Therapeutic Interventions** ■ Offer nutritional supplements ■ Record oral intake ■ Provide tube feedings: A. Start dilute feedings slowly B. Observe for adverse effects of feedings ■ Cleanse and inspect skin around the tube entry site daily ■ Provide total parenteral nutrition (TPN): A. Infuse solution continuously B. Report any signs of infection to physician ■ Maintain asepsis of TPN access device	■ Patient will attain adequate nutritional intake as evidenced by stable weight and physiologic parameters

Patient Education

- Discuss importance of and need for adequate nutrition
- Encourage family to bring in food if dietary prescription allows
- Encourage family to be available during mealtime
- If visual deficits are present, teach patient methods to compensate for deficits, e.g. scanning visual field by turning head
- If swallowing difficulties are present, teach patient and family methods to facilitate swallowing
- Instruct family to provide verbal support rather than feed patient
- Inform patient about need for nutritional support

REFERENCES

Anderson L, Dibble MV, Turkki PR, and others: Nutrition in health and disease, ed 17, Philadelphia, 1982, JB Lippincott Co.

Guyton AC: Textbook of medical physiology, ed 7, Phildelphia, 1986, WB Saunders Co.

Heimlich HJ: Rehabilitation of swallowing after stroke, Ann Otol Rhino Laryngol 92:357, 1983.

Horner J and Massey EW: Silent aspiration, Neurology 38:319, 1988.

Kaplan PE and Cerullo LJ: Stroke rehabilitation, Stoneham, Mass, 1986, Butterworth Publishers.

Mitchell M: Neuroscience nursing: a nursing diagnosis approach, Baltimore, 1989, Williams & Wilkins.

Mitchell PH, Hodges LC, Muwaswes M, and others: AANN's Neuroscience nursing, East Norwalk, Conn, 1988, Appleton & Lange.

Whitney EN and Cataldo CB: Understanding normal and clinical nutrition, St. Paul, 1983, West Publishing Co.

Williams SR: Nutrition and diet therapy, ed 5, St. Louis, 1985, Times Mirror/Mosby College Publishing.

Wirth FP and Ratcheson RA: Neurosurgical critical care, Baltimore, 1987, Williams & Wilkins.

Wright AJ: An unusual but easily treatable cause of dysphagia and dysarthria following stroke. Brit Med J 291:1412, 1985.

Chapter 9

Alterations in Elimination

After a stroke, alterations in bladder and bowel functioning are not uncommon. Changes in bladder and bowel function can result from medications, disrupted neurologic pathways between elimination organs and the brain, and other stroke-related deficits, such as visual, perceptual, and motor losses that make it difficult for the person to reach the commode in sufficient time. In addition, stroke-related changes may be concomitant with preexisting bladder and bowel problems brought on by other chronic illnesses, by surgery, or as a result of aging. Because these elimination problems are complex, this chapter will address four areas: stroke-related factors that influence bladder and bowel elimination, normal bladder and bowel elimination (an overview), alterations in elimination secondary to stroke, and nursing assessment and interventions to promote healthy bladder and bowel functioning and to minimize complications that may occur.

Before examining the specific effects on the bladder and bowel after a stroke, it is important to discuss more general deficits that affect elimination and are commonly seen in stroke patients. By assessing these general factors the nurse will have a more complete understanding of the causes of problems the patient is having with elimination and will be able to identify the appropriate interventions. General factors associated with altered urinary and bowel elimination in stroke patients include impaired mobility, cognitive impairment, aphasia, altered emotional status, and preexisting and/or concomitant urinary problems.

Impaired mobility affects bladder and bowel elimination in a variety of ways. A loss of mobility makes it difficult for the person to get to the bathroom independently and may result in urinary incontinence (Brocklehurst and others, 1985; Romanowski and others, 1988). Being immobilized in bed or using the bedpan in the supine position makes it difficult to effectively expel urine, resulting in incomplete bladder emptying (Lorenze and others, 1959). Additionally, loss of fine motor skills on the affected side may make it difficult for the patient to manipulate clothing or the urinal and to perform necessary hygiene tasks after bowel and/or bladder elimination. Decreased mobility is also associated with constipation in stroke patients (Kaplan and Cerullo, 1986) during their hospitalization and after discharge.

Studies of incontinence in the elderly have found mental confusion to be a common precipitating factor of incontinence (James, 1979; Romanowski and others, 1988). Even if the person is mobile, confusion may impair the ability to express the need to use the bathroom and to use the facilities properly. The nurse must carefully assess any cognitive impairments to determine the level at which the patient is capable of participating in toileting and the appropriate interventions to resolve the problems.

An altered sensation of bladder or bowel fullness may make it difficult for patients to feel bladder or bowel fullness and/or to be aware of their needs to use the bathroom. Decreased vision may cause the person to have difficulty locating the bathroom, resulting in incontinence (Romanowski and others, 1988; Ruff and Reaves, 1989).

Aphasia has been associated with increased urinary incontinence probably because the aphasic person cannot communicate the need to use the bathroom or any problems or concerns about elimination. The patient may be embarrassed at needing assistance with this part of his care and be unable to communicate this need. A timely nursing assessment to determine the interventions needed to facilitate appropriate elimination patterns will prevent unnecessary frustration and embarrassment for the patient.

Stroke-related mood changes may have primary or secondary effects on a patient's elimination patterns. The stroke patient may be depressed. Stroke-related depression may also have an effect on patients' response to treatment for incontinence (Burgio and others, 1985). Altered mentation may result in a stroke patient losing motivation for control. This loss of motivation may result in the patient not responding to the sensory stimuli of bladder distention and reflex emptying without cortical inhibition (Lorenze and others, 1959). Secondarily, feelings of embarrassment about being dependent on others may make it difficult for stroke patients to ask for help. Inability to ask for help may result in incontinence or unsafe toileting behaviors.

After a stroke, a patient may have difficulty chewing or swallowing (see Chapter 8) and/or difficulty independently ingesting food or fluids. These difficulties put the stroke patient at risk for secondary bladder and bowel alterations related to changes in nutritional status. Possible problems include dehydration and constipation. When one becomes dehydrated, this decreases the signal of the full bladder to stimulate voiding. Because one stimulus for voiding is bladder fullness, an adequate ingestion of fluids is necessary for healthy bladder functioning. Constipation is a common complication after a stroke for some patients because of immobility and/or a change in dietary habits as a result of swallowing problems or the change in environment. A secondary effect when one becomes constipated is that the bladder neck may become obstructed, resulting in the person having difficulty voiding (Ruff and Reaves, 1989).

Because many stroke patients are elderly, they may have elimination problems that existed before the stroke. For example, an estimated 19% of men and 38% of women 60 years and older living in the community have some degree of involuntary urine loss (Diokno and others, 1986). Other common preexisting urinary tract problems include prostatic hypertrophy, loss of pelvic floor muscle tone (in women), infection, and cicatricial urethritis (in women). Some potential preexisting age-related bowel problems include constipation, diarrhea, diverticulitis, bowel inflammation, and bowel problems related to laxative abuse. A complete nursing assessment will distinguish preexisting problems from stroke-related alterations in elimination.

These general factors may have a significant impact on a stroke patient's elimination processes. However, evaluating general factors alone does not provide the nurse with sufficient information upon which to base assessment and interventions. It is crucial that the nurse understand basic anatomy and physiology of bladder and bowel elimination and the potential alterations after a stroke.

URINARY ELIMINATION

Central Nervous System Influence on the Lower Urinary Tract

Several parts of the brain are believed to play a role in regulating bladder function. These include areas in the cerebral cortex, brain stem, cerebellum, basal ganglia, thalamus, hypothalamus, and limbic system (Fig. 9-1). While the exact role of each area of the brain is not clearly delineated, early animal studies and preliminary studies in humans suggest that damage from stroke in any of these areas could alter normal bladder functioning.

Frontal. Two regions in the frontal lobes of the cerebral cortex are believed to innervate the bladder and the periurethral striated muscle (Hald and Bradley, 1982). The bladder is innervated by the

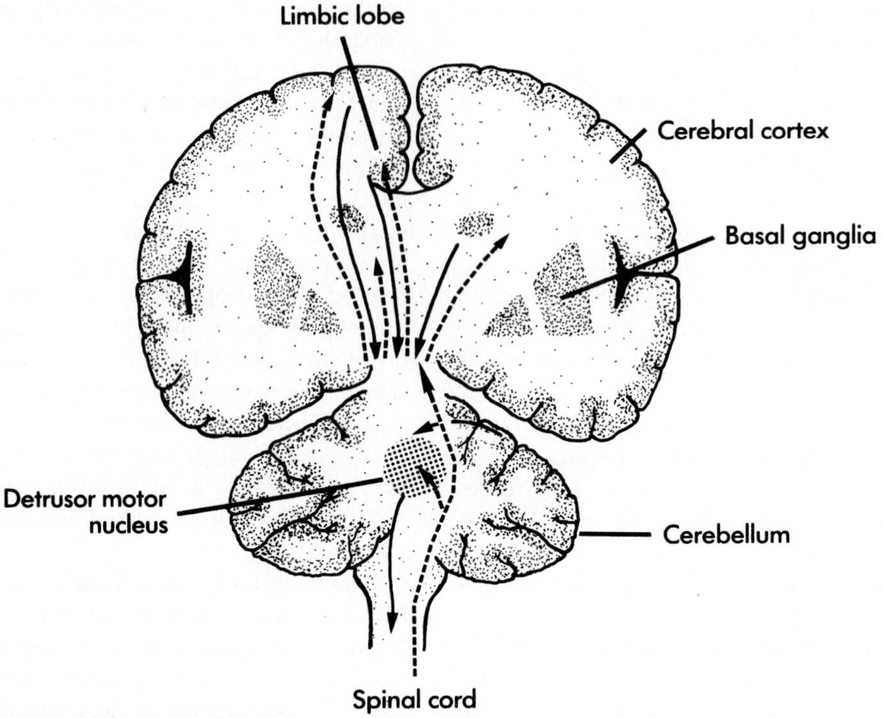

Fig. 9-1 Parts of the brain involved in regulating bladder function.

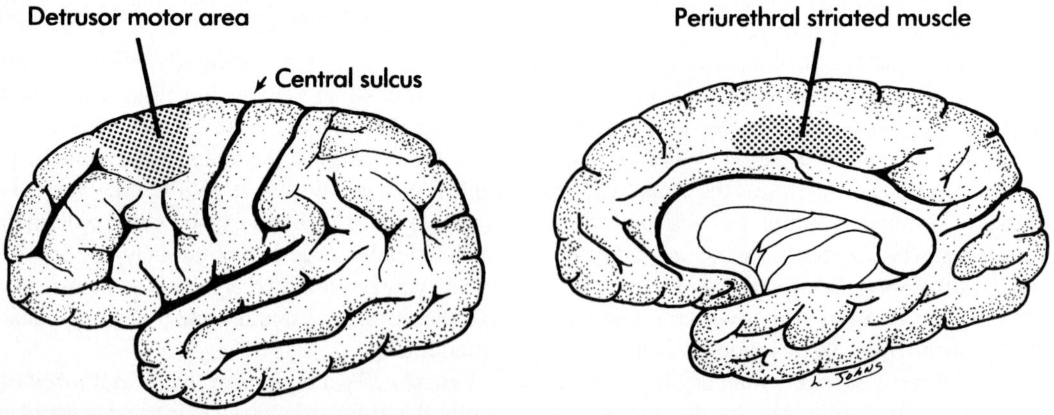

Fig. 9-2 Areas in the cerebral cortex believed to control detrusor muscle and periurethral striated muscle.

detrusor motor area, located in the superomedial area of the frontal lobes and the genu of the corpus callosum (Fig. 9-2). Detrusor motor area neurons cut across the basal ganglia and terminate in the pons. Another area of the cortex is believed to innervate the periurethral striated muscle: it is located on the medial aspect of the sensorimotor cortex (Fig. 9-2). Axons that originate from neurons in this area pass through the internal capsule and brainstem, continuing to the lateral corticospinal tracts in the spinal cord. Damage to these areas in the frontal lobes could result in an overactive detrusor reflex, resulting in urinary incontinence and urgency (Wein and others, 1987).

Brainstem. The brainstem, specifically the anterior pontine region, contains nuclei that facilitate impulses to the bladder. This area of the anterior pons is called Barrington's center, which facilitates normal reflex contraction of the detrusor muscle. Input into Barrington's center comes from all other parts of the brain. Destruction of this center in animals causes permanent urinary retention (Barrington, 1925).

Cerebellum and basal ganglia. The cerebellum receives sensory input from the bladder and pelvic floor muscles and is believed to inhibit the lower urinary tract. This inhibitory effect acts by regulating the rate and force of muscle contractions and by coordinating contraction of the detrusor muscle and reciprocal relaxation of the periurethral striated muscle during voiding (Hald and Bradley, 1982). Also having an inhibitory influence are the nuclei of the basal ganglia. These nuclei are believed to inhibit detrusor reflex contractions. Damage to these areas secondary to stroke could interrupt the inhibitory effects, resulting in urinary incontinence.

Thalamus, hypothalamus, and limbic system. The role of the thalamus, hypothalamus, and limbic system in bladder function is still being investigated. However, the following relationships are hypothesized. The thalamus is the relay station through which all input comes to higher centers and probably receives sensory input from the urinary bladder. The hypothalamus may influence aspects of micturition and defecation that are mediated by the autonomic nervous system. The limbic system is believed to inhibit or facilitate bladder activity, depending on what part of the limbic system is stimulated. Damage to these areas by stroke could alter urinary elimination.

Spinal cord. The micturition center in the spinal cord is located at sacral nerve segments 2 to 4. From these segments come the nerves that extend to most striated muscles of the pelvic floor, including the periurethral and anal sphincters. Through the spinal pathways nerve impulses travel to and from the brain. Via the spinothalamic tracts, pain, temperature, and touch impulses from the lower urinary tract travel to the brain. Via the posterior columns, proprioceptive impulses from the bladder muscle and periurethral striated muscle travel to the brain. At the sacral level of the cord motor impulses generated in the pons descend and synapse on motor neurons in the intermediolateral cell column. The reticulospinal tracts innervate the detrusor muscle and the corticospinal tracts innervate the periurethral striated muscle (Hald and Bradley, 1982).

In summary, voluntary urinary elimination is coordinated by cerebral pathways that transmit signals to and from the brain. A center that inhibits urinary elimination is located in the midbrain. Fibers that facilitate this are located in the pontine region and the posterior hypothalamus. Fibers in the cerebral cortex are mainly inhibitory but can, at times, be excitatory (Guyton, 1987). In general, lesions above the pons are associated with a hyperactive detrusor muscle; but they do not disrupt coordination between bladder and pelvic floor muscles. Lesions below the pons and above the sacral micturition center may result in uncoordinated contraction of the detrusor and pelvic floor muscles; this could result in simultaneous contraction of both muscle groups, and difficulty voiding (Gray and Dougherty, 1987).

Understanding the impact of brain control on urination will help the nurse to accurately assess urinary function after stroke and determine the appropriate interventions.

Lower Urinary Tract Structure and Function

Urine produced in the kidneys travels down the ureters to collect in the bladder. The bladder is a spherical, hollow organ made of smooth muscle. The main smooth muscle layer of the bladder is divided into the detrusor and the trigone. The detrusor makes up the bulk of the bladder wall. The trigone is that area of smooth muscle lying between the ureteral opening and the vesicourethral junction. The bladder neck and proximal urethra make up a physiologic "internal sphincter" of smooth muscle rich in elastic fibers. While not a true "sphincter," this area increases in tone when urine is stored in the bladder and facilitates maintaining the tone of the bladder wall. A true sphincter, the striated muscle urethral/periurethral sphincter, surrounds the urethra in females and the posterior urethra in males. This sphincter plays a definite role in actively preventing incontinence (Hald and Bradley, 1982).

There are two basic functions of the lower urinary tract: (1) filling the bladder and storing urine, and (2) actively expelling urine from the bladder. During bladder filling, the intravesicular pressure in the bladder rises slowly. As the bladder fills, stretch receptors in the bladder wall are stimulated and muscle contractions begin. For the bladder to fill properly and be able to store urine, the following conditions must be met (Wein and others, 1987):

1. The bladder must accommodate increasing volumes of urine at a low intravesical pressure and with appropriate sensation.
2. The bladder outlet must be closed at rest and remain closed during increases in intraabdominal pressure.
3. There must be no involuntary bladder contractions.

The normal micturition reflex consists of a cycle of (1) rapid and progressive increase in pressure; (2) a period of sustained pressure; and (3) return of the pressure to the basal tonic pressure to the bladder. The first urge to void is normally felt when the bladder contains about 150 ml. Reflex contraction of the bladder occurs when the bladder fills to between 300 to 400 ml. Voluntary urination probably occurs as a result of the pelvic floor muscles relaxing and tugging on the detrusor muscle to initiate contraction. For the bladder to empty properly, the following conditions are necessary (Wein and others, 1987):

1. The bladder musculature must contract in a coordinated fashion and contractions must be of ample magnitude.
2. There must be a simultaneous lowering of resistance of the smooth muscle and external sphincter.
3. There can be no anatomic obstruction.

Normally, a person is able voluntarily to contract the perineal muscles and external sphincter to prevent urine from passing down the urethra or to interrupt the flow of urine. A person learns (at toilet training) to maintain the external sphincter in a contracted state to delay urination.

Peripheral nervous system control of urination is primarily through parasympathetic and somatic nerve fibers. When the micturition reflex becomes strong enough and the fluid pressure in the bladder exerts pressure on the bladder neck, the reflex travels to the sacral spinal cord, where the micturition reflex is mediated. Sensory signals are transmitted to the sacral segments of the spinal cord via the pelvic nerves (afferent); nerve impulses travel back to the bladder through the parasympathetic fibers in pelvic and pudendal nerves (efferent) (Fig. 9-3). At these nerve impulses, the bladder contracts and the external sphincter relaxes. Relative to the parasympathetic nervous system, the sympathetic nervous system plays a minor role in influencing lower urinary tract function. It is suspected that a spinal sympathetic reflex through the efferent limb of the hypogastric nerve may inhibit bladder contractility and facilitate the filling and storage phase of micturition (Wein and others, 1987).

While the micturition reflex is an automatic spinal cord reflex, it can be inhibited or facilitated by centers in the brain. Centers in the brain exert final control on micturition mainly by:

1. Partially inhibiting micturition at all times

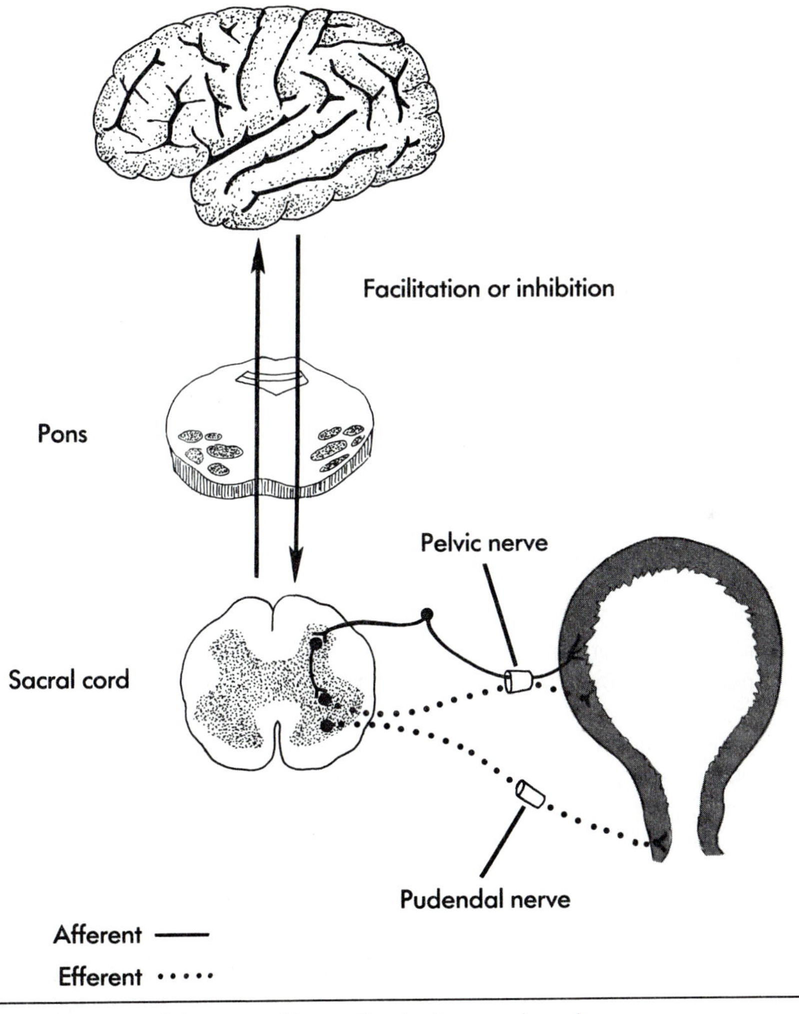

Fig. 9-3 Mediation of the micturition reflex in the sacral cord.

except when one desires to urinate.
2. Contracting the external sphincter during the micturition reflex until it is possible to urinate.
3. Facilitating the micturition reflex in the sacral cord and inhibiting contraction of the external sphincter so that urination can occur.

Effects of Stroke on Urinary Elimination

The nurse can be alerted to alterations in urinary elimination in stroke patients by a variety of symptoms. These urinary symptoms may signal a preexisting problem made worse by the stroke; bladder dysfunction specifically resulting from the stroke; or impending complications resulting from lack of early diagnosis and treatment of the initial problem. Symptoms might include one or more of the following: frequency, dysuria, burning on urination, urge incontinence, and/or urinary retention. This discussion will be limited to the types of alterations in urinary elimination most likely to occur in stroke patients.

The International Continence Society defines the following terms:

Incontinence—a condition in which involuntary loss of urine is a social or hygienic problem and is objectively demonstrable (Bates and others, 1979).

Urge incontinence—involuntary loss of urine associated with a strong desire to void (Bates and others, 1979). Signs usually include relatively little warning to void and incontinence is often a large volume. In stroke patients with urge incontinence, the detrusor muscle is usually overactive and urethra and bladder sensation are normal (Wein and others, 1987).

Two other types of incontinence are relevant to stroke patients:

Functional incontinence—involuntary loss of urine in spite of normal urinary tract function (Diokno, 1983). This type of incontinence in stroke patients may be due to alterations in mobility, speech, cognition, sensation, perception, and to psychologic and/or environmental factors.

Transient incontinence—altered urinary tract function of various types due to conditions of acute illness such as confusion, immobilization, and fecal impactions, and related treatments such as medications or altered hydration (Palmer, 1985).

FUNCTIONAL CLASSIFICATION OF BLADDER AND URETHRA*

DETRUSOR
Normal
Overactive
Underactive

URETHRA
Normal
Overactive
Underactive

SENSATION
Normal
Hypersensitive
Hyposensitive

*Based on the International Continence Society Classification
From: Fourth report on the standardization of terminology of lower urinary tract function, Br J Urol 53:333, 1981.

Altered urinary function specifically brought on by stroke might be due to abnormal sensation, an overactive or underactive sphincter, an overactive or underactive bladder, or combinations of these problems. A classification of bladder and urethral function by the International Continence Society is presented in the box above.

Stroke patients might also experience urinary retention, frequency, dysuria, and burning on urination. Urinary retention is the inability to empty urine from the bladder. In stroke patients, urinary retention is likely due to an underactive detrusor muscle and/or dyssynergy between the detrusor and the external urinary sphincter. Frequency, dysuria, and burning on urination may be due to an overactive detrusor muscle resulting in frequent bladder contractions, difficult voiding resulting from bladder-sphincter dyssynergy, or urinary tract infections. Urinary frequency can also occur in patients who have a normal bladder and sphincter.

The most common problem documented in stroke patients is detrusor instability (Khan and others, 1981; Tsuchida and others, 1983). One study of urinary incontinence after stroke found that 85% of previously continent stroke survivors had detrusor instability or an overactive bladder (Borrie and others, 1986). The overactive bladder contracts frequently and spontaneously with little force, probably because of loss of cortical inhibition. While the bladder is overactive, the urinary sphincter may be normal, underactive or overactive. Some patients with frontal lobe lesions have been noted to have a normal sphincter but frequent bladder contractions (Khan and others, 1981) resulting in frequency, urge incontinence, or frequency associated with dysuria (Lorenze and others, 1959).

In patients with an underactive sphincter and frequent bladder contractions, the external sphincter reflexively relaxes during uninhibited bladder contractions. Symptoms noted in these patients are frequency and urge incontinence (Tsuchida and others, 1983).

Another poststroke possibility is an overactive bladder with an uncoordinated sphincter. That is, the detrusor muscle of the bladder and the external sphincter are not contracting in synchrony to facilitate voiding (dyssynergia). This may result in urinary retention, urge incontinence, frequency, and frequency accompanied by dysuria. Dyssynergia has been documented in some patients with lesions of the parietal lobe and basal ganglia areas and in patients with multiple, bilateral stroke lesions (Khan and others, 1981).

Few research studies have investigated poststroke alterations in urinary elimination. Poststroke urinary incontinence has been investigated to measure incidence and urodynamic changes in stroke patients. Incidence of urinary incontinence was reported to be between 51% to 60% (Borrie and others, 1986; Brocklehurst and others, 1985) during the first 2 weeks poststroke with a steady decline in incidence in one study to 32% at 4 weeks and 21% at 12 weeks poststroke (Borrie and others, 1986). A longitudinal study (n = 135) reported an incidence of incontinence of 6% between 9 and 50 weeks poststroke (Brocklehurst and others, 1985). It is unclear whether this reported decline was due to spontaneous recovery or to interventions by the health care team. While the incidence of incontinence is quite high during the acute stroke period, incontinence does not affect the majority of stroke patients as time goes on. However, certain physiologic changes in the lower urinary tract of stroke patients have been documented by urodynamic studies.

In urodynamic studies, a majority of incontinent stroke patients have abnormal urodynamic findings. Patients with frontal and internal capsule lesions or a putaminal lesion of the brainstem tended to have hyperactive bladders resulting in frequency, urgency and/or incontinence (Tsuchida and others, 1983). Researchers suggest that patients with frontal lobe lesions accompanied by parietal or internal capsule involvement also have altered sphincter function (Khan and others, 1981 and Tsuchida and others, 1983). Stroke lesions in the dominant cortex seem to more often result in incontinence than in lesions of the nondominant cortex (Khan and others, 1981); and no relationships were found between incontinence and the subject's sex or other lesion locations. Further urodynamic studies using larger samples are necessary to more clearly define the relationships between bladder dysfunction and stroke lesion.

In summary, stroke patients potentially may experience frequency with or without incontinence, dysuria, urge incontinence, or urinary retention. The type of urinary dysfunction that they experience will be influenced by the location of the stroke lesion, possibly the side of the lesion, whether it is a first or multiple stroke and other deficits that the stroke has caused, such as immobility, aphasia, altered sensation and cognition, and/or mood changes. Also, preexisting alterations in urine elimination must be considered in the nurse's assessment of the stroke patient.

Assessing Bladder Function

When caring for the stroke patient, the nurse must thoroughly assess the patient's bladder function in acute care, in postacute care, and in the

NURSING EVALUATION OF BLADDER FUNCTION

Nursing History

Previous urine elimination patterns/habits

Problems with urine elimination since stroke (onset, duration, symptoms)

Activities, behaviors that make the problem worse/better

Amount and pattern of fluid intake (voiding diary)

Amount, pattern, consistency of output (voiding diary)

Past medical history (including surgeries, childbirth, chronic illnessess, any prestroke urinary dysfunction, major infections)

Current medications

Patient's affective response that may influence elimination (modesty, depression, anger, frustration)

Place for elimination (bedpan, commode, bedside commode)

Physical assistance required for elimination (for walking, standing and sitting balance, hygiene, handling clothing)

Assistive devices needed (e.g., cane, walker, reachers, elevated commode seat, grab bars)

Other stroke-related deficits that may influence urinary function (e.g., aphasia, altered mobility, cognition, or mood)

Psychosocial concerns of patient, family, significant other

Community resources and future life style (affects on one's ability to continue hospital-initiated routine)

Physical Examination

Neurologic examination (vision, mental status, emotional state, motor abilities including manual dexterity, gait, sitting/standing balance, transferring, ambulation)

Abdominal examination (auscultate for bowel sounds, note scars, distension, palpate for tenderness)

Urogenital examination (skin condition, signs of infection, discharge, urine specimen, rectal check for impaction and for prostate [in males])

rehabilitation setting. Because the patient's bladder function may change, an ongoing assessment is crucial. Subjective and objective data are collected by obtaining a nursing history and doing a physical examination. Components of each are listed in the box above. As part of the nursing history, the nurse should complete a voiding diary, which logs the frequency and timing of urination and fluid intake (Fig. 9-4). The voiding diary is a valuable tool that enables the nurse to document frequency and amount of urine output, fluid intake, location of voiding (i.e., bed, bedside commode, bathroom), patient's awareness of the urge to void and whether or not the patient had any incontinence. To obtain an accurate picture of the patient's voiding patterns the nurse should compile the voiding diary for a 1 to 2 week period. The nursing history (including the health history, voiding diary, and the physical examination) should be completed on all patients as part of urinary function assessment after stroke.

It is not uncommon for alterations in urinary elimination (incontinence or retention) to be induced by medications. Drugs that disrupt the alpha- and beta-adrenergic receptors of the urinary tract can affect continence. Alpha-adrenergic antagonists such as antihypertensive drugs cause relaxation of the bladder neck and may result in urinary frequency, urgency, and dysuria. Some antihypertensives, such as methyldopa (Aldomet), can cause postural hypotension and, secondarily, unsafe ambulation to the commode.

Other types of medications affecting urinary elimination include diuretics, skeletal muscle relaxants, sedatives/hypnotics, and anticholinergics (Romanowski and others, 1988). Because diuretics increase the frequency and volume of urine, this medication may worsen urge incontinence. One study noted urge incontinence was more common in patients taking diuretics than in patients not taking diuretics (Shimp and others, 1988). Skeletal muscle relaxants such as baclofen (Lioresal), dan-

VOIDING DIARY

PATIENT'S NAME ______________________ DATE ______________

TIME OF VOID	LOCATION OF VOID 1=BEDPAN 2=URINAL 3=BEDSIDE COMMODE 4=TOILET 5=BED (INCONTINENT)	DID YOU HAVE A LEAKING EPISODE BEFORE VOIDING? S=SMALL M=MEDIUM L=LARGE N=NONE	IF LEAKING EPISODE, ACTIVITY AT THE TIME?	DID YOU FEEL THE URGE TO VOID? Y=YES N=NO D=DON'T KNOW	AMT/TYPE OF FLUID INTAKE (CC)	COMMENTS
____ AM						
____ AM						
____ AM						
____ AM						
____ AM						
____ AM						
____ AM						
____ AM						
____ AM						
____ AM						
____ AM						
____ AM						
____ PM						
____ PM						
____ PM						
____ PM						
____ PM						
____ PM						
____ PM						
____ PM						
____ PM						
____ PM						
____ PM						
____ PM						

Fig. 9-4 Sample voiding diary.

trolene sodium (Dantrium), and diazepam (Valium) may cause incontinence because they relax the external urinary sphincter and decrease tone and resistance to the bladder outlet. Sedatives and hypnotics alter mental alertness and may decrease cortical inhibition, causing a patient to be inattentive and unresponsive to bladder cues (Willington, 1983). Anticholinergics and other medications with anticholinergic effects may cause difficult voiding and/or urinary retention because they inhibit bladder contractions. In summary, when assessing urinary tract function, it is important for the nurse to record current medications and to monitor medication effects in an ongoing manner.

If the stroke patient is incontinent or has other symptoms of urinary dysfunction, additional information can be obtained from a more extensive physical examination, laboratory tests and urodynamic evaluation and by measuring post-void residuals. These observations will guide the nurse to select the appropriate interventions.

Interventions

While approximately 23% to 51% of patients experience alterations in urinary elimination after stroke (Lorenze and others, 1959; Brocklehurst and others, 1985; Borrie and others, 1986), these alterations usually occur during the acute care period. Altered urinary elimination is often manifested by urge incontinence and sometimes by urinary retention. Following acute care, a significant number of stroke patients with urinary tract problems recover their normal functioning; the percentage of stroke patients whose recovery is spontaneous vs. recovery as a result of some intervention is unknown. Similarly, the number of stroke patients who sustain long-term alterations in urinary tract function is also unknown. Further research is needed in these areas. However, it is important for the nurse to be aware of potential alterations and to identify appropriate nursing interventions to treat alterations that do exist. Voiding dysfunctions may be subtle, and the long-term impact of urinary problems on health and on a patient's ability to participate in a rehabilitation program are significant.

Alterations most commonly experienced by stroke patients include urinary frequency, dysuria, urge incontinence, and urinary retention. It is important to note that alterations in urinary tract function may be complex and encompass etiologies that are stroke-related and problems that may have existed before the onset of the stroke. For example, patients in one study reported a 17% incidence of prestroke urinary incontinence (Borrie and others, 1986). Thus the nurse must carefully assess all aspects of the patient's voiding patterns to accurately describe the problem and identify the cause. Often a combination of treatment approaches will most effectively treat the alterations.

Treatments for bladder dysfunction in stroke patients can be divided into three general categories: treatments that facilitate urine storage, treatments that facilitate bladder emptying, and treatments directed at alleviating functional, psychologic and/or environmental causes.

Treatments to facilitate storing urine in the bladder. One of the most common urinary elimination problems that stroke patients experience is that of difficulty holding urine in the bladder. Symptoms of this type of urinary dysfunction include frequency with or without incontinence, dysuria, and urge incontinence. The goals of treatment to facilitate urine storage are to increase the bladder's ability to hold urine and decrease the number of incontinent episodes. Treatments used to achieve this goal include habit training, bladder retraining, prompted voiding, Kegel exercises, biofeedback, contingency management, and medications. Often, these treatments are used in combination.

Habit Training. Habit training is a behavioral strategy that involves putting the patient on a voiding schedule. This voiding schedule usually consists of toileting the person every 2 to 4 hours, whether the urge to void is present or not. If the patient is consistently dry at the timed interval, the interval is lengthened; if the patient is incontinent, the interval between voiding is shortened. The goal of habit training is to keep the patient dry. Habit training is used to treat frequency and urge incontinence related to an overactive detrusor muscle and may be combined with other treatments, such as medications, Kegel exercises, contingency management, and monitoring fluids. Nursing interventions essential to this strategy include: keeping a voiding record, monitoring fluid intake, evaluating patient's ability to request help with toileting or to use the bathroom independently, and strongly reinforcing the appropriate behavior. While no studies have been done on the effectiveness of this method specifically in stroke patients, some studies report habit training has been successful in treating incontinence in rehabilitation patients and the elderly (Clay, 1978; Sogbein and others, 1982; Spangler and others, 1984).

Bladder Retraining. Another behavioral strategy is bladder retraining, also called bladder training or bladder drill. Based on Frewen's bladder drill concept, patients are encouraged to resist the urgency, to postpone voiding, and to urinate by the clock rather than as a response to the urge (Burgio and Burgio, 1986). The rationale for this method is that urinary urgency may perpetuate urinary frequency, resulting in more frequent urination and a reduction in bladder capacity (Frewen, 1978, 1980). Thus, by increasing the time between voiding, the patient improves the ability to suppress bladder contractions and gradually returns to a normal pattern of voiding and normal bladder function. Nursing interventions include keeping the toileting schedule consistent; letting patients know when you'll be back to assist them with toileting; communicating clearly; giving positive reinforcement for accomplishing the desired behavior, and encouraging the patient to participate and manage his own program. Recent research on bladder retraining in elderly persons demonstrates an 82% success rate in decreasing incontinent episodes (Burton and others, 1988). Because this approach requires patient motivation and cooperation, a prerequisite is that one not be cognitively impaired. Bladder retraining may be used in combination with medications.

A variation of bladder retraining that emphasizes patient involvement is called *prompted voiding*. In this method the patient is checked hourly and asked about the need to void. The nurse assists the patient to the bathroom if the urge to void is felt. If not, the patient is approached at the next interval. Ideally, patients schedule their own voiding intervals and keep a record of their progress. The goal is to avoid incontinence and assist the patient to develop control. Research supports the use of prompted voiding as a behavioral strategy to reduce incontinence in nursing home residents (Creason and others, 1989; Hu and others, 1989).

Kegel Exercises. Kegel exercises (Kegel, 1948) were designed to strengthen the pubococcygeal muscles by having the person voluntarily tighten the perineal muscles. When effectively doing the Kegel exercises, patients increase pelvic striated muscle tone, which helps increase the bladder outlet resistance, thus facilitating urine storage. Patients are taught to contract these muscles at least 10 times, 3 times daily (morning, afternoon and evening), as though to interrupt the flow of urine, while tightening the vaginal muscles, perineum, and rectum as if stopping a bowel movement. While these exercises are most effective in treating stress incontinence (McCormick and others, 1988), Kegel exercises, when combined with biofeedback, have also helped to decrease urinary incontinence in elderly patients with urge incontinence (Baigis-Smith and others, 1989). By combining the Kegel exercises with biofeedback, the person receives immediate feedback on how effectively the exercises are being performed. Feedback is important to ensure the patient is doing the exercises correctly and to keep her motivated.

Biofeedback. Biofeedback is a behavioral strategy in which the patient receives feedback on her response to pelvic exercises initiated to improve bladder function. To accomplish this, a diagnostic device called a perineometer is inserted into the vagina or rectum to record electrical activity of the pubococcygeus (PC) muscle. This device displays audio and visual feedback to the patient, indicating how successful she is in tensing the PC muscle. Researchers suggest that using biofeedback to augment Kegel exercises provides more effective treatment of urge incontinence than using the exercises alone (Baigis-Smith and others, 1989). Biofeedback was successfully used to treat urinary incontinence in a small sample of stroke patients with overactive detrusor muscles, impaired bladder sensation, and poor sphincter control. In combination with sphincter exercises and habit training, biofeedback resulted in all subjects achieving continence within 6 months (Middaugh and others, 1989).

Contingency Management. Another approach traditionally used for functional or urge incontinence is contingency management. In this approach, the patient is rewarded to reinforce appropriate toileting behaviors and punished for unsuccessful toileting behaviors. Rewards can be verbal praise, attention, social approval, added privileges, and tokens to purchase needed items. Punishments can be verbal disapproval, withheld privileges, and withdrawal of tokens. A critical nursing intervention is to give positive reinforcement for the desired behaviors in a consistent manner for contingency management to be effective. Contingency management has been combined with habit training and bladder retraining for a more comprehensive treatment approach. It is important to note that studies using contingency management have primarily been done with elderly psychiatric patients (Grosicki, 1968; Pollack and Liberman, 1974; Wagner and Paul, 1970) and report limited success. Effective use of contingency management for incontinence after stroke has not been studied.

Finally, medications may be used in conjunction with the aforementioned treatments to facilitate the ability to store urine in the bladder. Types of medications most commonly used include: anticholinergics/antispasmodics and antidepressants/alpha-adrenergics. Anticholinergic/antispasmodics inhibit bladder contractility, increase bladder capacity, and control symptoms of urgency. Improvement in symptoms is usually seen within several days of starting the medication. Common drugs of this type used to treat urge incontinence are propantheline bromide (Probanthine), oxybutynin chloride (Ditropan), flavoxate hydrochloride (Urispas), and dicyclomine hydrochloride (Antispas). Nursing interventions when administering these medications include observing and documenting common side effects such as constipation, blurred vision, tachycardia, dry mouth, confusion or excitement, increased intraocular pressure, and urinary retention. Orthostatic hypotension is seen in patients taking high doses of Probanthine because of the strong ganglionic blocking properties of this medication. Nurses should monitor intake and output and assess postvoid residuals to detect urinary retention (Griffin, 1983).

Antidepressant/alpha-adrenergic medications are sometimes used to treat urge incontinence. While the exact mechanism of action is uncertain, it is believed that these medications increase bladder capacity and sphincter tone. Effects of the medication on incontinence may not be seen for several weeks. A drug of this type used to treat urinary incontinence is imipramine hydrochloride (Tofranil). Adverse effects of this medication include drowsiness, tachycardia, excess sweating, orthostatic hypotension, constipation, mucous membrane dryness, and cardiac conduction disturbances. Nursing interventions for administering this medication include observing and recording side effects. It should be noted that because imipramine has caused complications in stroke patients, this population should be carefully monitored (Lipsey and others, 1984).

In summary, several strategies are available to manage alterations in urinary function resulting from difficulty storing urine. Nursing strategies include habit training, bladder retraining, prompted voiding, Kegel exercises, biofeedback, and contingency management. In addition, medications may be prescribed by the physician based on a complete nursing and medical evaluation. A relevant nursing diagnosis for patients with this type of alteration is:

Urge incontinence resulting from an overactive detrusor muscle. The stroke patient may experience urge incontinence at each voiding or only episodically. While the patient has a physiologic cause (detrusor overactivity) for the incontinence, additional factors such as preexisting urinary tract problems, and concomitant stroke-related deficits (i.e., altered bladder sensation, mobility, and speech) make it crucial for the nurse to accurately assess the patient's circumstances surrounding the incontinence and to customize interventions to patient needs. For example, for two patients who are on a habit training program, one with mild urge incontinence may ambulate to the bathroom with assistance, while the other may need a bedside commode because of more severe urge incontinence and altered mobility. Possible behavioral interventions to decrease the frequency of incontinent episodes include habit training, bladder retraining, prompted voiding, instruction in Kegel exercises (combined with biofeedback when possible), and/or contingency management. The nurse should discuss appropriate interventions with the patient and/or family, based on the severity of the problem and on the patient and environmental factors (i.e., patient preference, ability to participate in treatment, compatibility with patient's lifestyle, resources available, and expertise of the staff in implementing the program). Interventions should be selected to promote safety and optimize independence in self-care.

Treatments to facilitate bladder emptying. Another potential problem with urinary elimination that stroke patients may experience is difficulty emptying the bladder. As mentioned earlier, this may be caused by an underactive detrusor muscle and/or dyssynergy between the detrusor and the external urinary sphincter. Symptoms can include urinary retention, frequency, and frequency accompanied with dysuria. The goal of treatment is to facilitate voiding by decreasing outlet resistance at the bladder neck and external sphincter, and/or increasing bladder contractions. Treatments used to facilitate bladder emptying in stroke patients include medications and intermittent catheterization.

Medications used to facilitate bladder emptying fall into two general categories: those that increase contractility of the bladder and those that decrease outlet resistance of bladder at the level of the bladder neck or the external sphincter. Medications that increase the contractility of the bladder include parasympathomimetic agents. One drug, bethanecol (Urecholine) chloride, stimulates cholinergic receptors of the bladder wall, eliciting tension in the bladder smooth muscle to decrease bladder capacity and promote bladder emptying. Potential side effects of cholinergic medications include flushing, sweating, salivation, nausea, vomiting, diarrhea, abdominal cramps, headache, bradycardia, bronchospasm, hypotension, and difficulty with visual accommodation. Nursing interventions for administering this medication include monitoring vital signs, observing for difficulty breathing, monitoring intake and output, and giving the drug on an empty stomach to reduce the possibility for gastrointestinal distress.

Medications that reduce bladder outlet resistance can work at the level of the bladder neck or the external urinary sphincter. Medications that affect the bladder neck include alpha-adrenergic agonists. These medications promote bladder emptying by blocking alpha-adrenergic receptors in the smooth muscle of the bladder neck and proximal urethra, which decreases the resistance to urine leaving the bladder. The goal is to increase the flow of urine and decrease the amount of residual urine in the bladder. Drugs used to decrease outlet resistance at the bladder neck include: phenoxybenzamine (Dibenzyline), prazosin hydrochloride (Minipress), methyldopa (Aldomet), and clonidine (Catapres) (Barett and Wein, 1987). Potential adverse effects include orthostatic hypotension, nasal congestion, inhibited ejaculation, tachycardia, miosis, nausea, vomiting, diarrhea, and sedation. Nursing interventions when administering these medications including giving the medication with milk in divided doses to reduce gastric irritation (Mulrow, 1985) and evaluating the patient for postural hypotension. The patient who experiences postural hypotension should be directed to dangle his legs at the bedside before standing and should be accompanied by the nurse when ambulating.

Medications that decrease outlet resistance at the level of the external sphincter include skeletal muscle relaxants and alpha-adrenergic antagonists. These drugs promote relaxation of the external sphincter and the pelvic floor muscles; thus, by reducing spasticity of the external sphincter and the dyssynergy between bladder and sphincter, this facilitates voiding. Three drugs that may be used to treat spasticity in stroke patients are baclofen (Lioresal), dantrolene sodium (Dantrium) and diazepam (Valium) (Kaplan and Cerullo, 1986). Baclofen is thought to decrease the reflex activity in the spinal cord, resulting in relaxation of the external sphincter. Potential side effects of baclofen include drowsiness, insomnia, rash, pruritus, dizziness, weakness, and urinary incontinence.

Dantrolene sodium also relaxes the external urinary sphincter, decreasing tone and resistance to the bladder outlet. While this drug has no autonomic side effects, it may induce such severe generalized weakness that it compromises its therapeutic benefits (Barrett and Wein, 1987). Other side effects of dantrolene sodium include euphoria, dizziness, diarrhea, and liver toxicity. This drug may have limited effectiveness in elderly stroke patients.

In general, diazepam has not been found to be effective in decreasing dyssynergy secondary to neurologic disease (Barrett and Wein, 1987). However, this centrally acting muscle relaxant may be used when the etiology of the urinary retention is obscure and other treatments have been ineffective. Because it produces generalized sedation, diazepam is believed to work in some situations by promoting relaxation of the pelvic floor muscles, thus facilitating voiding. Nursing interventions for all skeletal muscle relaxants include observing and recording side effects, spacing the medication as much as possible to promote alertness during the day, and making sure the patient is not performing high risk activities when drowsy. One final intervention, intermittent catheterization, may be used alone or in combination with medication.

Intermittent catheterization (IC) may be indicated after stroke if the patient is unable to void or has high residual urine volume because of detrusor-sphincter dyssynergia. Usually IC is not used until medication is either ineffective or not tolerated by the patient. If IC is the treatment of choice, the nurse will need to assess the patient to determine the level of participation that the patient is capable of. Crucial factors that determine whether the patient will do self-catheterization or whether this will be done by a caregiver include the patient's mental status, existing motor and sensory deficits, available resources, and the patient's preferences and feelings about this part of her care. Difficulties with fine motor coordination, vision, problem-solving, and a reluctant attitude may interfere with the patient's ability to do self-catheterization. If the patient is willing to do self-catheterization despite motor and sensory deficits, the nurse and occupational therapist should collaborate to identify the optimal positioning, necessary equipment, and modifications that are needed. The nurse must assess all factors for each patient and evaluate alternative resources.

The process of IC consists of inserting a straight catheter into the urethra approximately every 4 to 6 hours to drain urine from the bladder. The frequency of IC is individual for each patient and is determined by the patient's residual volume of urine. The underlying rationale for IC is that (1) an overdistended bladder decreases blood flow to the tissue and weakens that tissue to bacterial infection; and (2) emptying the bladder often by frequent catheterization prevents or cures infection (Lapides, 1974). In acute and postacute care and usually in rehabilitation, IC is done by the nurse using sterile technique. However, to prepare patients for discharge, those who require IC should be taught to use clean technique at home. Patients doing self-catheterization assume a comfortable position, which can be in bed, sitting in a wheelchair, sitting on the commode, or standing in front of the commode. Females need apply no lubricant to the catheter before inserting it; on the other hand, because of a longer urethra, males need to apply water soluble lubricant to the catheter before insertion to prevent traumatic urethritis (Lapides, 1974). After self-catheterization, patients are taught to rinse the soiled catheter in warm soapy water and store it in a plastic bag. While handwashing with soap and water is encouraged before starting the procedure, patients should *never* forego catheterization if this is not possible (Lapides, 1974). The emphasis is on frequency rather than sterility. While intermittent catheterization is strongly preferred to an indwelling catheter, the patient either may not have the ability for self-catheterization and not have a caregiver to assist him.

In some situations, indwelling catheters may be inserted to continuously drain urine from the bladder. From the standpoint of patient health, indwelling catheters should only be used as a last resort because of the high incidence of catheter-related infections. Within 24 hours after placement of an indwelling catheter, 50% of patients have urinary infections; and within 4 days, 98% to 100% of patients with open indwelling catheters have urinary infections (Andriole, 1975). Additionally, longterm use of indwelling catheters in patients with spinal cord injuries suggests there is a higher incidence of complications such as pyelonephritis, calculi formation, cystitis, penoscrotal fistula (males), and bladder carcinoma (Jacobs and Kaufman, 1978). Nursing care of a patient with an indwelling catheter includes anchoring the catheter to the patient to prevent trauma to the urethra; encouraging fluid intake of at least 3000 ml per day to minimize urinary stasis, calculi formation, and infection; cleaning the perineum twice daily (females); and *always* keeping the urine collection bag below the level of the bladder. The catheter should *never* be clamped because this causes stasis and backflow of urine into the bladder (Freed, 1982).

A nursing diagnosis relevant to the patient with

this type of alteration in urinary elimination is:

Urinary retention because of dyssynergy between the detrusor and external urinary sphincter. Possible nursing interventions to facilitate bladder emptying include monitoring the patient's response to medications and intermittently catheterizing the patient to empty the bladder. If the stroke patient's urinary retention is managed solely by medication, the nurse should take care to space the medication out evenly throughout the day and monitor the patient's response to the medication. Keeping a voiding diary helps to monitor intake and output, record voiding volumes, identify frequency of voiding, and alert the nurse to incontinent episodes. The nurse should monitor the patient for side effects of the drug or signs that the dosage is inappropriate. Incontinent episodes indicate that the medication or dosage may need to be changed. Educating the patient and family about drug therapy will facilitate their understanding and enable them to consistently follow the medication routine at home. Medication cards may be appropriate for the stroke patient with cognitive or sensory deficits to provide the critical information needed to take the drug at home. The nurse can design index cards showing the pill with a brief description of the purpose, dosage, and times for taking the medication. Special needs the patient has because of visual, speech, or cognitive deficits may influence the size of the print, the color of ink, the depth at which the information is presented, and whether all the medications are put on one large card or each one on individual cards.

Nursing interventions for the patient who requires intermittent catheterization begin with diagnosing that the patient has urinary retention. Frequently nurses are the first to detect urinary retention when they note that the stroke patient is not voiding regular and sufficient amounts, or the patients complains of burning or straining to urinate. It is appropriate to catheterize the patient after voiding to determine the amount of postvoid residual (PVR) in the bladder and report this to the physician. When starting IC the nurse must educate the patient and/or caregiver about why and how this should be done and, as the time for discharge approaches, where to get supplies in the community. Adequate time should be provided for the patient and/or family to learn the procedure and to give return demonstrations to the nurse. If the stroke patient's dominant hand is weak, adaptive devices for positioning and/or manipulating the equipment may be necessary to allow independence with this part of care. Lights or mirrors can help the patient with visual or other sensory deficits manipulate the equipment and carry out the procedure appropriately.

Treatments for functional incontinence. While a stroke may provide a physiologic cause for altered urinary tract function, not all urinary tract problems are due to brain damage. Stroke patients may experience functional incontinence, which has been defined as involuntary loss of urine in spite of formal urinary tract function. As discussed earlier, possible causes of functional incontinence in stroke patients include altered mobility, altered communication, altered cognition, sensation and/or perception, and psychologic and/or environmental causes. Strategies to manage each of these will be discussed briefly.

When impaired mobility is the cause of urinary incontinence, it is important for the nurse to create a safe and healthy environment for the patient to carry out toileting activities. The nurse must assess the patient's mobility in bed, transferring activities, ambulation, and fine motor skills. The goal of nursing intervention is to assist the patient to safely compensate for motor deficits that interfere with toileting, while enabling the patient to be as independent as possible. Nursing interventions include collaborating with the physical and occupational therapists to identify the patient's motor skills and needs for adaptive equipment as they relate to urinary elimination on the unit and at home; encouraging the patient to use remaining motor skills and compensatory behaviors learned in therapy to transfer onto the bedpan, commode, or bedside commode; evaluating the patient's ability for toileting hygiene and assist him as needed; evaluating the patient's ability to manipulate clothing (snaps, zippers, waistbands) and encouraging family or friends to bring clothes the patient can easily use; and discussing a schedule for toileting and assisting the patient as needed. Identifying appropriate interventions depends on the nurse obtaining an accurate nursing history of incontinent episodes and precipitating factors and having the patient actively involved in planning strategies with the nurse whenever possible.

Other causes of functional incontinence in stroke patients might be alterations in communication, cognition, sensation, or perception. The patient may have expressive or receptive aphasia, making communication with the nurse difficult or impossible. Strategies for the nurse include identifying the aphasia type (collaborating with the speech therapist if possible), allowing plenty of time for the patient to speak (i.e. if expressive aphasia), and determining alternative ways for the patient to express her needs. Cognitive, sensory, and perceptual deficits may compound other stroke-related deficits, making it difficult for the patient to perceive bladder fullness, to interpret the sensation of fullness, and to initiate appropriate voiding behaviors, resulting in functional incontinence. Sensory deprivation has also been noted to result in incontinence (Brocklehurst, 1973). Because of the variation from one patient to another, it is crucial for the nurse to carefully assess each patient to determine the nature of problems and identify appropriate interventions.

Functional incontinence after stroke may be due to psychological difficulties such as anxiety, depression, and dependence. While no studies have investigated this in stroke patients, some psychologic mechanisms of incontinence in the elderly population are thought to be due to regression, dependency, rebellion, insecurity, and attention-seeking (Willington, 1976; McCormick and others 1988). Examples of nursing interventions directed at alleviating psychologic causes include assessing reasons for the behavior; reinforcing positive behaviors; encouraging the patient to express feelings; be a good listener; educating the patient in constructive problem-solving; modeling honesty and openness in your communication with the patient; and facilitating realistic goal-setting. Accurate assessment of the patient will facilitate identifying effective nursing interventions.

Environmental obstacles in the hospital may make it difficult for the patient to safely maneuver from the bed to the bathroom. Some of these obstacles include excess furniture or equipment in the patient's room, inconveniently located equipment (e.g., bedside commode, walker, cane), insufficient light, lengthy distances to the bathroom (e.g., bathroom is in the hallway), and ill-placed or broken call lights (Anichini, 1985; McCormick and others 1988). Nursing interventions should be directed at removing all obstacles and organizing the patient's environment to promote safe access to the bathroom.

A nursing diagnosis relevant to the patient with this type of alteration in urinary elimination is:

Functional incontinence resulting from difficulty ambulating to the bathroom. Because stroke patients with functional incontinence have normal lower urinary tract functioning, interventions for functional incontinence are directed at alleviating patient and/or environmental causes for the incontinence. When a stroke patient has difficulty walking to the bathroom, the nurse must assess the extent of the patient's impaired mobility with the physical therapist to determine if ambulation is a realistic goal. If ambulation is possible, the nurse should walk with the patient to the bathroom with the appropriate ambulation devices (e.g., cane or walker). Until the patient is safe walking at night, it may be appropriate to put a bedside commode near the bed to minimize ambulating and the danger of falling when the patient is sleepy. If ambulation is not realistic at that time, the nurse should accompany the patient who is in a wheelchair to the bathroom and help with transfer onto the commode. Whenever possible, the patient should be sitting on a commode to void; using the bedpan in a supine or semi-Fowler's position does not facilitate complete bladder emptying. The stroke patient with a weak upper extremity will need help to manage clothing and personal hygiene. In addition, environmental barriers in the room and bathroom should be kept at a minimum. These barriers impede independence in self-care and sometimes can even be dangerous for the stroke patient with neglect and other sensory and perceptual deficits. Adequate lighting and mirrors can help the patient compensate for deficits. Educating the patient and family about safety and obstacles in the home that impede continence will help the patient to achieve independence and will help the family to understand the needs of the patient.

To summarize, while patients may experience alterations in urinary function after stroke, these changes are often temporary. The most common bladder-related problems are urge and functional incontinence. Less commonly, patients may experience difficulty voiding and/or urinary retention because of detrusor-sphincter dyssynergia. Research supports the effectiveness of different strategies and suggests that patients with altered urinary function have many options by which to manage or eliminate urinary dysfunction. Collaborating with the physician regarding potential medications or with the physical or occupational therapist for adaptive equipment may enhance the effectiveness of all nursing interventions. Educating the patient and family or caregiver about the underlying mechanism of incontinence and the rationale for the selected interventions is fundamental to successful treatment and consistent home management. A more complete list of nursing diagnoses related to altered urinary function, along with interventions and expected outcomes after stroke, are listed in the care plan on p. 159.

BOWEL ELIMINATION

Central Nervous System Influence on the Lower Gastrointestinal tract

While control of bladder elimination by higher centers has been the focus of considerable research, the role of central nervous system control of bowel elimination has not been described in depth. It is believed that the brain influences bowel function primarily by cortical inhibition. Interaction between the neural plexuses that innervate the gastrointestinal tract is controlled by the central nervous system, which influences the motor and secretory activities of the gastrointestinal tract. A recent study suggests that urinary and fecal incontinence can occur as a result of bilateral lesions of the putamen (Klutzow and others, 1989). However, precise details of central nervous system influence and control on bowel function are not clearly understood.

Spinal cord. The defecation reflex center is located in the sacral cord at level S3-5. This reflex is activated when the bowel becomes distended, stimulating stretch receptors. Afferent impulses travel up to the spinal cord at the sacral level, triggering a parasympathetic response and creating the urge to defecate (Fig. 9-5).

Lower Gastrointestinal tract structure and function

The basic gastrointestinal tract consists of the mouth, esophagus, stomach, small intestine, and large intestine. Gastrointestinal tract functions are aided by other structures in the body, including the salivary glands, gallbladder, and portions of the liver and pancreas. The function of the gastrointestinal tract is to change ingested food and nutrients into a form in which the body can use. The process includes digesting and transporting materials through the gastrointestinal tract, absorbing necessary nutrients and water, and eliminating waste products. To promote adequate lower gastrointestinal tract function, the upper gastrointestinal tract must also be functioning well. For example, chewing and swallowing must be intact. Difficulties with chewing and swallowing may occur after stroke because of loss of muscle control in the face, neck, larynx, pharynx, and damage to cranial nerves V, IX, X, and XII (see Chapter 8).

When food in the stomach is mixed with gastric secretions it is called *chyme*. The chyme passes from the stomach through the pyloric sphincter into the small intestine where most digestion and absorption occurs. The small intestine is made up of three segments: the duodenum, the jejunum, and

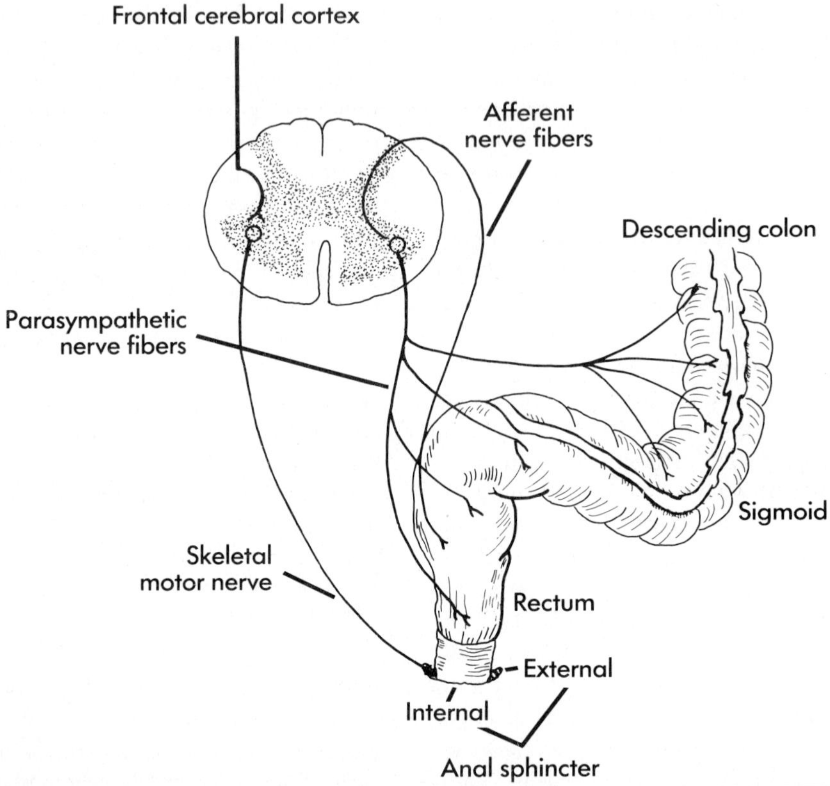

Fig. 9-5 Schematic representation of the defecation reflex.

the ileum. The movement of chyme is facilitated by rhythmic segmental movements of the small intestine that are greater in the proximal than in the distal segments. More frequent contractions in the proximal portion of the small intestine help to move the chyme downward.

The movement of chyme from the small intestine into the large intestine is facilitated by a series of reflexes. In the small intestine these include the *gastroileal reflex,* the *iliogastric reflex,* the *intestino-intestinal reflex,* and the *peristaltic reflex.* The gastroileal reflex increases contractions in the ileum, stimulated by gastric emptying, that move the chyme through the ileocecal sphincter into the large intestine. Unlike the gastroileal reflex, the ileogastric reflex, stimulated by gastric distension, results in the decrease in contractions and gastric motility in the ileum. The intestino-intestinal reflex occurs when overdistension in one segment relaxes the smooth muscle in the rest of the intestine, resulting in complete cessation of motor activity (Vander and others, 1980). Finally, the peristaltic reflex is a set of coordinated contractions of the small intestine that are triggered by distension of the intestinal wall. Reflexes, mediated by the nervous system, are influenced by endocrine factors and help the chyme move from the small intestine into the large intestine.

The large intestine is composed of four parts: the ascending colon, the transverse colon, the descending colon, and the sigmoid colon. The function of the large intestine is to absorb water and electrolytes and to compact the chyme into feces. Compared with the small intestine, motility in the large intestine is decreased, thus enabling more water absorption by the epithelium. Approximately 1 to 3 times per day, a wave of contraction (mass movement) occurs in the colon. Reflexes that facilitate the movement of colonic chyme into the anal canal include the gastrocolic reflex and the defecation reflex. The gastrocolic reflex occurs when the stomach and duodenum become distended, typically after a meal, resulting in an increase in mass movements in the colon. The defecation reflex occurs when the rectum becomes distended and transmits impluses via parasympathetic fibers to the spinal cord. Impulses are sent back to the colon to initiate strong peristalsis, relaxation of the internal sphincter, and constriction of the external anal sphincter, resulting in the urge to defecate (Guyton, 1982). The defecation process is complex and involves reflex and voluntary actions. Reflex actions are processed in the sacral spinal cord but mediated by higher centers. Voluntary actions include relaxing the pelvic floor muscles and external anal sphincter and increasing intrathoracic and intraabdominal pressure by taking a deep breath and closing the glottis (Berne and Levy, 1988).

Muscles in the small and large intestines are innervated by the autonomic nervous system in a complex network of fibers called the *enteric nervous system* (Patton and others, 1989). Made up of Meissner's plexus, Auerbach's plexus, and other neurons of the gastrointestinal tract, this network helps to integrate the motor and secretory activities of the gastrointestinal system. The enteric nervous system is innervated by sympathetic and parasympathetic fibers. The celiac, superior and inferior mesenteric, and hypogastric plexuses provide sympathetic innervation to various segments of the gastrointestinal tract, inhibiting the transmission of nerve impulses and motor activity, except for stimulating some sphincters to contract (Berne and Levy, 1988). Parasympathetic innervation above the level of the transverse colon is supplied by branches of the vagus nerve. The rest of the colon receives parasympathetic fibers from the pelvic nerves via the hypogastric plexus. Parasympathetic input typically activates motor (except sphincters) and secretory activities in the intestinal tract.

In summary, lower gastrointestinal tract function is controlled both by the central nervous system, and the enteric nervous system resulting in both reflex and voluntary control. Any disruption in these processes either locally or centrally could result in altered bowel function.

Effects of Stroke on Bowel Elimination

Stroke patients may experience alterations in bowel function as a result of brain damage accompanied by loss of cortical inhibition; as a consequence of other stroke-related deficits (i.e., sensorimotor losses, aphasia, mood changes, altered cognition); or as a complication of untreated ineffective bowel elimination. Possible alterations in bowel elimination include incontinence, constipation, and diarrhea.

Although it is rare, incontinence can occur with unilateral or bilateral damage to the paracentral branch of the anterior cerebral artery (Fig. 9-6) (Berman and others, 1980; Chusid, 1976). Damage to the superomedial part of the middle frontal lobe, the anterior end of the cingulate gyrus, the white matter between these areas, and the genu of the corpus callosum is probably responsible for causing transient or permanent alterations in urination and defecation (Andrew and Nathan, 1964). Fecal incontinence may also occur in stroke patients who have lost cortical inhibition, resulting in uninhibited contractions of the bowel (Patrick and others, 1986).

The most common bowel problems after stroke are constipation and impaction (Hirschberg and others, 1976; O'Brien and Pallett, 1978; Lal, 1986). Risk factors for constipation include inactivity, low-roughage diet, limited fluid intake, postponing defecation, and patient and family knowledge deficit about how and why a bowel program is necessary. Constipation can be prevented if the nurse assesses bowel function early and starts the patient on an appropriate bowel program. If constipation does develop, it must be diagnosed and

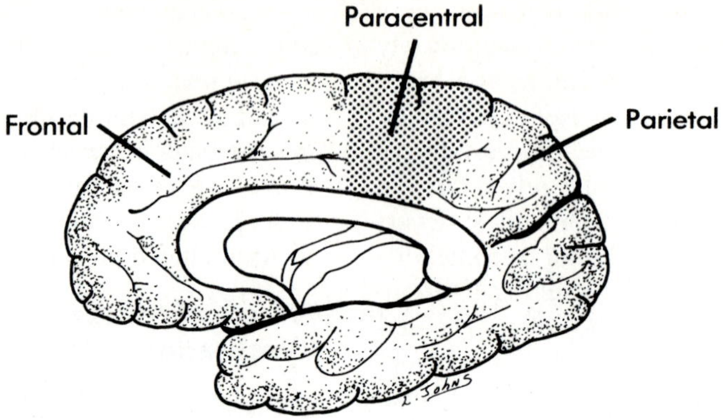

Fig. 9-6 Medial view of the right cerebral hemisphere. Area of the brain supplied by the paracentral branch of the anterior cerebral artery.

treated early, or the patient may develop a fecal impaction.

If a patient develops a proximal impaction, she may be incontinent of small, frequent stools or diarrhea. Thus when a patient is incontinent, it is important to assess overall bowel function to determine whether the problem is due to loss of cortical inhibition or is an actual symptom of a fecal impaction. In spite of the potential seriousness of undetected bowel dysfunctions, alterations in bowel function usually improve with time. However, during the acute care, postacute care, and rehabilitation periods after stroke, it is essential that the nurse continually assess and monitor the patient for actual and potential changes in bowel function.

Assessing bowel function

To prevent complications (constipation and impaction) and a significant delay in the patient's rehabilitation after stroke, nursing assessment of bowel function must begin in the acute care period. Adequate bowel function is necessary to maintain and promote health. One study noted that the normal range of bowel movements in healthy, active people was between three bowel movements per day and three per week (Connell and others, 1965). Unfortunately, because of the often life-threatening situations that may occur duing the acute care period, maintaining adequate bowel function is often a lower priority. While constipation and fecal impaction are not usually life threatening, these complications are costly in terms of patient comfort and health, often adding preventable expenses (x-rays, laxatives, enemas), and postponing the patient's active participation in a rehabilitation program.

When caring for the stroke patient, the nurse collects subjective and objective data by obtaining a nursing history and performing select aspects of a physical examination. Components of each are listed in the box on p. 153. It is important to note that not all aspects of assessment will be relevant at all times. For instance, during acute care, the focus should be on assessing when the patient's last bowel movement was and what risk factors are present for constipation and making sure that the patient has a regular bowel movement. In addition to that part of the assessment, the rehabilitation nurse may focus on evaluating effectiveness of the program, evaluating the patient's ability for independence, and identifying necessary community resources and supplies. Therefore, at each phase of the patient's recovery, nursing assessment of bowel function provides unique and valuable information.

The nurse should assess bowel function in an ongoing manner to identify patterns and problem

NURSING EVALUATION OF BOWEL FUNCTION

NURSING HISTORY

Previous bowel habits (include stool consistency, frequency, episodes of incontinence, personal habits to facilitate defecation)
Problems with bowel elimination since stroke (onset, duration, symptoms)
Amount and pattern of fluid intake (voiding diary)
Amount and pattern of output (voiding diary)
Dietary intake (include frequency and content of meals and snacks)
Past medical history (including diverticulitis, ulcerative colitis, hemorrhoids, and any sphincter disturbances)
Current medications (including laxatives and suppositories)
Patient's affective response that may influence elimination (modesty, depression, anger or frustration)
Place for elimination (bedpan, commode or bedside commode)
Physical assistance required for elimination (for walking, standing and sitting balance, hygiene, handling clothing)
Assistive devices needed (cane, walker, reachers, elevated commode seat or grab bars)
Other stroke-related deficits that may influence bowel function (aphasia or altered mobility, cognition, or mood)
Patient, family, or significant other coping with loss of function
Psychosocial concerns of patient, family, significant other
Community resources and future life-style (impact on one's ability to continue hospital-initiated routine)

PHYSICAL EXAMINATION

Neurologic examination (vision, mental status, emotional state, motor abilities including manual dexterity, gait, sitting and standing balance, transferring, ambulation)
Abdominal examination (auscultate for bowel sounds, note scars, distension, palpate for tenderness)
Rectal examination (skin condition, signs of infection, discharge, anal reflex, saddle sensation, bulbocavernous reflcx, rectal check for impaction)

areas and to determine the effectiveness of the current bowel program. One way of doing this is to use a bowel movement record (Fig. 9-7). This record allows systematic recording of daily information throughout the stroke patient's hospitalization, provides the nurse with valuable information, and is useful as a teaching tool to educate the patient about his bowel patterns.

When assessing stroke patient's bowel function, it is important to understand the cause of the altered bowel function to determine the most appropriate interventions. It may be possible that normal bowel function can be restored simply by adding a high fiber diet and more fluids; however, sometimes more invasive procedures are required, such as removing a fecal impaction and administering enemas or routine suppositories. Only a thorough and ongoing assessment of bowel function will provide the nurse with necessary information to determine appropriate interventions.

Interventions

Alterations in bowel function that stroke patients experience include constipation, fecal impactions, functional incontinence, or, less commonly, diarrhea or incontinence resulting from loss of cortical inhibition. For a discussion on management of functional incontinence, refer to the earlier section in this chapter.

Constipation commonly occurs after a stroke be-

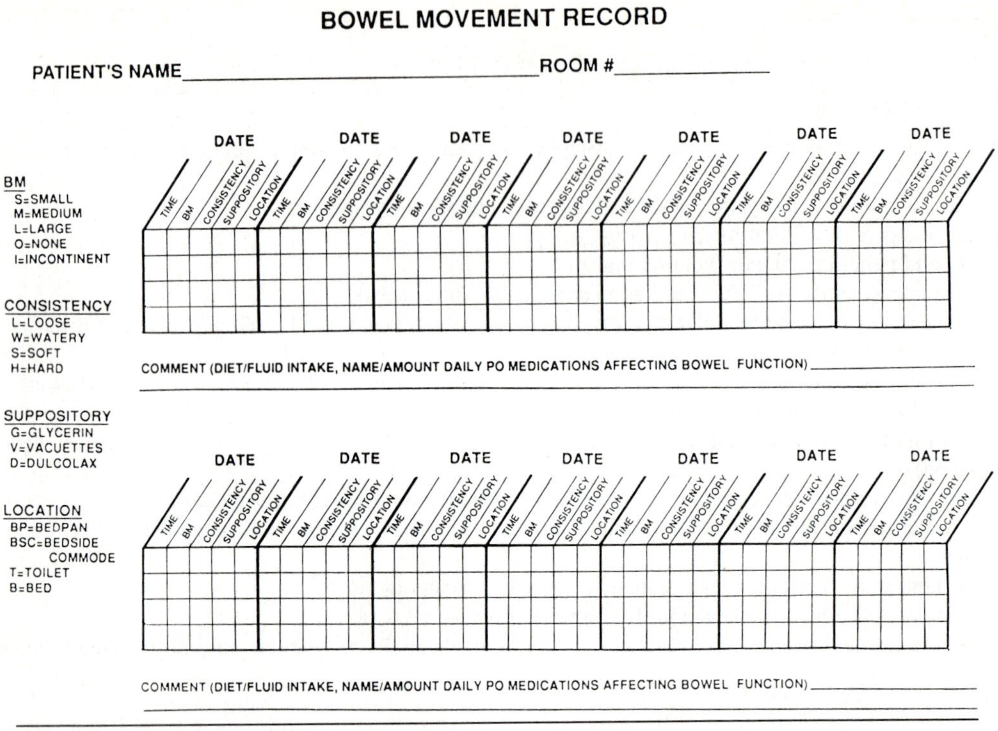

Fig. 9-7 Record allows daily documentation of bowel patterns.

cause of a combination of factors, including changes in diet and fluid intake, immobility, altered cognition, difficulty communicating, as a side effect of medications. The primary way to prevent and treat constipation is to start the patient on a bowel program. A bowel program has two main objectives: to establish bowel evacuations at regular, timed intervals and to prevent constipation and fecal impactions (Rusk, 1977). Bowel programs differ, depending on the etiology of bowel dysfunction. Stroke patients typically have an uninhibited bowel with normal peripheral innervation, normal saddle sensation, and a normal or increased bulbocavernous reflex (Rusk, 1977; Cannon, 1981). Therefore a bowel program for the stroke patient would include all of the following: exercise, increased fluids and fiber, a stool softener and/or suppository as needed, and a consistent habit time. Additional components of a bowel program identified by Dittmar (1989) include starting with a "clean bowel," exercise, privacy, and positioning. The following general principles facilitate a successful bowel program and promote healthy bowel elimination:

1. Fluid intake should be at least 2 liters per day.
2. If possible, the patient should always be sitting in the upright position to have a bowel movement; this allows gravity to facilitate peristalsis.
3. The patient should have at least the equivalent of two heaping teaspoons of bran or dietary fiber per day (Sodeman, 1989).
4. When scheduling the timing of the bowel program (time of day and frequency), consider patient's previous habits and be consistent.
5. Take advantage of the gastrocolic reflex; help the patient to the bathroom after meals (especially breakfast).
6. Exercise increases muscle tone and strength,

and facilitates gastric motility. Encourage patients' participation in activities as the patient's endurance permits.

The patient's bowel program may include some type of oral or rectal medication. Oral medications may be bulking agents, emollients, stimulants, saline cathartics, or osmotic agents. Rectal medication may be in the form of suppositories or enemas. Bulking agents work by producing bulk in the digestive tract that stimulates intestinal motility. When taking bulking agents, the patient must drink an adequate amount of water, otherwise the bulk may cause an intestinal obstruction. In general, bulking agents are least harsh and the most useful to manage constipation in the older stroke patient.

Emollients provide lubrication and have a detergentlike effect, allowing water to enter the feces and soften the stool and preventing straining during defecation. Emollients can be used if the patient has difficulty taking a bulking agent.

Stimulants cause irritation to the mucosa and can produce formed or diarrhea stool, depending on the type of stimulant taken. Stimulants may be used occasionally for acute constipation, but, in general, they should not be used for a routine bowel program. Saline cathartics and osmotic agents work by drawing water into the intestine to purge and cleanse the bowel, producing watery diarrhea stool. These agents should be used only after less harsh laxatives have been tried. Because of their potent action on the intestinal tract and the resulting diarrhea, these drugs can cause fecal incontinence in the stroke patient if the patient has sensorimotor losses and/or needs assistance to the bathroom. In general, stimulants, saline cathartics, and osmotic agents can cause loss of bowel control because of increasing intestinal motility and should not be used as part of a regular bowel program.

Finally, a rectal suppository may be used as part of a routine bowel program. Glycerin, bisacodyl, and CO_2 suppositories are commonly used to stimulate defecation. When inserting the suppository, it is important to insert it into the colon, past the internal sphincter, making sure the suppository is in contact with the intestinal wall. If the suppository is inserted into the stool, it will not be effective. Suppositories, bulking agents, and stool softeners are helpful components of a bowel program.

Two general rules for treating altered bowel elimination are (1) to start with the least harsh medication and (2) to give the bowel program an adequate trial before introducing changes. If many changes are introduced at once, it is difficult to evaluate which interventions are effective and which are not. Once a reliable pattern of bowel elimination has developed, it may be possible to decrease the dosage of the bulking agent or emollient, or to decrease the frequency of using suppositories. As the stroke patient becomes more active and increases dietary intake and fluids, it is likely the intestinal motility will increase and bowel elimination will return to normal. For this reason, the nurse should discuss this with the patient and evaluate the bowel program regularly.

In combination with stroke-related constipation, patients may experience altered bowel function from prescription or over-the-counter drugs. Common prescription medications that cause constipation in the elderly include opiates, anticholinergics, and antacids (Sodeman, 1989). Opiates used to treat chronic and acute pain and diarrhea can alter bowel habits. Drugs with anticholinergic effects are widely used in the elderly population and have an effect on the central nervous system, and also direct effects on the smooth muscle of the intestinal tract. This direct effect on the intestine can cause constipation or diarrhea. Anticholinergics used to treat Parkinson's disease, urinary incontinence, and depression are listed in the box on p. 156. Finally, antacids containing aluminum and calcium are common causes of constipation. Patients needing the antacid can relieve constipation by using an antacid that contains magnesium and has a cathartic action (Sodeman, 1989).

Fecal impactions are serious because they disrupt regular bowel function and can even obstruct the bladder neck to cause urinary retention (Freed, 1982; Newman, 1989; Wyman, 1988). Resulting from prolonged constipation, a fecal impaction occurs when a large mass of hard stool becomes

DRUGS WITH ANTICHOLINERGIC EFFECTS

MANAGEMENT OF PARKINSON'S DISEASE

Trihexyphenidyl (Artane)
Benztropine (Cogentin)

MANAGEMENT OF INCONTINENCE

Propantheline (Pro-Banthine)
Oxybutynin (Ditropan)
Dicyclomine (Bentyl)
Flavoxate (Urispas)
Imipramine (Tofranil, SK-Pramine, Janimine)

MANAGEMENT OF DEPRESSION

Tricyclic
- Amitriptyline (Elavil, Endep, Etrafon, Limbitrol, Triavil)
- Doxepin (Sinequan, Adapin)
- Imipramine (Tofranil, SK-Pramine, Janimine)
- Desipramine (Norpramin, Pertofrane)
- Protriptyline (Vivactil)
- Nortriptyline (Pamelor)
- Amoxapine (Asendin)

Tetracycline
- Maprotiline (Ludiomil)

Other
- Trazodone (Desyrel)

From Sodeman S et al., *Geriatric gastroenterology,* Philadelphia, 1989, WB Saunders Co.

lodged, usually in the rectum, and the patient is unable to pass the stool mechanically. The bowel becomes very distended, and sometimes loose stool flows around the impacted feces. While diarrhea can have different etiologies, the nurse should always evaluate the patient with diarrhea for an impaction. Elderly stroke patients are particularly susceptible to developing impactions that are usually caused by a decrease in dietary intake, dietary fiber, and physcial activity; depression; impaired sensation in the rectal vault because of laxative abuse or confusion; and inaccessible toilet facilities, resulting in inattention to the defecation reflex (Sodeman, 1989).

Treatments for an impaction start with doing a rectal digital examination and breaking of the impaction with the gloved finger if possible. Other treatments that might be necessary include mineral oil, magnesium citrate, bisacodyl tablets, a phosphate buffered laxative, and using oil retention enemas to soften the stool so it can be passed. If the patient tires easily, it may be necessary to repeat the digital examination and enemas for 2 or 3 days to avoid exhausting the patient (Hirschberg, and others 1976). Once the impaction is removed, the goal is to prevent future impactions. This is best accomplished by monitoring the patient's bowel movements with a bowel movement record, providing adequate fluid and dietary fiber, providing timely access to the toilet as needed, and assisting the patient to exercise. Patients may also benefit from a stool softener twice daily.

Though less common, diarrhea or fecal incontinence can occur after stroke. Although diarrhea may be caused by antibiotic therapy or by supplemental feedings, it should be evaluated because it can be serious if prolonged. As mentioned earlier, diarrhea can be a cause of fecal incontinence because the patient may be experiencing expulsive and frequent stools. The stroke patient may also experience fecal incontinence with formed stool. Treatments for fecal incontinence include establishing a regular bowel program, and in some cases, biofeedback. The components and advantages of a regular bowel program have already been discussed. Biofeedback was found to be effective as a treatment for fecal incontinence in postobstetric and postsurgical patients (MacLeod, 1987), and in the elderly (Whitehead and others, 1985).

The use of biofeedback in the elderly is most relevant to this discussion. Patients with fecal incontinence were placed in three treatment groups: a bowel program group, a sphincter exercises and no biofeedback group, and a sphincter exercises combined with biofeedback group. Patients using exercise and biofeedback demonstrated a 75% decrease in incontinence for 77% of the patients in that group. At 6 months, improvements were maintained for 60% of the patients; at one year, for 42% of the patients. While depression was not consistently related to outcome, altered mental status was. Two patients had severe dementia and were unable to follow the directions necessary for the biofeedback intervention (Whitehead and others, 1985). While biofeedback for fecal incontinence has not been evaluated for use in stroke patients specifically, this study using biofeedback in fecally incontinent geriatric patients is promising. Biofeedback may be a useful treatment for fecal incontinence after stroke.

In summary, bowel problems after stroke are common. Common bowel problems are constipation and fecal impactions; less common is incontinence. These alterations may be due to a loss of cortical inhibition; they may be a secondary effect of other stroke-related deficits (sensori-motor losses, aphasia, mood changes, or altered cognition); or due to complications resulting from ongoing ineffective bowel elimination. The best treatment is to make an ongoing assessment, establish a regular bowel routine, and prevent complications. Nurses play a major role in managing altered bowel function in stroke patients. A nursing diagnosis relevant to the stroke patient with altered bowel elimination is:

Alteration in bowel elimination: constipation. Since constipation is a common alteration in bowel function among stroke patients, all patients should be on a bowel program. The bowel movement record and the nursing assessment form the nursing data base to record the patient's history and bowel patterns; this data base provides the foundation and rationale for the patient's bowel program. Bowel programs can be as simple as increasing fluids and dietary fiber, or they may be more complex and consist of routine rectal suppositories with or without oral medications. General considerations in carrying out a bowel program with the stroke patient are for the patient to sit upright on the commode whenever possible to promote adequate emptying; for the bowel program to take place at a convenient and regular time, not conflicting with other activies (e.g., therapy, visitors); and to ensure that the patient has adequate time for evacuation. Because of other stroke-related deficits, the patient may take a little longer to use the bathroom; if an inadequate amount of time is allowed, the patient may feel frustrated and anxious. If the patient is hurried, she may be unsafe in walking or transferring in and out of the wheelchair. The nurse should observe the patient's affect and problem-solving skills when encountering environmental barriers and when compensating for deficits. Alterations in mentation may cause the patient to be impulsive, to exercise poor judgment, and to have difficulty sequencing steps to solve problems. Nursing interventions should focus on helping the patient achieve regular and adequate bowel elimination and on promoting a safe level of independence in self-care.

Another nursing diagnosis relevant to the stroke patient with altered bowel elimination is:

Uninhibited bowel elimination due to loss of cortical inhibition. Nursing interventions to promote bowel continence include putting the patient on a bowel program to achieve a consistent and predictable time for evacuation. If the stool is too soft or loose, what little bowel control the patient does have may not be utilized. Some factors that may cause loose stool include tube feedings, too much dietary fiber, overmedication with stool softeners or harsh laxatives, or a preexisting fecal impaction. Once the consistency of stool is regulated, a regular time of evacuation will facilitate bowel control and minimize episodes of incontinence. The nurse should assist the patient as he feels the urge to defecate, and the patient should use the commode whenever possible to promote more complete emptying. The nurse must educate the patient and family about the importance of a regular bowel movement and signs of complications; this will help them to follow through with the program at home and to minimize accidents.

Additional nursing diagnoses for altered bowel function are listed in the care plan on p. 159. Through nursing assessment and interventions, it is likely that stroke patients will be able to reestablish regular, healthy bowel habits.

NURSING CARE PLAN

Nursing Diagnosis	Interventions	Expected Outcomes
Urinary Elimination, Altered Patterns related to an overactive detrusor muscle **Defining Characteristics** ■ Urinary urgency ■ Frequency (voiding more often than every 2 hrs) ■ Bladder contractions/spasm ■ Nocturia (more than twice per night) ■ Voiding in small amounts (less than 100 ml) ■ Inability to reach the toilet in time	**Ongoing Assessment** ■ Assess preexisting urinary tract problems ■ Assess history of current problem (including onset, symptoms, frequency and timing of incontinent episodes, reasons for incontinence, nocturia) ■ Assess typical urinary elimination patterns and habits ■ Determine current medications ■ Determine location for elimination (bed, commode) ■ Determine assistive devices and/or physical assistance needed (i.e., for walking, balance, hygiene, manipulating clothing) ■ Assess other stroke-related deficits (e.g., aphasia, altered mobility, cognition, sensation, perception, mood) ■ Assess psychosocial concerns of patient, family, caregiver ■ Perform physical examination and/or evaluate physical findings ■ Monitor or evaluate results of voiding diary for 1 week ■ Monitor lab results (urinalysis, culture, and sensitivity) ■ Monitor or evaluate postvoid residuals ■ Monitor results of urodynamic tests **Therapeutic Interventions** ■ Evaluate patient and implement appropriate behavioral strategy(ies) (habit training, bladder retraining, prompted voiding, Kegel exercises combined with biofeedback when possible, contingency management)	■ The patient will have regular voiding episodes with complete bladder emptying ■ The patient will have minimal to no incontinent episodes ■ The patient and family will describe factors that influence urge incontinence ■ The patient and family will understand medications, actions, dose, and potential side effects ■ The patient and family will identify strategies to minimize or eliminate incontinent episodes ■ The patient and family will identify potential problems of urge incontinence and strategies for dealing with these problems

Continued.

NURSING CARE PLAN — cont'd

Nursing Diagnosis	Interventions	Expected Outcomes
	■ Maintain voiding diary for assessment and ongoing evaluation ■ Decrease fluid intake in late afternoon and evening ■ Decrease caffeine intake ■ Position upright for voiding whenever possible ■ Use bedside commode or urinal to increase accessibility of receptacle ■ Provide privacy ■ Collaborate with patient, family, and team members regarding home routine and equipment needed ■ Evaluate program effectiveness in ongoing manner; increase patient and family involvement as soon as possible	

NURSING CARE PLAN — cont'd

Nursing Diagnosis	Interventions	Expected Outcomes
Urinary retention related to dyssenergy between the detrusor and external urinary sphincter **Defining Characteristics** ■ Bladder distension ■ Small, frequent voidings or no voidings ■ Sensation of bladder fullness ■ Dribbling ■ Residual urine ■ Dysuria ■ Overflow incontinence	**Ongoing Assessment** ■ Assess preexisting urinary tract problems ■ Assess history of current problem (including time of onset, symptoms, reasons for difficulty voiding, presence of incontinence) ■ Assess typical urinary elimination patterns and habits ■ Determine current medications ■ Determine location for elimination (bed, commode) ■ Determine assistive devices needed (e.g., cane, walker, reachers, elevated commode seat, grab bars) ■ Determine physical assistance needed (i.e., for walking, balance, hygiene, manipulating clothing) ■ Assess other stroke related deficits (e.g., aphasia, altered mobility, cognition, sensation, mood) ■ Assess perceived need to urinate or feelings of bladder fullness; feelings of incomplete bladder emptying ■ Assess psychosocial concerns of patient, family, caregiver ■ Percuss or palpate bladder to assess for distension ■ Monitor or evaluate results of voiding diary for 1 week ■ Monitor lab results (urinalysis, culture and sensitivity) ■ Monitor or evaluate postvoid residual amounts ■ Monitor results of urodynamic tests	■ The patient will have regular voiding episodes with complete emptying ■ The patient and family will describe factors that influence urinary retention ■ The patient and family will understand medications, actions, dose, and potential side effects ■ The patient and family will identify strategies to minimize or eliminate urinary retention ■ The patient and family will identify potential complications of urinary retention and strategies for dealing with these

Continued

NURSING CARE PLAN — cont'd

Nursing Diagnosis	Interventions	Expected Outcomes
	Therapeutic Interventions ■ Maintain voiding diary for assessment and ongoing evaluation ■ Promote consistent fluid intake; avoid large amounts of fluid at one time, especially in late afternoon or evening ■ Position upright for voiding whenever possible ■ Establish timed voiding schedule, consult with physician about catheterizing patient for postvoid residuals ■ Catheterize patient for postvoid residuals within 5 min after voiding ■ Consult with physician for appropriate medication; administer medications as therapeutically as possible (i.e., timing and spacing of doses) ■ Monitor patient response to medications ■ Evaluate patient's fine motor skills and ability for self-catheterization ■ Provide privacy ■ Evaluate program effectiveness in ongoing manner; increase patient and family involvement as soon as possible ■ Collaborate with patient, family, and team members regarding home routine and equipment needed	

NURSING CARE PLAN — cont'd

Nursing Diagnosis	Interventions	Expected Outcomes
Incontinence, Functional related to deficits in mobility, sensation, and/or cognition and altered environment **Defining Characteristics** ▪ Urge to void or bladder contractions sufficiently strong to result in loss of urine before reaching an appropriate receptacle	**Ongoing Assessment** ▪ Assess preexisting urinary tract problems ▪ Assess history of current problem (including onset, symptoms, frequency and timing of incontinent episodes, reasons for incontinence, nocturia) ▪ Assess typical urinary elimination patterns and habits ▪ Assess other stroke related deficits (e.g., aphasia, altered mobility, cognition, sensation, mood) ▪ Determine current medications ▪ Determine location for elimination (bed, commode) ▪ Determine assistive devices needed (i.e., cane, walker, reachers, elevated commode seat, grab bars) ▪ Determine physical assistance needed (i.e., for walking, balance, hygiene, manipulating clothing) ▪ Assess psychosocial concerns of patient, family, caregiver ▪ Perform physical examination and evaluate physical findings ▪ Monitor or evaluate results of voiding diary for 1 week ▪ Monitor lab results (urinalysis, culture, and sensitivity) ▪ Monitor or evaluate postvoid residuals ▪ Monitor results of urodynamic tests	▪ The patient will have regular voiding episodes with minimal to no incontinence ▪ The patient and family will describe the relationship between stroke-related deficits and functional incontinence ▪ The patient and family will describe factors that influence functional incontinence ▪ The patient and family will identify strategies to minimize or eliminate incontinent episodes ▪ The patient and family will identify potential problems of functional incontinence and strategies for dealing with these problems

Continued.

NURSING CARE PLAN — cont'd

Nursing Diagnosis	Interventions	Expected Outcomes
	Therapeutic Interventions ■ Remove obstacles and organize patient's room and bathroom to promote safe and easy access ■ Discuss with the patient a voiding schedule and implement appropriate strategies ■ Maintain a voiding diary for assessment and ongoing evaluation ■ Decrease fluid intake in late afternoon and evening ■ Decrease caffeine intake ■ Place in upright position for voiding whenever possible ■ Use bedside commode or urinal to increase accessibility of receptacle ■ Provide privacy ■ Collaborate with physical, occupational, and speech therapists as needed to assist patient with compensatory behaviors ■ Model open communication with the patient; encourage the expression of feelings; be a good listener ■ Collaborate with patient, family and team members regarding home routine and equipment needed ■ Evaluate program effectiveness in ongoing manner; increase patient and family involvement as soon as possible	

NURSING CARE PLAN — cont'd

Nursing Diagnosis	Interventions	Expected Outcomes
Constipation related to inactivity, low roughage diet, limited fluid intake, medication . . . **Defining Characteristics** ■ Hard, forced stools ■ Reported feeling of pressure or fullness in rectum ■ Straining to have a bowel movement ■ Decreased activity level ■ Diminished frequency of bowel movements	**Ongoing Assessment** ■ Assess preexisting bowel problems ■ Assess history of current problem (including onset, duration, symptoms) ■ Assess typical bowel elimination patterns and habits ■ Assess pattern of fluid and dietary intake ■ Determine current medications ■ Determine location for elimination (bed, commode) ■ Determine assistive devices needed (e.g., cane, walker, reachers, elevated commode seat, grab bars) ■ Determine physical assistance needed (i.e., for walking, balance, hygiene, manipulating clothing) ■ Assess other stroke related deficits (e.g., aphasia, altered mobility, cognition, sensation, mood) ■ Assess ability of patient to participate in bowel program ■ Assess psychosocial concerns of patient, family, caregiver ■ Auscultate bowel sounds, check for bowel distension, perform rectal check for fecal impaction ■ Monitor or evaluate results of bowel movement record for one week	■ The patient will have regular bowel movements at predictable times ■ The patient and family will describe factors that influence constipation ■ The patient and family will understand medication, actions, dose, and potential side effects ■ The patient and family will identify strategies to minimize or eliminate constipation ■ The patient and family will identify potential problems of constipation and strategies for dealing with these problems

Continued.

NURSING CARE PLAN — cont'd

Nursing Diagnosis	Interventions	Expected Outcomes
	Therapeutic Interventions ■ Remove impactions before starting bowel program ■ Maintain bowel movement record for assessment and ongoing evaluation ■ Promote consistent and adequate fluid intake ■ Promote adequate intake of dietary fiber ■ Establish regular toileting schedule (after meals preferred) ■ Position upright for defecation whenever possible ■ Evaluate patient's fine motor skills and ability for self-care (toileting hygiene, suppository insertion if necessary) ■ Develop exercise routine with patient if physical condition permits ■ Consult physician for appropriate medication; administer medications as therapeutically as possible (i.e., timing and spacing of doses) ■ Monitor patient response to medication ■ Provide privacy and adequate time for toileting ■ Model open communication; encourage patient to talk about feelings ■ Evaluate program effectiveness in ongoing manner; increase patient and family involvement as soon as possible ■ Collaborate with patient, family, and team members regarding home routine and equipment needed	

NURSING CARE PLAN — cont'd

Nursing Diagnosis	Interventions	Expected Outcomes
Bowel Incontinence related to loss of cortical inhibition **Defining Characteristics** ■ Involuntary stools ■ Lack of awareness of need to defecate ■ Inability to inhibit defecation ■ Urgency ■ History or evidence of smearing	**Ongoing Assessment** ■ Assess preexisting bowel problems ■ Assess history of current problem (including onset, duration, symptoms, timing and frequency of incontinent episodes) ■ Assess typical bowel elimination patterns and habits ■ Assess pattern of fluid and dietary intake (including supplemental feedings, dietary fiber) ■ Determine current medications (evaluate frequency and current doses of laxatives, stool softeners) ■ Determine location for elimination (bed, commode) ■ Determine assistive devices and/or physical assistance needed (i.e., for walking, balance, hygiene, manipulating clothing) ■ Assess other stroke-related deficits (e.g., aphasia, altered mobility, cognition, sensation, mood) ■ Assess ability of patient to participate in own bowel program ■ Assess psychosocial concerns of patient, family, caregiver ■ Auscultate bowel sounds, perform rectal check for fecal impaction ■ Monitor or evaluate results of bowel movement record for one week	■ The patient will have regular bowel movements at predictable times ■ The patient will have minimal to no incontinent episodes ■ The patient and family will describe factors that influence bowel incontinence ■ The patient and family will understand medications, actions, dose, and side effects ■ The patient and family will identify strategies to minimize or eliminate incontinent episodes ■ The patient and family will identify potential problems of bowel incontinence and strategies for dealing with these problems

Continued.

NURSING CARE PLAN — cont'd

Nursing Diagnosis	Interventions	Expected Outcomes
	Therapeutic Interventions ■ Remove any impactions before starting bowel program ■ Maintain bowel movement record for assessment and ongoing evaluation ■ Promote consistent and adequate fluid intake ■ Promote adequate intake of dietary fiber ■ Establish regular voiding schedule (after meals preferred) ■ Position upright for defecation whenever possible ■ Evaluate patient's fine motor skills and ability for self-care (toileting hygiene, suppository insertion if necessary) ■ Develop exercise routine with patient if physical condition permits ■ Consult physician for appropriate medication; administer medications as therapeutically as possible (i.e., timing and spacing) ■ Monitor patient response to medications ■ Provide privacy and adequate time for toileting ■ Evaluate program effectiveness in ongoing manner; increase patient and family involvement as soon as possible ■ Collaborate with patient, family, and team members regarding home routine and equipment needed	

NURSING CARE PLAN — cont'd

Nursing Diagnosis | **Interventions** | **Expected Outcomes**

Patient Education

- Educate about normal urinary tract function and ways to maintain healthy function
- Provide description and rationale for selected behavioral strategies, including fluid control, medications, catheterization, and regualr voiding
- Educate about signs, symptoms, and actions to take for urinary tract complications, skin problems
- Educate about actions, dose, and potential side effects of medications
- Educate patient and family about self-catheterization (proper technique, complications, maintenance of supplies)
- Educate about the impact of physical, psychologic, and environmental factors on incontinence
- Educate patient in constructive problem-solving and setting realistic goals
- Educate about normal bowel functions and factors influencing bowel function (including relationship of meals, fluids, gastrocolic reflex, stimulant beverages, exercise, and medications)
- Educate family about voiding program
- Educate about potential problems of constipation and strategies for dealing with complications

Other Relevant Nursing Diagnoses

- Total incontinence
- Altered patterns of urinary elimination
- Alteration in bowel elimination: neurogenic (reflexic) bowel
- Alteration in bowel elimination: diarrhea

REFERENCES

Anchini MA, Mulrow M, and Griggs WP: Alterations in urine elimination: incontinence (funded by the Retirement Research Foundation), Chicago, 1985, Rehabilitation Institute of Chicago.

Andrew J and Nathan PW: Lesions of the anterior frontal lobe and disturbances of micturition and defecation, Brain 87:233, 1964.

Andrews K, Brocklehurst BR, and Laycock PJ: The recovery of the severely disabled stroke patient, Rheumatol Rehabil 21: 225, 1982.

Andriole VT: Hospital-acquired urinary infections and the indwelling catheter, Urol Clin North Am 2:451, 1975.

Autry D and others: The voiding record: an aid in decreasing incontinence, Geriatr Nurs 5:38, 1984.

Baigis-Smith J, Smith DA, Rose M and others: Managing urinary incontinence in community-residing elderly persons, Gerontologist 29:229, 1989.

Barrett DM and Wein AJ: Voiding dysfunction: diagnosis, classification, and management. In Gillenwater JY, Grayhack JT, Howards SS and others, editors: Adult and pediatric urology, vol 1, Chicago, 1987, Year Book Medical.

Barrington FJ: The effect of lesions of the hind and midbrain on micturition in the cat, Q J Exp Physiol 15:181, 1925.

Bates P, Bradley WE, Glen E and others: Standardization of terminology of lower urinary tract function, J Urol 121:551, 1979.

Berman SA, Hayman LA and Hinck VC: Correlation of CT cerebral vascular teritories with function: anterior cerebral artery, AJR 135:253, 1980.

Berne RM and Levy MN: Physiology, ed 2, St. Louis, 1988, The CV Mosby Co.

Borrie MJ, Campbell AJ, Caradoc-Davies TH, and others: Urinary incontinence after stroke: a prospective study, Age and Ageing 15:177, 1986.

Brocklehurst JC: A textbook of geriatric medicine and gerontology, London, 1973, Churchill Livingstone Inc.

Brocklehurst JC, Andrews K, Richards B and others: Incidence and correlates of incontinence in stroke patients, J Am Geriatr Soc 33:540, 1985.

Buchan AMJ: Gastrointestinal motility. In Patton HD, Fuchs AF, Hille B, and others, editors: Textbook of Physiology, ed 21, Philadelphia, 1989, WB Saunders Co.

Burgio KL, Whitehead WE and Engel BT: Urinary incontinence in the elderly, Ann Intern Med 103:507, 1985.

Burgio KL and Burgio LD: Behavioral therapies for urinary incontinence in the elderly, Clin Geriatr Med 2:809, 1986.

Burton JR, Pearce L, Burgio KL and others: Behavioral training for urinary incontinence in elderly ambulatory patients, J Am Geriatr Soc 36:693, 1988.

Cannon B: Bowel function. In Martin N, Holt NB, and Hicks D, editors: Rehabilitation Nursing, New York, 1981, McGraw-Hill Inc.

Chusid JG: Neuroanatomy and functional neurology, ed 16, Los Altos, Ca, 1976, Lange Medical.

Clay EG: Incontinence of urine: a regime for retraining, Nursing Mirror 146:23, 1978.

Connell AM, Hilton C, Irvine G and others: Variation of bowel habit in two population samples, Br Med J 2:1095, 1965.

Creason NS, Grybowski JA, Burgener S and others: Prompted voiding therapy for urinary incontinence in aged female nursing home residents, J Adv Nurs 14:120, 1989.

Currie CT: Urinary incontinence after stroke, Br Med J 293:1322, 1986.

Ditmar S: Rehabilitation nursing, St. Louis, 1989, The CV Mosby Co.

Diokno AC: Practical approach to the management of urinary incontinence in the elderly, Compr Ther 9:67, 1983.

Diokno AC, Brock BM, Brown MB, and others: Prevalence of urinary incontinence and other urological symptoms in the non-institutionalized elderly, J Urol 136:1022, 1986.

Freed SZ: Urinary incontinence in the elderly, Hosp Pract 17:81, 1982.

Frewen WK: An objective assessment of the unstable bladder of psychosomatic origin, Br J Urol 50:246, 1978.

Frewen WK: The management of urgency and frequency of micturition, Br J Urol 52:367, 1980.

Gray M and Dougherty MC: Urinary incontinence-pathophysiology and treatment, J Enterostomal Therapy 14:152, 1987.

Grosicki JP: Effect of operant conditioning on modification of incontinence in neuropsychiatric geriatric patients, Nurs Res 17:304, 1968.

Griffin D: Urinary incontinence in the elderly, Postgrad Med 73:143, 1983.

Guyton AC: Human physiology and mechanisms of disease ed 3, Philadelphia, 1982 WB Saunders Co.

Guyton AC: Basic neuroscience: anatomy and physiology, Philadelphia, 1987, WB Saunders Co.

Hald T and Bradley WE, editors: First report on standardization of terminology of lower urinary tract function, In The urinary bladder: neurology and dynamics, Baltimore, 1982, Williams & Wilkins.

Hirschberg GG, Lewis L, and Vaughan P: Rehabilitation ed 2, Philadelphia, 1976, Lippincott.
Hu T, Igou JF, Kaltreider L, and others: A clinical trial of a behavioral therapy to reduce urinary incontinence in nursing homes, JAMA 261:2656, 1989.
James MH: Disorders of micturition in the elderly, Age Ageing 8:286, 1979.
Kaplan PE and Cerullo LJ: Stroke Rehabilitation, Boston, 1986, Butterworth Publishers.
Kegel AH: Progressive resistance exercises in the functional restoration of the perineal muscles, Am J Obstet Gynecol 56:238, 1948.
Khan Z, Hertanu J, Yang WC and others: Predictive correlation of urodynamic dysfunction and brain injury after cerebrovascular accident, J Urol 126:86, 1981.
Klutzow FW, Gleason D, Lancaster HK and others: Incontinence associated with bilateral lesions of putamen, Arch Neurol 45:168, 1989.
Kuru M: Nervous control of micturition, Physiology Review 45:425, 1965.
Lal S: Physiatric complications in stroke syndromes. In Kaplan PE and Cerullo LJ, editors: Stroke rehabilitation, Boston, 1986, Butterworth Publishers.
Lapides J: Neurogenic bladder, Urol Cli North Am 1:81, 1974.
Lipsey JR, Robinson RG, Pearlson GD and others: Nortriptyline treatment of post-stroke depression: a double-blind study, Lancet 1:297, 1984.
Lorenze EJ, Simon HB and Linden JL: Urologic problems in rehabilitation of hemiplegic patients, JAMA 110:1042, 1959.
McCormick KA, Scheve AA, and Leahy E: Nursing management of urinary incontinence in geriatric inpatients, Nurs Clin North Am 23:231, 1988.
MacLeod JH: Management of anal incontinence by biofeedback, Gastroenterology 93:291, 1987.
Middaugh SJ, Whitehead WE, Burgio KL and others: Biofeedback in treatment of urinary incontinence in stroke patients, Biofeedback Self Regul 14:3, 1989.
Newman DK: The treatment of urinary incontinence in adults, Nurse Pract 14:21, 1989.
O'Brien MT and Pallett PJ: Total care of the stroke patient, Boston 1978, Little, Brown & Co. Inc.
Ouslander JG and Kane RL: The cost of urinary incontinence in nursing homes, Med Care 22:69, 1984.
Patrick ML, Woods SL, Craven RF and others: Medical-surgical nursing: pathophysiological concepts, Philadelphia, 1986, JB Lippincott.
Pollock DD and Liberman RP: Behavior therapy of incontinence in demented inpatients, Gerontologist 14:488, 1974.
Romanowski GL, Shimp LA, Balson AB and others: Urinary incontinence in the elderly: etiology and treatment, Drug Intell Clin Pharm 22:525, 1988.
Ruff CC and Reaves EL: Diagnosing urinary incontinence in adults, Nurse Pract 14:8, 1989.
Rusk HA: Rehabilitation medicine, ed 4, St. Louis, 1977, The CV Mosby Co.
Shimp LA, Wells TJ, Brink CA and others: Relationship between drug use and urinary incontinence in elderly women, Drug Intell Clin Pharm 22:786, 1988.
Sodeman WA: Normal colon function and aging. In Sodeman WA, Saladin TA, and Boyd WP, editors, Geriatric gastroenterology, Philadelphia, 1989, WB Saunders.
Sogbein K and Awad SA: Behavioral treatment of urinary incontinence in geriatric patients, Can Med Assoc J 127:863, 1982.
Spangler PF, Risley TR, and Bilyew DP: The management of dehydration and incontinence in nonambulatory geriatric patients, J Appl Behav Anal 17:397, 1984.
Tsuchida S, Noto H, Yamaguchi O and others: Urodynamic studies on hemiplegic patients after cerebrovascular accident, Urology 21:315, 1983.
Vander AJ, Sherman JH, and Luciano DS: Human physiology, New York, 1980, McGraw-Hill Inc.
Wade DT and Hewer RL: Outlook after an acute stroke: urinary incontinence and loss of consciousness compared in 532 patients, Q J Med 56:601, 1985.
Wagner BR and Paul GL: Reduction of incontinence in chronic mental patients, J Behav Ther Exp Psychiatry 1:29, 1970.
Wein AJ, Levin RM, and Barrett DM: Voiding function: relevant anatomy, physiology, and pharmacology. In Gillenwater JY, Grayhack JT, Howards SS and others, editors: Adult and pediatric urology, vol 1, Chicago, 1987, Year Book Medical.
Whitehead WE, Burgio KL, and Engel BT: Biofeedback treatment of fecal incontinence in geriatric patients, J Am Geriatr Soc 33:320, 1985.
Williams ME and Pannill FC: Urinary incontinence in the elderly, Ann Inter Med 97:895, 1982.
Willington FL: Incontinence in the elderly, London, 1976, Academic Press.
Wyman JE: Nursing assessment of the incontinent geriatric outpatient population, Nurs Clin North Am 23:169, 1988.

Chapter 10

Alterations in Sensation and Perception

KAREN FERGUSON

Altered sensory and perceptual abilities often present as some of the more subtle consequences of a devastating event, such as stroke. It takes careful examination to discover the extent of perceptual loss following a cerebrovascular event. Yet it is well documented that a significant perceptual deficit adversely affects rehabilitation outcome (Kaplan and Hier, 1982; Anton and others, 1988). The strategies the nurse selects in caring for these patients and their families can have a major effect on the patient's recovery. The purpose of this chapter is to describe perceptual deficits seen after stroke in order to increase the nurses' awareness of the effect these syndromes have on patients and how nursing strategies can be tailored to minimize the associated disabilities.

Anatomy of normal sensory-perceptual mechanisms, from the periphery to the cortex, is presented. Stroke-related perceptual deficits—apraxia, agnosia, and neglect, among others—are described in terms of suspected causal mechanism, impact on function, and research on trends in diagnosis and treatment. In the final section, nursing assessment, diagnoses, and interventions are discussed and a suggested nursing care plan is offered.

SENSATION vs PERCEPTION

The definitions of sensation and perception are sometimes interchanged. *Taber's Medical Dictionary* defines *sensation* as a feeling or awareness of conditions within or without the body resulting from the stimulation of sensory receptors (Thomas, 1985). *Perception* is a more abstract concept. It is the process of deriving *meaning* from sensory impressions. Perceptual awareness occurs primarily at the cortical level while sensation requires an intact pathway from the periphery all the way to the cerebral cortex. The syndromes discussed in this chapter will highlight what can go wrong when a vascular insult destroys part of the pathway.

ANATOMY

The parietal lobe is that region of the brain that contains the sensory cortex. Here, sensory information is received and interpreted and connections are made to other parts of the brain to effect an action in response to the original sensory input. However, all sensory and perceptual deficits that can occur in stroke cannot be explained by a simple anatomy lesson about the parietal lobe. There are a multitude of parietal and extra-parietal structures and pathways that interconnect in intricate ways to comprise one's perceptual awareness. Information must first be received from the environment, converted to electrical impulses, and carried up the spinal cord for ultimate processing in the brain.

Initial Receiving of Information

Our interpretation of stimuli, both external and internal (i.e., from our own bodies), begins with contact between these stimuli and sensory receptors located throughout our bodies. These receptors are

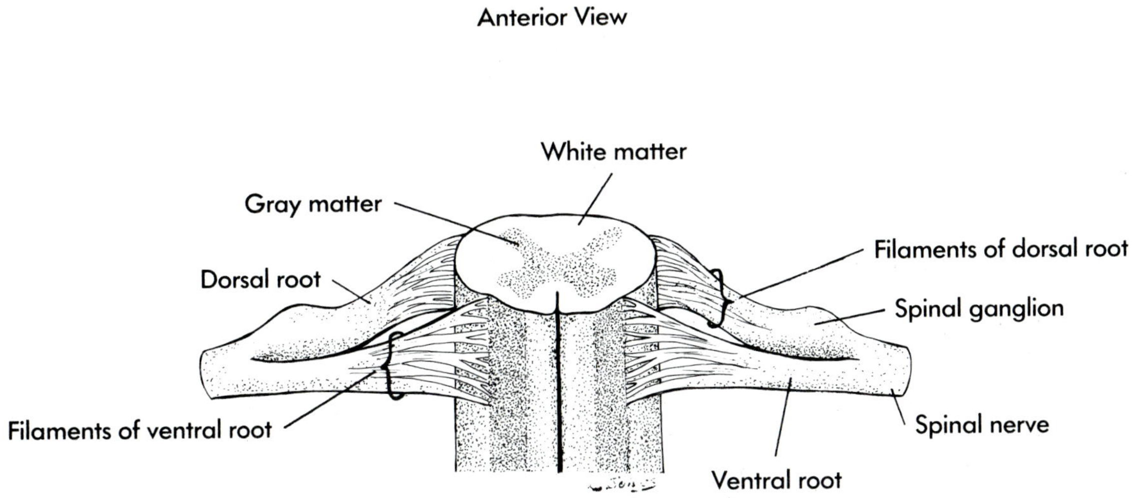

Fig. 10-1 Dorsal roots of the spinal cord.

found in skin, mucous membranes, tendons, muscles, and viscera. Receptors are thought to be specific to a form of sensibility; e.g., cold, heat, light touch, and joint position. The receptors for pain are not well differentiated. Pain receptors are actually free nerve endings that are sensitive to chemical, mechanical, and thermal stimuli (Kelly, 1985). They are termed *nociceptors*.

Receptors can be grouped into three categories that distinguish the sources of stimuli: exteroceptive, proprioceptive, and interoceptive. *Exteroceptive* systems respond to external stimuli, namely vision, audition, and skin sensation. *Proprioceptive* systems are sensitive to the body's position in space and to the relative position of body parts to each other. Finally, *interoceptive* systems interpret internal body events, such as blood pressure and blood glucose concentration (Martin, 1985). Interoceptive signals do not reach consciousness and are not addressed in this chapter. Vision and hearing will be presented separately.

The Pathway from Periphery to Center

Once the sensory receptor has been stimulated, the information is translated into electric impulses that travel via peripheral nerves. Peripheral nerves join together into spinal nerves as they approach the spinal cord. The sensory cell bodies are located in the dorsal roots of the spinal cord. The spinal nerves each have a dorsal root by which afferent (sensory) impulses enter the cord and a ventral root by which efferent (motor) impulses leave the cord (Fig. 10-1). The sensory cell bodies are located in the spinal ganglion of the dorsal roots. Each sensory dorsal root is responsible for innervating a specific peripheral region of skin called a *dermatome*. The familiar dermatome map of the anterior and posterior skin surfaces is provided in Fig. 10-2. The boundaries of the dermatomes may differ slightly, depending upon the sensation (e.g., pain vs light touch) being examined. Although dermatomal maps appear quite well demarcated, there can be considerable overlap of adjacent dermatomes.

The Pathways up the Spinal Cord

Once the dorsal root has received the sensory stimulus, the spinal cord functions to carry the impulse to higher centers for the purposes of perception, arousal, and motor planning. There are two major ascending systems for somatic information

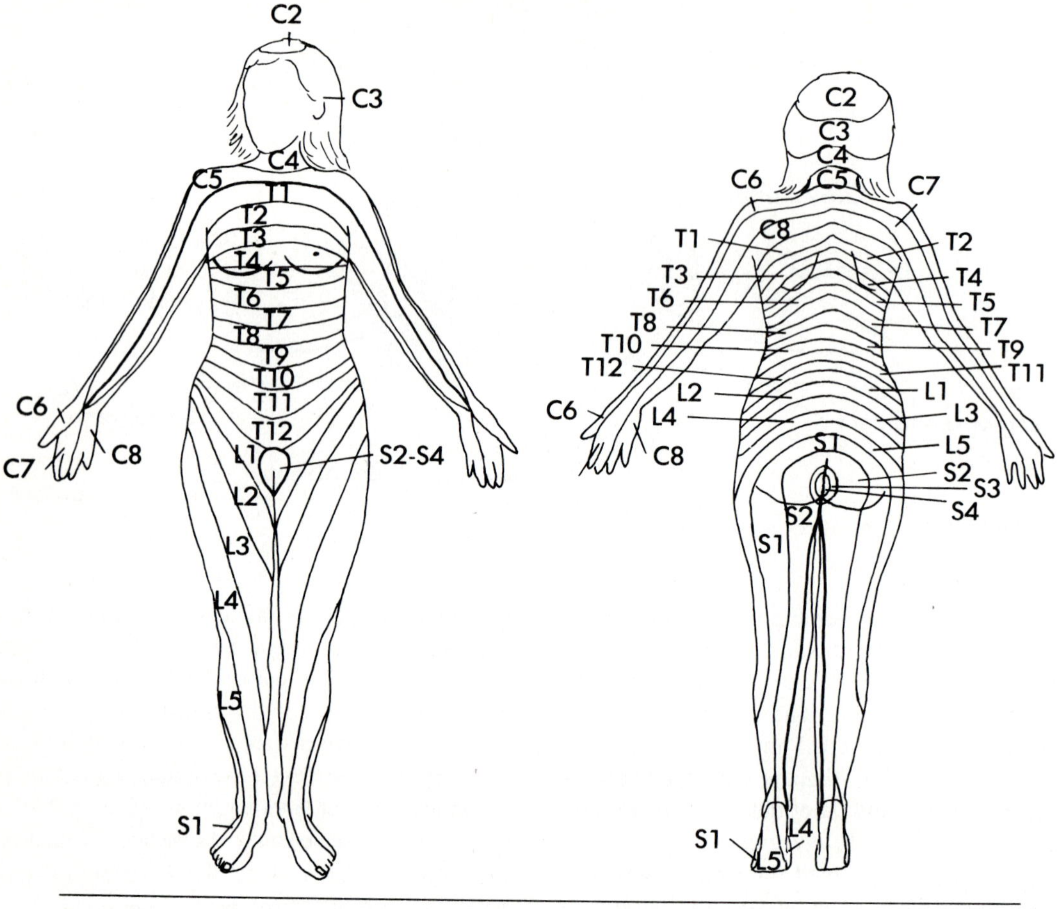

Fig. 10-2 The dermatome map of anterior and posterior skin surfaces.

(Fig. 10-3). One carries pain, temperature, and crude touch (*anterolateral system*). It originates in the dorsal horn of the cord, crosses (decussates) to the opposite side within a few segments, then travels upward to synapse at various points of the brainstem's reticular system (which acts as a first-order arousal, or activating, system) and then to nuclei of the thalamus, a complex relay center.

The other main ascending tract is called the *dorsal column-medial lemniscal system*. Tactile sensation, vibration sense, and proprioception consume most of the functions of the dorsal columns. This tract does not cross over until it reaches the medulla in the brainstem. All fibers, whether from upper or lower extremities, terminate in the lower medulla in the dorsal column nuclei. As fibers leave these medullary nuclei, they cross midline in a bundle known as the *medial lemniscus* and continue on to the thalamus.

The Relay Center

Virtually all afferent pathways are relayed through the thalamus, a deep brain structure that serves as a "connecting station" of nuclei between the spinal cord and cerebral cortex. The thalamic nuclei specific to the somatic sensory projections are the ventral posterior lateral nucleus, the posterior nuclear group, and the intralaminar nuclei

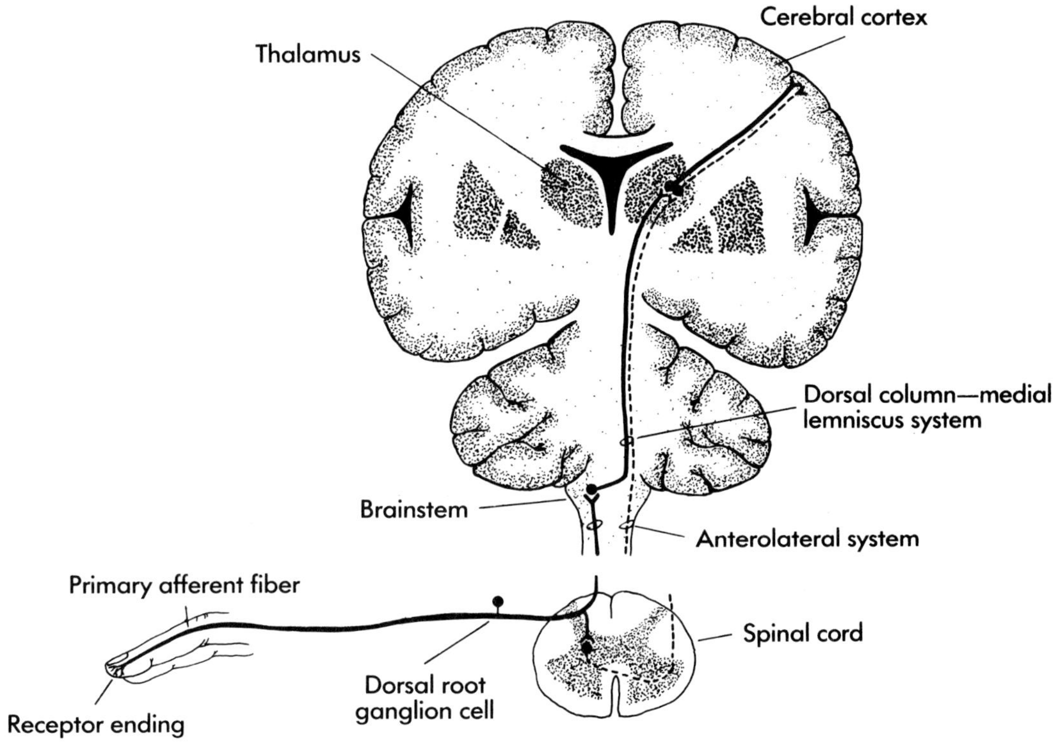

Fig. 10-3 The two major ascending systems for somatic information: the anterolateral system and the dorsal column-medial lemniscal system.

(Fig. 10-4). The relationship of the thalamus with the cortex is shown in Fig. 10-3. These nuclei have very little interconnection with one another, so information projected to the cortex is fairly stimulus-specific.

Additionally, most thalamic nuclei tend to have preferred cortical projection sites (Mesulam, 1985), which may help "prepare" the cortex by focusing incoming stimuli. The ventral posterior nucleus of the thalamus regulates the flow of both sensory input and motor feedback to the cerebral cortex through inhibitory interneurons (Kelly, 1985). It is this regulatory function that defines the thalamus as a true relay center; i.e., it is not merely a "way-station" indiscriminantly projecting information to the cortex. Thus integration and correlation of input from the periphery occurs at the level of the thalamus, without yet conscious appreciation of the input. The exception to this is pain, which will be discussed in the section about central pain.

The Final Sensory Destination—A Cellular Perspective

The cerebral cortex controls conscious awareness of the incoming stimuli. The cortex specializes in sensation, motor coordination, and higher cognitive functions. The two main varieties of cortical neurons are defined by their shapes—pyramidal and stellate. The differences in axon and dendrite anatomy between the two types account for their specialization of roles. *Pyramidal cells* tend to have long axons and few dendrites, making them well designed for transmitting motor signals downward. *Stellate cells,* on the other hand, are round with many short dendrites in a stellar shape around the

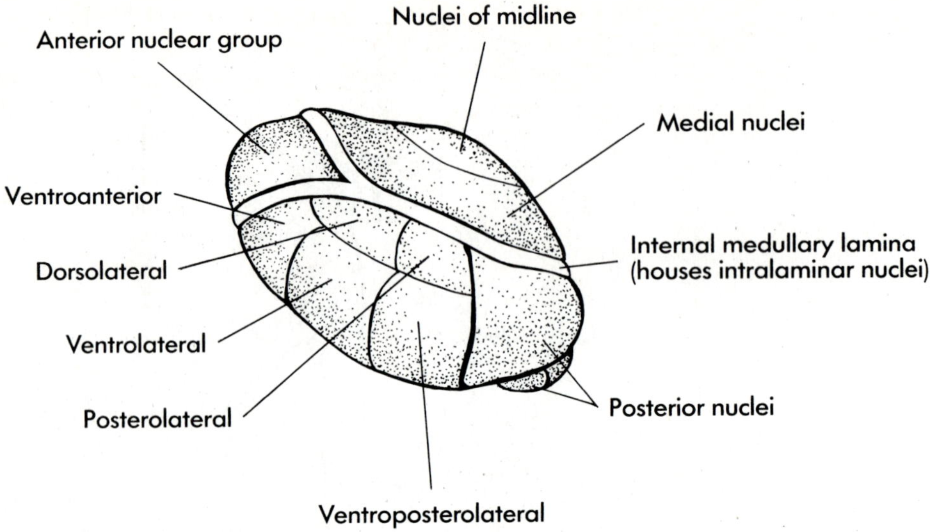

Fig. 10-4 Thalamic nuclei specific to the somatic sensory projections.

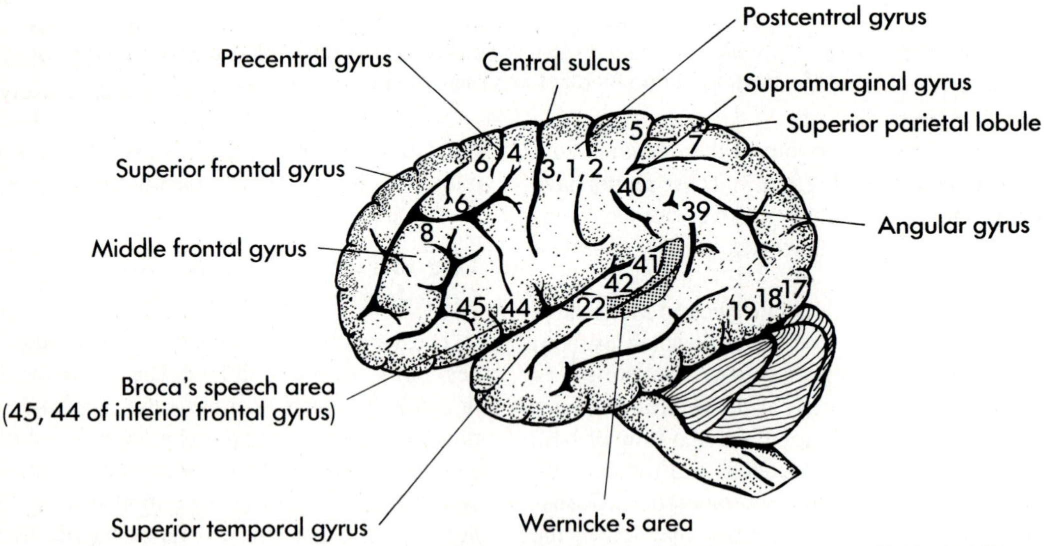

Fig. 10-5 Brodman's map of the human cerebral cortex.

cell body. These cells are therefore particularly sensitive to incoming information from thalamic afferent projections. Their axons are short and more effective for local intracortical processing of sensory input. Though both cells are located in each cortical layer, their ratios differ, depending upon the primary function of the layer.

There are six identified layers of the cerebral cortex. In brief, the most superficial (layer I) is mostly supportive glial cells with some axonal processes. Layers II and III are mostly small pyramidal cell layers projecting to other cortical layers. It is layer IV that is rich in stellate cells, receiving most of the afferent input from the thalamus. Layer V has the largest pyramidal cells, with axonal projections down the spinal cord. Finally, layer VI houses neurons that transmit impulses back to the thalamus. Layer IV is thus the main cortical sensory receiving zone and is more prominent in the primary and association sensory cortices than in any other cortical region.

The Final Sensory Destination—A Functional Perspective

The cerebral hemispheres are divided into four major lobes, named for the overlying bones of the skull: parietal, frontal, temporal, and occipital. Although each lobe has certain characteristic functions, there is considerable overlap. Brodman's classic map of the human cerebral cortex has been known to scholars for nearly a century (Kelly, 1985). A modification of the original map, which originally identified 52 unique regions, is provided in Fig. 10-5. Each number represents a structural area of the brain, although there is no systematic relationship among the numbers. The primary sensory cortex located in the postcentral gyrus is represented by Brodman's regions 3, 1, and 2.

The primary cortex receives and processes the raw, gross information transmitted via afferent fibers from the lower brain. Body parts are represented along the postcentral gyrus in proportion to how much sensory input they transmit. For example, the index finger representation is much larger than that of the lower leg, even though the finger is a much smaller body part. This disproportionate body part representation along the postcentral gyrus is characterized as the *sensory homunculus* (Fig. 10-6).

The primary sensory cortex is not the end of the line for communication of sensory input. Conscious understanding can only be attached to the input by means of extensive synaptic connections within sensory association areas, referred to as association cortex. Association cortex is not directly involved in processing isolated sensory input but rather in the integration of multiple sensory modalities. Experimental electrical stimulation to these areas does not elicit overt sensory responses. The functions of the association cortex are to link the primary sensory cortices to each other and to link the sensory and motor cortices to one another (Kupfermann, 1985).

Cerebral functions of the highest order—thought and perception—are attributed to the association cortex. Studies over the last few years suggest the association areas are not quite as extensive as they were once believed to be. Instead, some of the "designated" association areas are actually higher order sensory cortices (Kupfermann, 1985). The Brodman's areas that most closely represent the parietal association areas are 5 and 7. Areas 39 and 40 (the supramarginal and angular gyri) also serve as association areas, but their function is to interrelate somesthetic, visual, and sensory stimuli. Without an intact association cortex, incoming sensory stimuli has no meaning, a phenomenon not unlike hearing the words of an unknown language being spoken without expression.

The Special Senses

The pathways discussed thus far are for somatosensory information, i.e., sensation from the body. The special senses of vision, hearing, equilibrium, taste, and olfaction each has its own intricate receptor organs with complex neuronal connections for transmission to the sensory cortex. Refer to texts on neuroanatomy for further information about the intake of sensory information through the ears, eyes, nose, and mouth. A brief

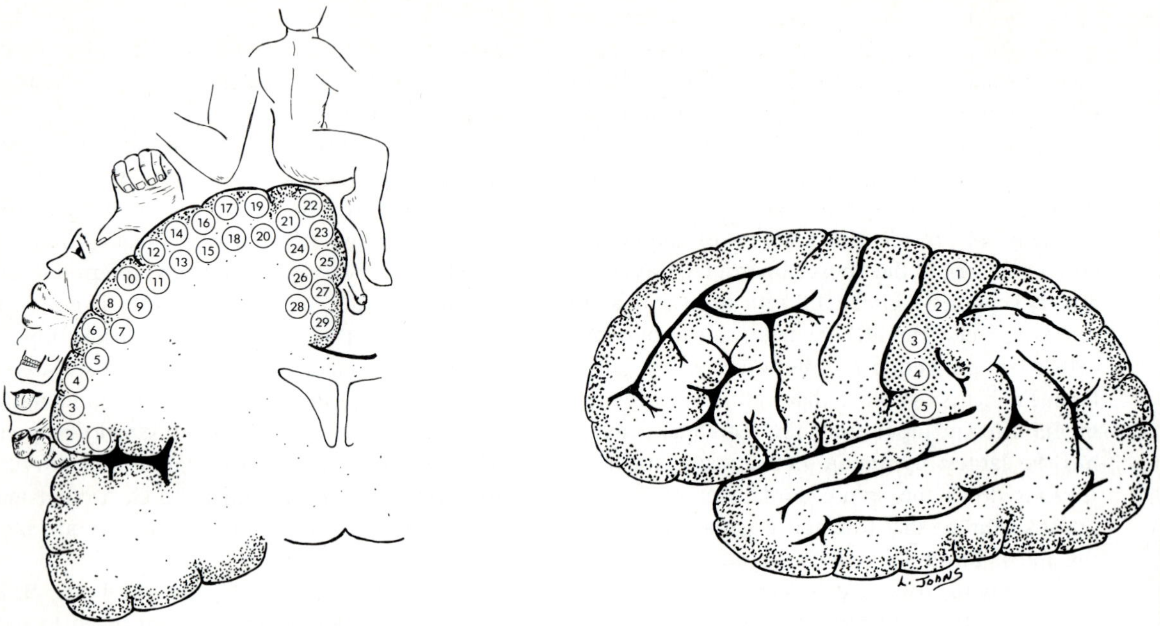

Fig. 10-6 The sensory homunculus.

discussion of the visual and auditory pathways is presented next.

Vision. Retinal cells receive external visual information, convert it photochemically into nerve impulses, then transmit those impulses via their axons into the *optic nerve* of each eye. The left and right optic nerve meet and partially decussate at the *optic chiasm*, located immediately in front of the pituitary gland. Only fibers from the nasal half of each retina cross to the contralateral brain. Fibers from the temporal half of each retina remain uncrossed at the chiasm. Behind the optic chiasm, the fibers are called *optic tracts* (Fig. 10-7). These fibers terminate in the *lateral geniculate bodies* of the thalamus and are projected from there as the *optic radiation* upon the primary visual cortex in each occipital lobe, which is represented on Brodman's map (Fig. 10-5) by area 17. The visual association cortex provides meaning to visual sensation and is represented by areas 18 and 19.

Hearing. The organ of Corti, housed in the cochlea, or inner ear, is the body's sound receptor.

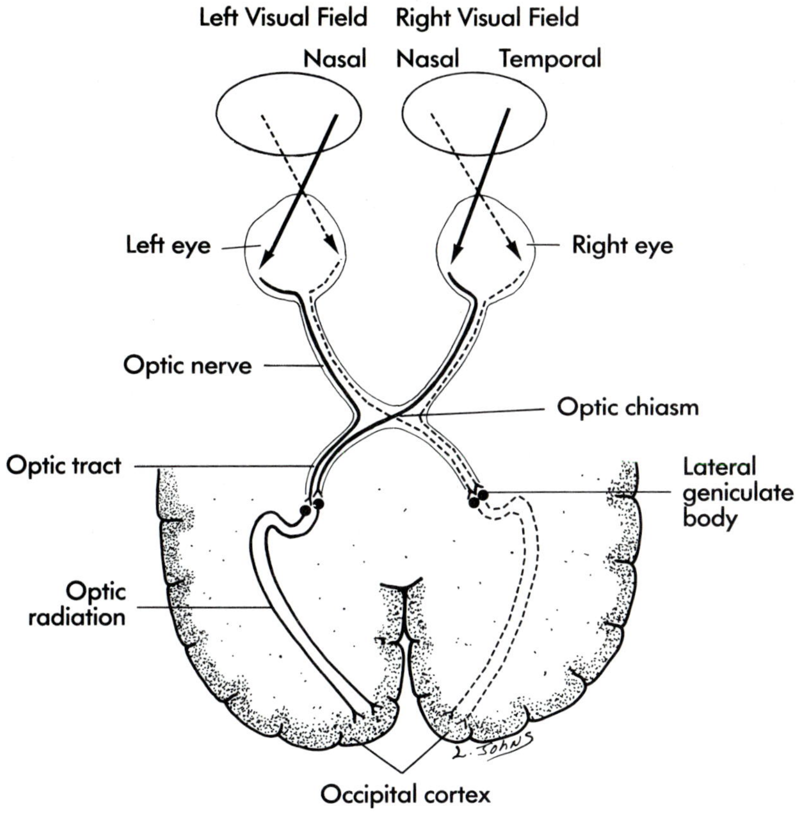

Fig. 10-7 The visual pathway: information is transmitted from the receptor organs (the eyes) to the sensory cortex.

Dendritic processes from the ganglion cells of cranial nerve VIII, the *vestibulocochlear (acoustic) nerve*, receive auditory information from the organ of Corti and transmit it to *cochlear nuclei* in the pons and medulla. These nuclei send out fibers, some of which cross to the other side of the medulla. (Vestibular information is carried in the same nerve from the ear to the brainstem but terminates in the vestibular nuclei of the pons and medulla.) Ascending axons from the cochlear nuclei send signals that eventually terminate in the *medial geniculate nucleus* of the thalamus, then to the primary auditory cortex, or Brodman's areas 41 and 42 (Fig. 10-5). The auditory association cortex interprets the meaning of sounds and is represented by area 22, with some input at areas 39 and 40 as well.

The Differences between Left and Right Cerebral Hemispheres

It was not until the late 1960s that anatomic asymmetries in the brain between the left and right temporal speech areas were reported (Geschwind and Levitsky, 1968). In one study, a central nervous system depressant (sodium amytal) was injected into either the right or left cerebral circulation while subjects were tested for language function. Research found that only 4% of right-handed and 15% of left-handed subjects had speech centers in the right hemisphere (Rasmussen and Milner,

1977). Interestingly, the same experiments yielded information about mood. Brief depression followed left hemisphere sodium amytal injection and brief euphoria followed injection into the right brain circulation.

Another experiment studying the recognition of emotional tone and content revealed that the two hemispheres extracted different aspects of the same stimulus, depending on whether it was presented to the right ear or to the left ear. Subjects wearing headphones listened to sentences being read in different emotional tones. The subjects were told to attend to a specific ear. It was concluded that the left ear (from which many fibers project to the right hemisphere) was superior to the right ear at recognizing emotional intonation of speech. The right ear (which projects to the left brain), as expected, had an advantage for recognition of verbal content of speech (Ley and Bryden, 1982). This study looked only at recognition, not *expression* of emotion.

The right hemisphere is involved to a greater extent than the left in integrating sensory input necessary to sustain postures (Mills and DiGenio, 1983). This may account for the difficulties some patients with right brain damage have in maintaining an erect sitting posture.

Another function that is weighted more heavily toward the right hemisphere is that of attention. It is this phenomenon that will be described in greater detail in the section on the syndrome of neglect. Heilman and Van Den Abell (1980) performed electroencephalograms on 12 right-handed college students while presenting them with visual stimuli from the left and right visual fields. The findings revealed that the left brain attended to stimuli from the right visual field, while the right brain attended to stimuli from *both* the left and right fields. It was concluded that the right hemisphere appears to be dominant for attention.

The anatomic specialization of the left temporal lobe for language functions is well known. Similar anatomic asymmetries exist between the right and left parietal lobes in the human (Eidelberg and Galaburda, 1984). A specific region of the *right* inferior parietal lobe has rich connections to the medial limbic area (a system of cortical and subcortical structures playing a major role in memory, motivation, and affect). These connections are not as highly developed in the left parietal lobe. It has been proposed that when humans developed language, synaptic space in the left hemisphere became dedicated to language function. The right brain then used its analogous synaptic space to develop nonlinguistic skills, such as spatial awareness and attention. Some perceptual capacity remained in the left hemisphere from residual synaptic space present before language developed (Mesulam, 1981).

The extent to which certain functions are lateralized within the brain is presented in Table 10-1. Cerebral functions are categorized as lower (somatic sensation and strength), middle (language interpretation, praxis, and perception), and higher (intellect, comprehension, information processing rate, and concentration). The lower level functions are strongly lateralized to the opposite limbs from very discrete cortical sites (the pre- and postcentral gyri). Refer once again to the sensory homunculus (Fig. 10-6). The middle cerebral level, with probable representation in the parietal lobes, differs in that it has bilateral functions influencing both lower-level hemispheres. There appears to be partial lateralization of function at this level. Language and praxis are weighted toward the left brain; visuospatial and tactile perception are weighted toward the right brain. The higher-level functions are diffusely represented, with no apparent lateralization between the hemispheres (Jones and others, 1989).

Depending on the extent of the insult, damage to the right hemisphere, then, has a high probability of affecting sensation and motor function in the left body. Perceptual problems are more likely to result than language problems. And alterations in intellect and concentration would be no more likely to occur from right brain damage than left brain damage. In right-handed individuals, the left hemisphere is usually considered the *dominant* hemisphere because of its specializations in the socially important functions of language and calculations.

Table 10-1 Lateralization of function within the brain

Level of function	Example of function	Lateralization
Higher	Intellect Compre-hension	None/Low
Middle	Language Perception	Moderate
Lower	Sensation Movement	High

Stroke

As described elsewhere in this book, the blood supply to the brain is fed from either the anterior (carotid) system or the posterior (vertebrobasilar) system. Each lobe receives blood from more than one major vessel. The parietal lobe is fed largely from the middle and anterior cerebral arteries.

Stroke occurs when the blood supply to a region of the brain is compromised and collateralization is either inadequate or unavailable. Strokes are of two types: infarcts and hemorrhages. Infarcts are twice as common, usually larger, and tend to affect more cortical grey matter than hemorrhages, which are often deep in the subcortical white matter of descending motor tracts. For these reasons, perceptual deficits from hemorrhagic strokes tend to be less common and show faster recovery than those from infarcts (Hier et al, 1983). The overall prevalence of perceptual deficits is not reliably known because of inconsistency in assessment and identification of certain deficits. Perceptual deficits are known to be much more prevalent following right hemisphere damage. Stroke is the most frequent cause of perceptual disorders (Anton, 1988).

SENSORY ALTERATIONS

Impaired Peripheral Sensation

Any or all of the classic modalities of vibration, pain, warmth, cold, pressure, and position sense are vulnerable to vascular insult at any level along the cerebral sensory pathway. Most of the sensory changes seen in stroke occur after damage to the fibers between the thalamus and the sensory cortex. While sensory changes are usually contralateral to the lesion, it has been reported that the right hemisphere is dominant for sensorimotor functioning of both sides of the body (Hom and Reitan, 1982). Sensory loss is often incomplete because of the multiple pathways carrying information to the cortex. However, if the lesion is large enough, most tactile sensibilities can be lost. Smaller subcortical lesions can also have a major effect on peripheral sensation. Two cases illustrate the range of effects stroke can have on sensation.

One is the case of a pure sensory stroke resulting from a small right pontine infarct. The pons is a brainstem structure through which motor and sensory fibers travel between the spinal cord and the cerebral cortex. The patient had numbness and tingling of the left side of the body, and diminished vibration and joint position sense. Pain and temperature were preserved, as were motor power and cognitive function (Hommel and others, 1989). The dorsal column–medial lemniscal system carries the affected stimuli (Fig. 10-3) crossing over in the lower brainstem (see earlier section on ascending sensory pathways). A less common sensory experience is that of a patient who developed unilateral pruritis following a right hemisphere stroke (Shapiro and Braun, 1987). While the hemiparesis and hemianesthesia gradually improved, a left-sided pruritis remained. Itch is believed to be transmitted via the pain and temperature pathways.

Functional effects. The patient who has lost pain and temperature sensibility is at risk of cutaneous injury. Loss of joint position sense can increase the risk of falls in the patient who does not adequately compensate with visual awareness of joint position. The loss of peripheral sensation can interfere with testing for other perceptual deficits. In the patient with a visual deficit, an additional tactile deficit precludes compensation by touch, leaving the patient at a distinct environmental disadvantage.

Assessment. Sensory changes are detected by bedside examination of the patient's responses to pinprick over various dermatomes (pain), gentle contact with a dull object or examiner's finger over same regions (light touch), and a vibrating tuning fork placed on distal bony prominences (vibration). Joint position sense is tested by having the patient, without looking, tell the examiner whether the toe (or finger) is being moved up or down. Testing for temperature awareness is usually unnecessary because these fibers are carried in the same tracts as pain fibers.

Treatment. Treatments that enhance peripheral sensory function are incorporated into therapies for perceptual deficits and will be discussed in the appropriate sections that follow.

Central Pain

On rare occasions, stroke patients will complain of severe spontaneous shooting pain, coldness, burning, or other vague but extremely unpleasant sensations (Kelly, 1985). There is an apparent physiologic "overreaction" to painful stimuli. The condition was first studied in patients who had lesions of the lateral thalamus. Motor deficits were also present in this series. Then, it was termed *thalamic pain syndrome*. Similar sensory changes are occasionally reported in neurosurgery patients who have undergone resection at various points along the nociceptor (pain and temperature) pathway, ironically, for the relief of chronic pain. Patients describe the pain as unlike anything they have ever experienced. There is often a strong emotional component to the pain. The condition, now known as *central pain*, can persist for years and can be refractory to treatment.

PERCEPTUAL ALTERATIONS

The major deficits to be examined are hemianopia, agnosias, apraxias, and neglect syndrome. Although presented here as separate entities, these deficits rarely occur in isolation from one another or from other sequelae of stroke. In fact, there is considerable variability in the literature regarding the classifications and even the definitions of many of the deficits.

Hemianopia

In hemianopia, one half of the visual field is missing. When it is the same half of each eye, it is known as *homonymous hemianopia* (HH). The patient sees only one half of his environment and may blame it on the eye on that side. For instance, if the patient cannot detect objects from his left visual field, he may assume his left eye is blind. In testing with alternate eyes closed, however, the field cut is perceived through *each* eye. A vascular lesion posterior to the optic chiasm, from the optic tract to the occipital cortex, can cause HH.

Functional effects. Although loss can occur in either hemisphere, the effects of left field loss are usually more significant because of the frequently concurrent left side neglect. Left side neglect is a phenomenon of inattention to the left side of the environment, regardless of visual ability. The effects of neglect are covered elsewhere. Even in the absence of neglect, hemianopia can pose a slight safety risk, and initially it can interfere with dressing, walking, and other ADLs, but it can be well compensated through education.

Assessment. Confrontation testing of visual fields (so named because the examiner "confronts" the patient face to face at close range) is the most common method of identifying HH. The patient is instructed to keep his eyes on the examiner's nose and report the minute he sees the examiner's finger or pen enter his field of vision. Or, the patients must count the total number of fingers the examiner is holding up. The examiner must ensure all fields are tested. Failure to recognize the object in one half of the visual field, with each eye tested separately, represents HH.

Treatment. Routinely used objects should be placed in the affected field of vision to encourage scanning past midline. Scanning is the conscious effort by the patient to rotate his head toward the affected (blind) side until objects from that side become visible within the intact field of vision. If, however, the patient cannot compensate, independence is enhanced with placement of objects in the intact field of vision. Patients with both left HH and neglect are extremely resistant to learning compensation techniques because of the lack of awareness of and attention to the left side. During the first few weeks following stroke, most patients experience substantial neurological improvement from initial hemianopia.

AGNOSIAS

The term *agnosia* derives from the Greek *gnosis*, or knowledge. Thus the literal translation of agnosia is "to be without knowledge." Agnosias are deficits in the ability to recognize previously familiar objects perceived by one or more of the senses, primarily vision, proprioception, audition, and tactile awareness. To accurately diagnose an agnosia, the patient must be alert, have no cognitive deficit, and have normal acuity of the involved sense. Visual, auditory, and tactile agnosias are described here. Agnosias dealing with body image will be covered in the section on the neglect syndrome.

Visual Agnosia

Visual agnosia is the inability to recognize an object by sight. *Prosopagnosia* (from the Greek *prosopon*, meaning "face") is a rare form of visual agnosia in which the ability to recognize both previously known and newly learned faces is lost. The syndrome is unique because the patient does not recognize certain members within a class. He may know he is looking at a building but be unable to recognize its facade as different from another. (For interesting reading, read Oliver Sacks' "The Man Who Mistook His Wife for a Hat" (1985), which describes a prosopagnosic patient.) The lesions causing prosopagnosia are thought to be the visual association cortices of *both* hemispheres. In other words, there is bilateral damage (Damasio, 1985). *Color agnosia* is another form of visual agnosia in which the patient cannot pick out a color on command but can identify that two objects are the same color. This lesion is more predominant in the left hemisphere, occipital lobe (Siev and others, 1986).

Tactile Agnosia

Also known as *astereognosis*, tactile agnosia is the inability to recognize objects or forms by touch even though tactile, proprioceptive, and thermal functions remain intact. When differences in material quality (e.g., rough or smooth) cannot be recognized by touch, it is called *ahylognosia*. Parietal lobe damage to either hemisphere can cause this deficit.

Auditory Agnosia

Recognition of the differences in sounds (words or other sounds) is impaired in auditory agnosia. The patient hears the sound but does not know what it means. A telephone ringing would not be differentiated from the sound of a dog barking. Hands clapping together may sound the same as words being spoken. This is different from Wernicke's aphasia, in which the patient cannot make sense of the spoken word (See Chapter 11), but recognizes the differences among speech, telephone ringing, dog barking, and so on. The patient with auditory agnosia, unlike the patient with Wernicke's aphasia, should be able to comprehend the *written* word because his language function remains intact. There is considerable controversy about the site of lesion producing auditory agnosia; the nondominant temporal lobe seems most likely (Benson, 1979).

Functional Effects. Clearly, ADLs will be more difficult for the patient with agnosias. The patient essentially loses the use of one of his senses, so he is required to learn many of the adaptive strategies employed by the blind or deaf. For example, the visually agnosic patient has to learn to identify objects by touch, smell, and sound. Agnosic patients may be mistakenly labeled as demented and not given full rehabilitation opportunity. Fortunately, pure agnosias are quite rare but, when combined with other effects of stroke, they can make life very difficult.

Assessment. To test for *visual agnosia,* the patient is shown several objects (including pictures of familiar faces) and asked to identify the named object and explain or demonstrate its use. The diagnosis can be made only if the patient has intact vision yet requires tactile or auditory input to identify the object. Testing for *auditory agnosia* is difficult because the patient may not understand directions unless they are written or gestured. Have the patient close his eyes and then tell you what sounds he hears as you clap your hands, whistle, or knock on a door. *Tactile agnosia* is easily tested at the bedside. With the patient's eyes closed, have him identify familiar objects as they are placed in his hand. Having a patient tell you the denomination of a coin placed in his hand tests for *ahylognosia* as well because he must feel for smooth or rough edges of the coin. Because this test requires intact tactile sensation of the hands, it often cannot be used for major strokes.

Treatment. In general, treatments routinely include training to compensate via preserved functions. The art of therapy lies in encouraging enough compensation to improve safety and quality of life without discouraging rehabilitation of the affected mode. Many of the treatment strategies proposed are based on theoretic constructs and have not undergone empiric testing. Conclusions cannot be drawn for treatment efficacy in those cases. Nurses can incorporate many of these strategies when assisting the patient in ADLs.

In attempts to stimulate new learning, the patient with visual agnosia is drilled about familiar objects, photographs, and colors. For patients with auditory agnosia, auditory drills are sometimes employed by SLPs, but response to treatment is poor. For patients with tactile agnosia, a sensory integrative approach stimulates touch and pressure receptors. One strategy is to vigorously rub the back of the affected hand, fingers, and forearm, and the ventral surface of the affected fingers with a rough cloth (Siev and others, 1986). As with visual agnosia, drills using various textures are considered effective.

APRAXIAS

The Greek derivative of apraxia is *prax*, meaning to do, to work, or to accomplish. Apraxia, also called *dyspraxia*, is the failure to perform either skilled or nonhabitual motor patterns in the presence of adequate muscle power, coordination, and sensation (Wyness, 1985). Four types of apraxia will be discussed: ideomotor, ideational, constructional, and dressing apraxias. Often, more than one apraxia is present. All are considered perceptual deficits frequently caused by stroke. The lesion is not necessarily confined to the right hemisphere. Left parietal damage can cause bilateral apraxia (Critchley, 1966). The suspected mechanism is a severing of connections between the site of formulation of a motor act and the motor association areas responsible for its execution.

Ideomotor and Ideational Apraxia

The patient who suffers from *ideomotor apraxia* fully understands the concept of the required motor task (i.e., he can describe and recognize it) but is unable to perform the act when asked. The problem lies in motor planning, the patient having lost the skilled sequence of movement. Because the kinesthetic memory patterns are preserved the patient may intermittently perform the act spontaneously. In *ideational apraxia*, the patient no longer comprehends the concept of the act so is unable to perform it either on command *or* spontaneously. She can no longer relate the words and visual imagery to a motor task and consequently is unable even to describe the act. The dominant (usually left) parietal lobe is the usual lesion site for both apraxias.

Constructional Apraxia

Constructional apraxia is an impairment in producing designs in two or three dimensions, whether by copying, drawing, or building. The deficit is present spontaneously and on command. The belief is that strokes to either hemisphere can result in constructional apraxia. Controversy exists about which hemisphere is dominant for this disorder. As will be described, its presentation differs slightly, depending upon the hemisphere. Patients with left-sided lesions may have aphasias that make testing difficult. They also are more likely to have lost use of their dominant (right) hand. Both of these conditions would preclude reliable testing. This type of apraxia, then, may just be more amenable to identification in the patient with right brain damage.

When present from right hemisphere damage, constructional apraxia is a disorder of spatial relations regardless of whether a visual field deficit is present. It appears that the patient lacks perspective about the exact location of a figure in space and the relationships of parts to one another. When asked to copy a simple drawing of a house, the patient with right brain damage may draw on the diagonal and make odd use of the space on the paper. The drawings are often quite complex but the pieces are not drawn in correct relation to one another. The front door, for example, may be found several inches away from the rest of the house (Fig. 10-8).

When present in patients with left hemisphere damage, there does not seem to be an associated spatial disturbance unless the patient *also* has a visual field cut. Instead, the disorder is one mostly of motor planning (Siev and others, 1986). The patients with left brain damage are more hesitant when starting the task and draw much more simplistic pictures than their cohorts with right brain damage (Fig. 10-8).

Dressing Apraxia

As its name implies, *dressing apraxia* is an inability to dress oneself even when motor power, coordination, and sensation are intact. Dressing apraxia is another disorder of spatial relations for both body parts and objects outside the body. It often occurs in the presence of constructional apraxia. The patient gets the orientation of clothes confused, putting items on inside out, backward, or upside down. There is often only gradual recognition of errors or no recognition at all. Lesions that cause dressing apraxia are commonly in the nondominant (usually right) hemisphere in the parietooccipital region.

Functional Effects. The apraxias are one of the least subtle causes of poor performance in ADLs. Obviously the patient with dressing apraxia cannot dress appropriately. Constructional apraxia has been associated with impairment in both dressing and grooming skills (Tsai and others, 1983). The inability to follow simple motor commands, as occurs in either ideational or ideomotor apraxia, is an obvious social handicap. As with the agnosias, the patient may present to the outside world as cognitively deficient.

Assessment. Though most testing is performed in occupational therapy, the nurse can observe and test patients on the unit during routine activities. To assess ideational and ideomotor apraxias, there are tests that grade responses to standardized commands by the therapist. Not all tests are sensitive enough to distinguish between the two apraxias. Constructional apraxia is screened by having the patient copy a two-dimensional figure, usually a house, clock face, or daisylike flower. One of these particular figures is chosen because each is simple and has enough symmetric components to act as a screening test for visual field deficit and neglect. If the drawing is abnormal, more complex, standardized tests may be implemented. Many of these tests use blocks to test three-dimensional abilities. Dressing apraxia is evaluated by asking the patient to remove, then to put on, his shirt and assessing the process and outcome.

Treatment. The basic component of treatment for ideational and ideomotor apraxias lies in practice that is supervised and encouraged by a skilled trainer. Nurses must ensure that the treatments they employ are consistent with physical and occupational therapies. The affected limb should be touched and moved as much as possible during a task to provide sensory feedback (Bobath, 1978). Many patients with limb apraxia should *not* have commands broken down into component steps. For example, the patient will find it easier to respond to "get up" than to the component commands of scooting forward, leaning, pushing against the bed, and, finally, standing up. This is because the former simple command allows the patient to respond on a more automatic level.

Have the patient with constructional apraxia practice copying designs. The temporary use of landmarks on the paper may help. Gradually in-

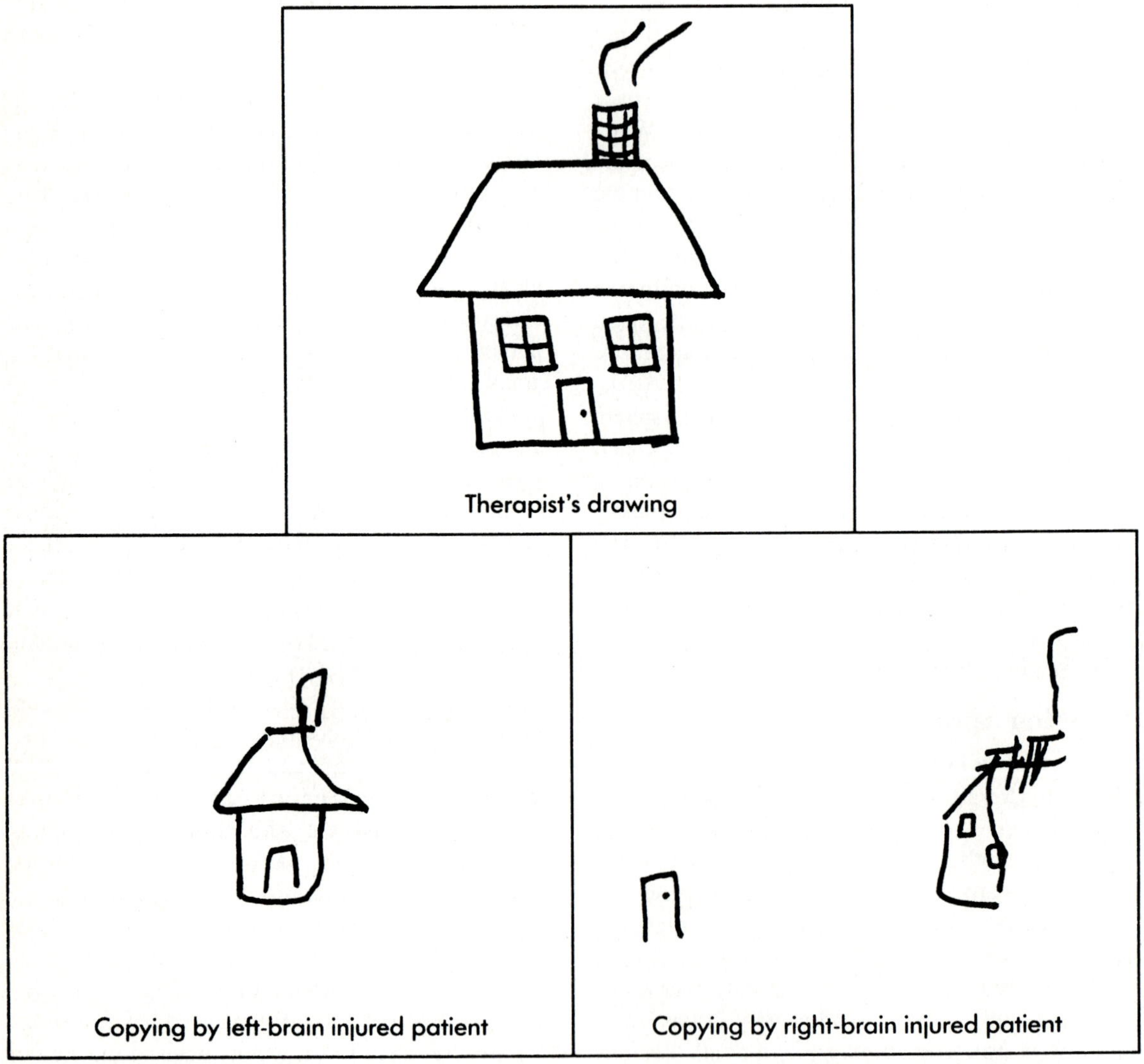

Fig. 10-8 Constructional apraxia. Differences in copying between left and right brain-injured patients.

crease the complexity or dimensions of the designs. Using other media besides paper and pencil will increase proprioceptive and kinesthetic input. Give the patient with dressing apraxia instructions and cognitive hints to make the task simpler. For instance, the patient can be taught correct initial placement of the clothing on the bed or her lap. Labels can be used to distinguish right side from wrong side. The fewer the manipulations of the garment, the better. Nurses can play an active role in the treatment and assessment of apraxias.

NEGLECT SYNDROME

Neglect of a portion of space or body is common following stroke, especially when the stroke involves the *right* cerebral hemisphere. It is a disorder of attention. Although neglect is thought to negatively affect rehabilitation outcome (Booth, 1982), problems of definition and assessment are hampering progress toward treatment of this disorder. Unilateral neglect, extinction, anosognosia, and somatognosia are disorders of attention that comprise the *neglect syndrome*.

Unilateral Neglect

Also called hemiinattention, left neglect, or hemineglect, or simply neglect, unilateral neglect (UN) is the inability to integrate and use perceptions from the left side of the body and/or the left side of the environment (Siev and others, 1986). It is an entity distinct from a visual field cut (such as hemianopia, which is previously described), although visual field cuts often accompany and compound the effects of unilateral neglect. Occurrence of UN is much more frequent after right hemisphere damage, as is explained in the anatomy of neglect section. Reliable figures on the occurrence of unilateral neglect are not available.

To the observer who has never before witnessed it, UN is an intriguing phenomenon. The patient will ignore the left, paralyzed half of his body while performing ADLs such as dressing and hygiene; e.g., the patient will stop after putting the right arm through the sleeve or shave only the right half of his face. If his UN involves hemispatial and hemibody inattention, he may ignore food on the left side of the plate, and words on the left side of a page.

Neglect of the left environment may also translate into errors on drawing and copying tasks. (Some authors believe neglect in drawing is not related to hemibody or hemispace neglect [Hier and others, 1983]). Much of the left side of a figure is omitted and the drawing may be positioned too far to the right of the page (Fig. 10-9). This differs from constructional apraxia, in which spatial relations are globally impaired (Fig. 10-8).

There is a wide spectrum of severity of neglect. Some authors consider them distinct types. In the more severe cases, it is not uncommon to find the wheelchair-bound, left hemiplegic patient bumping into walls on his left side as he wheels along a corridor. Peripheral sensory loss precludes the normal protective mechanisms afforded by tactile input. The patient is rarely concerned about injury to his left side and may even deny there is a problem with that side. (Denial of this type will be discussed separately.) In severe neglect, auditory, visual, and tactile stimuli may be ignored on the left. Prevalence data is unreliable because of problems with testing and defining neglect.

Extinction

Extinction is the phenomenon of inattention to a stimulus on the affected side when simultaneously presented with a similar stimulus on the unaffected side. Extinction can be visual, auditory, or tactile. For instance, when touched on the hands by the examiner, the patient with his eyes closed reports only the touch to the unaffected hand. This, of course, is a valid test only if the patient has intact tactile sensation on both hands. While the definition of extinction is clear cut, there is some controvery about how it fits into the neglect syndrome. Some consider extinction a mild form of neglect, while others consider extinction the primary deficit, with neglect being an extreme variant,

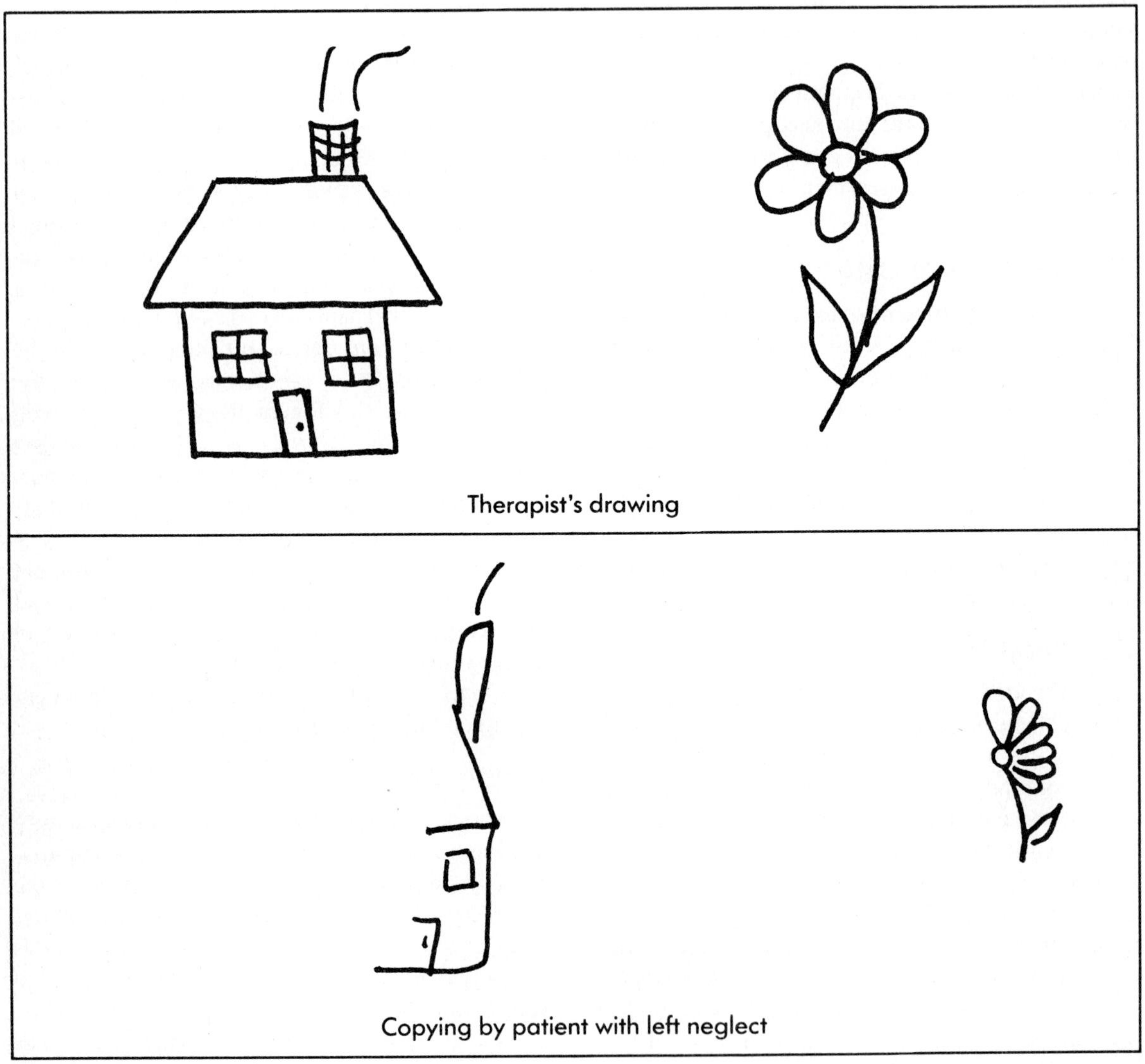

Fig. 10-9 Left neglect.

and still others consider the two as altogether separate entities (Hier and others, 1983). Most favor the first view.

Anosognosia

It was Babinski who coined the term *anosognosia* to describe a patient's unawareness of hemiplegia. Anosognosia is now considered by many to be a severe form of hemibody neglect. In its mildest form, there is simple unconcern for the paralysis, a phenomenon known as *anosodiaphoria*. Frequently, however, the patient adamantly denies the existence of paralysis. When challenged to the contrary, he makes vague excuses for his affected limbs (e.g., "That arm never did work too well."). The term *anosognosia* is usually applied to the denial phenomenon (Fisher, 1989). In its extreme form the patient denies ownership of the affected limb and may even be frightened by the sight of his own leg in bed. Patients have been known to attempt to push this "unknown" leg off the bed.

Somatognosia

Somatognosia is a body scheme disturbance in which the patient is unaware of his body structure and the relationship of its parts to each other (*soma* meaning body and *agnosia* meaning without knowledge). A patient so affected may confuse the sides of his body or may think the examiner's arm is his own. The lesion site is usually the parietal lobe of the dominant hemisphere.

The Anatomy of Neglect

Neglect is more frequent and severe following lesions to the right hemisphere. Recalling the earlier anatomy section of right-left brain differences, the right hemisphere was shown to assume the greater role in attention. Left hemisphere damage *can* result in right hemiinattention, but in most people the right hemisphere will compensate by increasing attention to the right. Compensation by the left hemisphere for left inattention is rare. Mesulam (1981) proposed a cortical network for directed attention and unilateral neglect. A summary of his concepts will aid in understanding the anatomy of neglect.

Lesions to the right inferior parietal lobe are frequent findings in cases of left neglect. However, attention is actually a function of an *integrated network* of four cerebral regions, each with its unique functional role. One of the four systems is the *reticular formation* in the brainstem, which functions as a first level arousal mechanism. A *limbic system* component attaches a motivational drive to the perception of external stimuli. A third component is the *frontal cortex*, where motor planning for eye movements (scanning, exploring, fixating) takes place. And the fourth component is the *posterior parietal cortex*, which acts as an "internal sensory map," integrating input through extensive synaptic connections between primary and association cortex (Mesulam, 1981).

Damage at any level of the four regions will yield a distinct form of neglect. Additionally, there does not appear to be a master center for neglect. Rather, a constellation of centers is more accurate (Vallar and Perani, 1986). Neglect has even been reported from right hemispheric thalamic strokes (Ferro and others, 1987). The anatomic substrate for neglect is diffuse and quite complex.

Functional Effects. In general, the neglect syndromes of unilateral neglect, extinction, anosognosia, and somatognosia have common functional effects. Patients cannot protect themselves from injury when they ignore stimuli from one side of their environment. The indifference to and/or denial of paralysis can lead to falls as the anosognosic patient tries to walk on his own. Perhaps the most significant impact of neglect, especially anosognosia, is that of hindrance to the patient's rehabilitation.

Assessment. There is no established standard for the accurate assessment of unilateral neglect. Bedside examination usually relies on confrontation tests such as described for HH. Therein lies the inaccuracy. The nonneglecting hemianopic patient will respond the same as the nonhemianopic patient with neglect. Drawing tests are often done in occupational therapy to identify a neglect, but some authors do not consider unilateral neglect on drawing to be true neglect (Hier and others, 1983).

There are many standardized tests available. Some involve bisecting lines or copying figures. Others require the patient to find and cancel all stars, lines, or capital letters from a maze of other figures. Scientific comparison of several of these tests was examined by Halligan and others (1989) who believed that the star cancellation test was the most sensitive indicator of visuospatial neglect. A sensitive computerized test of neglect and extinction has been described in the literature (Anton and others, 1988).

Extinction is tested by double simultaneous stimulation. The test for tactile extinction was mentioned earlier. In brief, the examiner simultaneously touches both hands of the patient, whose eyes are closed. The patient with tactile extinction will report only one hand being touched. The patient must have intact peripheral sensation in order to make this a valid test. Visual extinction can be assessed by confrontational testing, as described for hemianopia and neglect, but these two syndromes must be ruled out before a reliable diagnosis of extinction is made. Auditory extinction is not routinely tested but would require the patient to identify the source of a noise (e.g., finger snapping) when presented simultaneously to both ears.

There is no formal test for anosognosia. If the patient verbalizes his denial of obvious paralysis, the diagnosis is made. Otherwise, careful observation of the patient is necessary, especially as he performs his ADLs. This makes it a condition readily amenable to nursing assessment. Somatognosia is usually tested in occupational therapy by means of standardized tests that require the patient to point to body parts, answer questions about the interrelationships of body parts, or draw human figures.

Treatment. The principle of treatment of unilateral neglect and extinction is to encourage attention to the affected side through visual and tactile stimuli. Sitting at the patient's affected side will encourage attention to that side. The patient is instructed to watch himself as he touches his affected arm or leg with a rough cloth and even ice, if spasticity is not a problem. The patient also should move his arm through ROM exercises, using his unaffected hand. As is true for treatment of many perceptual deficits, the patient can practice with some of the standardized evaluation tests. Forced attention to the affected side is considered the best therapy for unilateral neglect. As always, compensation through visual scanning and other cues must be taught. Once again, communication among the treating professionals is mandatory to efficient team treatment.

The nature of anosognosia precludes any positive response to treatment. Keeping the anosognosic patient motivated for therapies in the face of his denial of disability is one of the greatest rehabilitation challenges. Therapies for somatognosia focus on the association of strong sensory input (usually tactile) with naming and movement of the body part. Drilling the patient on body relations is useful. Tasks requiring both hands or feet encourage normal movement and awareness of body parts.

OTHER BEHAVIORAL-PERCEPTUAL CONSEQUENCES OF STROKE

Many types of stroke-related disorders of behavior and perception have not been covered; selected definitions are presented in the box on p. 191.

ASSESSMENT

Many of the formal tests that diagnose the various perceptual disorders are conducted in the setting of occupational therapy. Nurses, however, are the only professionals who routinely observe the patient's abilities in dressing, undressing, washing, grooming, eating, toileting, and transferring 24 hours per day.

Assessments tend to have a greater sense of realism when performed outside of the clinical therapy area. For instance, an apraxic patient may have success in therapy with dressing but lose the ability

OTHER BEHAVIORAL-PERCEPTUAL CONSEQUENCES OF STROKE

Abulia: Extreme apathy seen following anterior cerebral artery stroke.

Agitated confusional state: Hyperactivity, restlessness, and easy distractibility associated with stroke to the inferior branch of the right MCA, the mirror area for Wernicke's aphasia in the left hemisphere (Caplan and others, 1986).

Allesthesia: Perception that stimuli delivered to the affected side was delivered to the unaffected side.

Anton's syndrome: Also called cortical blindness, this is a form of neglect in which the patient denies blindness.

Aprosodia: Lack of awareness of affective quality of speech; emotional aspect.

Autotopagnosia: An agnosia for body part recognition.

Figure ground deficit: The inability to distinguish the foreground from the background.

Form constancy deficit: The inability to recognize subtle variations in form (e.g., the difference between a water pitcher and a urinal).

Hemiakinesia: Failure to move the affected limb due to hemiinattention.

Impulsivity: The tendency to act quickly without forethought and without concern for safety, seen commonly in right-brain injured patients.

Motor impersistence: Failure to persist at motor tasks, such as eye closure.

Multi-infarct dementia: Stepwise deterioration in higher mental capacities as the result of multiple small strokes over time.

Right-Left disorientation: The inability to discriminate between right and left.

Simultanagnosia: A rare spatial analysis deficit in which the patient is unable to make meaning of an image in its entirety and sees and understands only a small fraction at a time. The patient literally cannot see the forest for the trees.

Topographic disorientation: Difficulty understanding and remembering relationships of places to one another; gets lost easily.

when trying the same task in the hospital room. Clothes laid out on the hospital bed may be more difficult to get to if there is little room to maneuver a chair next to the bed. Bedsheets may even be mistaken for, or obscure, clothes that are laid out. The patient with figure ground disorder is particularly affected if the color of the clothes is similar to that of the bedspread or sheets. If the patient is sitting on the bed, his balance may be affected by the softness in the mattress and the height of the bed precluding firm foot placement on the floor.

The nurse's assessment of the patient's performance in ADLs, especially eating, is often the first appreciation of neglect in the acute stages of stroke. The nurse will notice that the patient ate from only one half of the tray, or that he neglected to wipe food from one half of his face. As has already been mentioned, there is no established standard for the assessment of neglect. The patient will receive more formal testing in occupational therapy, but an ongoing responsibility of the nurse is to assess improvement and share this with the team.

To assess for tactile sensory loss, the nurse can use the techniques described in the earlier section on impaired peripheral sensation. It is not necessary from a nursing perspective to test vibratory sense, but joint position sense, which is carried in the same pathway as vibration, should be tested. Knowing whether a patient has a sense of joint position will aid in planning transfers and other ADLs.

The box above lists some other perceptual consequences of stroke. Some of these disorders are quite rare and may require sensitive standardized tests to identify them. However, many of these deficits can adversely affect a patient's performance of ADLs. The patient who frequently loses his way around the unit may have a topographical disorientation. A patient with form constancy deficit may mistakenly attempt to urinate into his water pitcher instead of the urinal. The agitated or impulsive patient may make unsafe transfers.

It is critical that nurses assume the responsibility of accurate assessment of their patients' problems so that appropriate early referrals are made and ongoing progress is measured. Sound assessments will dictate the best therapeutic interventions.

INTERVENTIONS

Several nursing diagnoses can be applied to the patient who suffers from sensory or perceptual deficits. Those that best address sensory loss, apraxia, agnosia, and neglect are (1) sensory/perceptual alterations: tactile, (2) unilateral neglect, and (3) alteration in visual-spatial relationships. Because the interventions for each of these diagnoses are directed at improving self-care and developing compensatory behaviors, a separate diagnosis of self-care deficit is not required. A sample nursing care plan for these three diagnoses follows on p. 194.

Sensory/Perceptual Alterations: Tactile

Stroke can affect a patient's ability to feel touch, pain, or temperature sensations because of a lesion along the sensory pathway to the cortex. The patient is at risk of cutaneous injury. If there is a concomitant hemineglect, it will require close nursing supervision to ensure that the patient does not injure herself. Nursing interventions for sensory loss include daily skin inspection to identify injury that may have gone unnoticed by the patient. Education of both the patient and family on safety practices is essential. When assisting with ADLs, especially bathing, the nurse should rub the affected skin with a cloth, her hand, or even the patient's good hand to stimulate sensory awareness. Motor function is also thought to be stimulated by sensory (especially postural) input and forms the basis for treatments using the Bobath technique (Bobath, 1978).

Unilateral Neglect

Most nurses who have worked on neurology, medical, and rehabilitation units have encountered the right brain–damaged patient who neglects both his left body and the left environmental space around him. When neglect of space and body is accompanied by any one of anosognosia, hemianopia, and tactile sensory loss, the patient is severely deprived of environmental and proprioceptive stimuli.

Nursing management of neglect must be communicated to the rest of the team. It is important that approaches are consistent between therapy and the nursing unit. Except for the use of standardized tests, nursing can implement any of the strategies suggested under treatment of unilateral neglect. The nurse should encourage the carryover of skills learned in therapy while assisting the patient with ADLs. Two valuable and often overlooked nursing contributions to a patient's rehabilitation are the reinforcement of learned skills and the modification of certain skills for environments outside the therapy areas. Patient and family education are a major part of the nurse's interventions.

Alterations in Visual-Spatial Relationships

Dressing and contructional apraxia constitute two of the most common disorders of visual-spatial relationships. Both cause significant limitations to independence in ADLs, especially when using skilled motor acts, such as those required for dressing. If ideational apraxia is also present, the patient will have additional deficits in hygiene and grooming.

Nursing interventions are many. In most cases, because the patient tends to encounter in his hospital room obstacles similar to those that he will encounter at home, the nurse is in an ideal position to conduct on the spot problem-solving education. Nurses can also provide valuable family education that can often be scheduled, or conducted spontaneously, more easily in the evening hours. Specific techniques for aiding the apraxic patient with ADLs are included in the nursing care plan on p. 194.

Nursing management of the stroke patient who suffers from sensory and perceptual deficits can be challenging. A sound knowledge of the anatomy and pathophysiology of the apraxias, agnosias, and neglect provide the basis for developing treatment strategies and research questions. Research into the sensitivity of nursing assessments of perceptual deficits can be conducted. Results may contribute to the development of standardized nursing assessment tools. Investigations that evaluate patients' responses to some of the nursing interventions mentioned earlier may introduce new findings applicable to many disciplines. In short, nursing research in the area of stroke-related sensory and perceptual alterations will make significant contributions to the science of stroke rehabilitation.

NURSING CARE PLAN

Nursing Diagnosis	Interventions	Expected Outcomes
Sensory/Perceptual Alterations (Tactile) related to altered sensory transmission and/or integration **Defining Characteristics** ■ Inability to discriminate various tactile sensations (e.g., pain, touch, joint position)	**Ongoing Assessment** ■ Assess patient's ability to sense light touch ■ Assess patient's ability to feel pinprick ■ Using patient's toes or fingers, assess ability to sense joint position ■ Check for hypersensitivity reactions **Therapeutic Interventions** ■ Perform regular skin inspections ■ Provide tactile stimulation to affected limbs using rough cloth or hand ■ Explain how the stimulus might feel (e.g., cool water, soft flannel) ■ Regularly move affected limbs ■ Enhance environment for optimum safety (e.g., improve lighting, remove sharp objects)	■ Patient and family will demonstrate skill in therapeutic interventions ■ Patient's skin remains free from injuries, including pressure ulcers ■ Patient will use learned compensatory methods

NURSING CARE PLAN — cont'd

Nursing Diagnosis	Interventions	Expected Outcomes
Unilateral neglect related to effects of disturbed perceptual abilities **Defining Characteristics:** ■ Consistent inattention to stimuli on affected side ■ Self care impaired (e.g., only washes half of face, leaves half of food on plate, dresses half of body) ■ Judgment appears impaired (e.g., no regard for safety of affected limbs) ■ May leave off half of figure when drawing ■ May not hear sounds as well from affected side ■ Has difficulty reading missing words from left of paper	**Ongoing Assessment** ■ Conduct sensory assessment (see preceding nursing diagnosis) ■ Perform visual fields confrontation test (i.e., nurse instructs patient to stare at her nose and report which hand is moving; nurse holds hands at different positions in patient's field of vision, randomly moves one hand or the other) ■ Observe patient's performance of ADL; note if dressing half of body, leaving half of food on plate ■ Observe patient's response to sounds from affected side ■ Conduct paper drawing test (e.g., instruct patient to draw a clock) ■ Observe for remarks of denial of hemiplegia (anosognosia) ■ Have patient point to various body parts (somatognosia) ■ Assess safety practices **Therapeutic Interventions** Acute phase (first 2 or 3 days only) ■ Approach patient from unaffected side ■ Ensure safe environment with call bell on unaffected side ■ Do not overestimate patient's abilities ■ Provide tactile stimulation to affected side ■ Place food in small quantities, arranged simply on plate Rehabilitation phase (ongoing) ■ Provide tactile stimulation to affected side (see above) ■ Approach patient from affected side, calling patient's name	■ Patient will incur no injuries ■ Patient will be able to cross midline with eyes and unaffected arm ■ Patient will observe and touch affected side during ADLs

Continued

NURSING CARE PLAN — cont'd

Nursing Diagnosis	Inteventions	Expected Outcomes
	■ Refer to affected side in conversation ■ Attach watch or bright bracelet to affected arm and encourage patient's attention to it ■ Place bright tape or shoelace on shoe covering affected extremity ■ Have patient touch affected side during ADLs ■ Offer olfactory stimulation (use of scented lotions on affected side of body) ■ Provide a mirror for visual cues with ADLs ■ Draw bright mark on left of paper when reading (gives cue to return for next line)	■ Patient will begin to wash, dress, and eat with attention to both sides ■ Patient will verbally acknowledge presence of hemiplegia

NURSING CARE PLAN — cont'd

Nursing Diagnosis	Interventions	Expected Outcomes
Alterations (visual-spatial) related to altered sensory reception, transmission, and/or integration **Defining Characteristics** ■ Inability to arrange objects in appropriate order ■ Inability to dress oneself (with intact motor system) ■ May get lost easily ■ Self care deficit (e.g., unable to use comb correctly, unable to wash face on request, unable to stand on request) ■ General inability to follow motor commands ■ Demonstrates right/left disorientation	**Ongoing Assessment** ■ Observe patient's skill in dressing ■ Observe patient's skill in performing other motor tasks, both spontaneously and on demand ■ Observe degree to which patient tends to confuse objects in space ■ Have patient copy house after observing nurse draw it (apraxic patient shows grossly distorted spatial relationships) ■ Have patient identify left and right **Therapeutic Interventions** ■ Provide time and supervision to practice dressing ■ Give cues to make dressing easier (e.g., have patient place shirt on lap in ready position) ■ Use labels to help identify correct side from wrong side of clothes ■ Have patient practice manipulating objects (e.g., pouring water into a glass) ■ Provide tactile stimulation to affected side ■ Do not give commands in component parts; instead give simple gross motor commands, such as "get up" (unless patient responds better otherwise) ■ Have patient practice drawing and copying figures ■ If patient has right/left disorientation, include commands referring to other cues (e.g., "Show me your *strong* left leg.")	■ Patient's dressing skills improve ■ Patient's other self-care skills improve ■ Patient is able to perform some tasks on command ■ Patient and family verbalize cognitive awareness of deficit

Continued

NURSING CARE PLAN — cont'd

Nursing Diagnosis	Interventions	Expected Outcomes

Patient Education

- Teach skin inspection
- Explain consequences of excess pressure on skin
- Teach patient to stimulate affected areas with unaffected hand
- Teach patient to check temperature of water with unaffected side before using (thermal screening)
- Teach compensatory strategies (e.g., patient must learn to look carefully at environment when planning activity to ensure safety; patient must learn to scan visual stimuli)
- Teach family therapeutic interventions
- Teach patient and family cognitive awareness of deficits
- Teach safety awareness
- Teach strategies to make dressing easier (e.g., laying out clothes on bed in orderly fashion)

REFERENCES

Anton HA, Hershler C, Lloyd P, and others: Visual neglect and extinction: a new test, Arch Phys Med Rehabil 69:1013, 1988.

Benson DF: Aphasia, alexia and agraphia, New York, 1979, Churchill Livingstone, Inc.

Bobath B: Adult hemiplegia, evaluation, and treatment, London, 1978, William Hennemann Medical Books, Ltd.

Booth K: The neglect syndrome, J of Neurosurg Nurs 14:38, 1982.

Caplan LR, Kelly M, Kase CS and others: Infarcts of the inferior division of the right middle cerebral artery: mirror image of Wernicke's aphasia, Neurology 36:1015, 1986.

Clark RG: Manter and Gatz's essentials of clinical neuroanatomy and neurophysiology, ed 5, Philadelphia, 1975, FA Davis, Co.

Critchley M: The parietal lobes, New York, 1966, Hafner Publishing Co.

Damasio AR: Disorders of complex visual processing: agnosias, achromatopsia, Balint's syndrome, and related difficulties of orientation and construction. In MM Mesulam: Principles of Behavioral Neurology Philadelphia, FA Davis Co., 1985.

Dannenbaum RM and Dykes RW: Sensory loss in the hand after sensory stroke: therapeutic rationale, Arch Phys Med Rehabil 69:833, 1988.

Eidelberg D and Galaburda AM: Inferior parietal lobule divergent architectonic asymmetries in the human brain, Arch Neurol 41:843, 1984.

Ferro JM, Kertesz A, and Black SE: Subcortical neglect: quantification, anatomy, and recovery, Neurology 37:1487, 1987.

Fisher CM: Neurologic fragments II: remarks on anosognosia, confabulation, memory, and other topics; and an appendix on self-observation, Neurology 39:127, 1989.

Geschwind N and Levitsky W: Human brain: left-right asymmetries in temporal speech region, Science 161:186, 1968.

Halligan PW, Marshall JC, and Wade DT: Visuospatial

neglect: underlying factors that test sensitivity, Lancet, 2:908, 1989.

Heilman KM and Van Den Abell T: Right hemisphere dominance for attention: the mechanism underlying hemispheric asymmetries of inattention (neglect), Neurology 30:327, 1980.

Hier DB, Mondlock J, and Caplan LR: Behavioral abnormalities after right hemisphere stroke, Neurology 33:337, 1983a.

Hier DB, Mondlock J, and Caplan LR: Recovery of behavioral abnormalities after right hemisphere stroke, Neurology 33:345, 1983b.

Hom J and Reitan RM: Effect on lateralized cerebral damage upon contralateral and ipsilateral sensorimotor performances, J Clin Neuropsychology 4:249, 1982.

Hommel M, Besson G, Pollack P, and others: Pure sensory stroke due to a pontine lacune, Stroke 20:406, 1989.

Jones RD, Donaldson IM, and Parkin PJ: Impairment and recovery of ipsilateral sensory-motor function following unilateral cerebral infarction, Brain 112:113, 1989.

Kaplan J and Hier DB: Visuospatial deficits after right hemisphere stroke, J Occup Ther 36:314, 1982.

Kelly DD: Central representations of pain and analgesia. In Kandel ER and Schwartz JH, editors: Principles of neural science, ed 2, New York, 1985, Elsevier Science Publishing Co., Inc.

Kupfermann I: Hemispheric asymmetries and the cortical localization of higher cognitive and affective functions, In Kandel ER and Schwartz JH editors: Principles of Neural Science, New York, 1985, Elsevier Sciences Publishing Co., Inc.

Ley RG and Bryden MP: A dissociation of right and left hemispheric effects for recognizing emotional tone and verbal content, Brain and Cognition 1:3, 1982.

Martin JH: Receptor physiology and submodality coding in the somatic sensory system, In Kandel ER and Schwartz JH, editors: Principles of neural science, ed 2, New York, 1985, Elsevier Science Publishing Co., Inc.

Mesulam MM: Principles of behavioral neurology, Philadelphia, 1985, FA Davis Co.

Mesulam MM: A cortical network for directed attention and unilateral neglect, Ann Neurol 10:309, 1981.

Mills VM and DiGenio M: Functional differences in patients with left or right cerebrovascular accidents, Phys Ther 63:481, 1983.

Rasmussen T and Milner B: The role of early left-brain injury in determining lateralization of cerebral speech functions, Ann New York Acad Sci 299:355, 1977.

Shapiro PE and Braun CW: Unilateral pruritus after a stroke, Arch Dermatol 123:1527, 1987.

Sacks O: The man who mistook his wife for a hat, and other clinical tales, New York, 1985, Harper & Row Publishers, Inc.

Siev E, Freishtat B, and Zoltan B: Perceptual and cognitive dysfunction in the adult stroke patient; a manual for evaluation and treatment, Thorofare, NJ, 1986, Slack, Inc.

Thomas CL, editor: Taber's cyclopedic medical dictionary, ed 15, Philadelphia, 1985, FA Davis Co.

Tsai LJ, Howe TH, and Lien IN: Visuospatial deficits in stroke patients and their relationship to dressing performance, J Formosan Med Assoc 82:353, 1983.

Vallar G and Perani D: The anatomy of unilateral neglect after right hemisphere stroke lesions: a clinical/CT scan correlation study in man, Neuropsychologia 24:609, 1986.

Wyness J: Perceptual dysfunction: nursing assessment and management, J Neurosurg Nurs 17:105, 1985.

Chapter 11

Alterations in Communication

Communication is a complex process that involves not only speech and language but also memory, reasoning, and emotions. A person's ability to communicate is crucial to any social interaction. Although nonverbal interaction plays a role, human communication is almost solely dependent on verbal interaction. Without the ability to adequately communicate, a person can be socially isolated.

Communication may not be impaired in every person with stroke. However, when communication impairments are present, the impairment can be catastrophic for the person and the family. To assist the nurse in the care of the person for whom stroke has resulted in a communication impairment, this chapter will clarify communication terms, review involved anatomy, describe assessment techniques and communication impairments, and discuss nursing interventions.

To understand communication impairment, the normal communication process must be understood. Communication involves a variety of functions, the two most prominent of which are language and speech. Language can be defined as the "symbolic formulation, vocal or graphic, of ideas according to semantic and grammatical rules for communication of thoughts and feelings." (Nicolisi and others, 1978). As the definition implies, language is learned and involves oral and written expression and auditory and reading comprehension. Language rules are initially acquired in the early years of life through passive exposure, assimilation, and trial and error. Refinement of basic language occurs during childhood, but language acquisition occurs throughout life.

Within this context, aphasia can be defined. *Aphasia* is the impairment of the ability to formulate or interpret language symbols. An acquired disorder, aphasia may affect any or all components of language, including expression and comprehension. Aphasia results from impairment of the language mechanism in the central nervous system. These mechanisms may be affected by a number of causes; one of the most common causes is stroke.

Speech, in contrast, is the "motor act of verbal expression" (Nicolisi and others, 1978) or the mechanical act of articulating language through the spoken word. Hence, speech is only one component of language. Two disorders of speech that may occur as a result of stroke are dysarthria and apraxia of speech. *Dysarthria* represents an alteration in speech sounds (phonation) that results from impaired muscle control of the speech mechanism. *Apraxia* refers to the loss of the ability to "program the positioning of speech musculature and sequencing of muscle movements" (Nicolisi and others, 1978), which results in an inability to convert an intended thought into speech. Although both disorders affect speech production, each has a different neuroanatomic correlate and, hence, different clinical characteristics.

Although stroke may affect memory, rarely does a stroke patient have an isolated difficulty recalling acquired language. However, new language acquisition may be impaired. Nonverbal language, such as that conveyed by body position or facial expression, may also be impaired by stroke. For

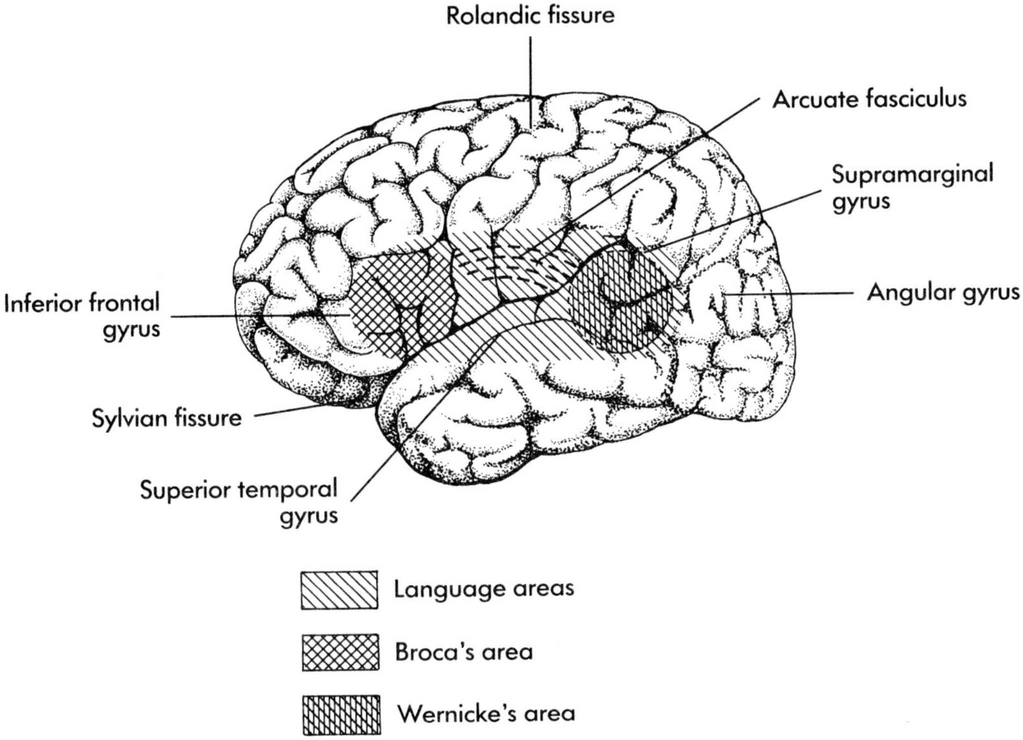

Fig. 11-1 Language areas of the brain.

example, facial droop or hemiparesis may make communication more difficult, even when speech or verbal language mechanisms are not impaired.

ANATOMY OF COMMUNICATION

Language and speech are primarily functions of the dominant cerebral cortex. (The left hemisphere is generally considered language dominant even in left-handed individuals.) However, subcortical areas in the nondominant hemisphere also play a role in language.

The frontal and temporal lobes are considered the language and speech areas (Fig. 11-1). Reception and comprehension of spoken language are functions of Wernicke's area (areas 41 and 42) and the primary auditory cortex, both of which are located in the superior temporal gyrus. The written word is interpreted in Wernicke's area with input from the primary visual cortex via the angular gyrus of the parietal lobe (area 39).

Broca's area (area 44), responsible for programming the motor-speech effort, is located in the inferior third frontal gyrus, adjacent to the precentral gyrus (motor strip). Broca's area lies proximal to the portion of the motor strip responsible for face, mouth, and movement. The arcuate fasciculus communicates information between Broca's and Wernicke's areas. Involvement of any of these areas results in some form of aphasia. In addition, infarcts in the dorsomedial portion of the thalamus have been noted to produce aphasia, probably because of connections with Broca's and Wernicke's areas also located in this area. Apraxia of speech results from isolated involvement of Broca's area or the adjacent motor strip.

Table 11-1 Clinical features of aphasia

Type	Involved anatomy	Expression	Auditory comprehension	Written comprehension	Naming	Word/phrase repetition	Ability to write
Broca's (motor, expressive)	Precentral gyrus, Broca's area	Nonfluent, telegraphic, may be mute	Subtle deficits	Subtle deficits	Impaired	Impaired	Impaired
Wernicke's (receptive, sensory)	Superior temporal gyrus	Fluent but content inappropriate	Impaired	Impaired	Severely impaired	Impaired	Impaired
Global (mixed)	Frontal-temporal area	Nonfluent	Severely impaired	Impaired	Severely impaired	Impaired	Severely impaired
Conductive (central)	Arcuate fasciculus	Fluent	Intact	Intact	Impaired	Severely impaired	Impaired
Anomic (amnesic)	Angular gyrus	Fluent	Intact	Intact	Severely impaired	Intact	Subtle deficits
Transcortical sensory (TCSA)	Periphery of Broca's and Wernicke's areas (watershed zone)	Fluent	Impaired	Impaired	Impaired	Intact	Severely impaired
Transcortical motor (TCMA)	Anterior, superior, or lateral to Broca's area	Nonfluent, speech initiation difficult	Intact	Subtle deficits	Impaired	Intact	Impaired

Speech is a function of the nervous system and peripheral structures. Neurogenic control of the speech mechanisms occurs through several cranial nerves:

- Trigeminal (CN V)—the motor component of this nerve is responsible for palatopharyngeal and mandibular movements.
- Facial (CN VII)—responsible for lip and cheek movement.
- Vagus (CN X)—innervates intrinisic laryngeal muscles to produce phonation; also responsible for palatopharyngeal movements.
- Hypoglossal (CN XII)—responsible for tongue movement.

Damage to the lower pons or medulla of the brainstem, internal capsule disruption of corticobulbar tracts, or dysfunction of the extrapyramidal system (especially the cerebellum) may affect function of these cranial nerves, resulting in dysarthria.

There is an affective component of language (known as *prosody*) that involves intonation, accent, timing, emotions, and attitudes. This language component appears to be mediated by the right hemisphere and probably mirrors left hemispheric language function. Stroke involving the right hemisphere may produce changes in affective language known as *aprosodia*.

An important point to note is that rarely is an isolated portion of the speech or language mechanism involved. Rather, diffuse areas may be affected, resulting in overlapping deficits. For example, apraxia may coexist with an aphasia. A second important point to note is that any communication impairment may occur along a continuum from mild to severe. Severity of the deficit is generally related to the severity of damage.

EFFECTS OF STROKE ON COMMUNICATION

Major communication disorders include aphasia, apraxia, and dysarthria, each with characteristic alterations in language or speech. There is no universally accepted classification system for communication impairment; however, most systems classify disorders according to anatomic lesion. Two important points to remember are that (1) the impairment may vary from mild to severe and that (2) changes in the impairment occur over time.

Aphasia

Aphasia disorders affect all language modalities. Aphasias are classified by involved anatomy, behavioral speech attributes, and fluency of speech (Table 11-1). Fluency refers to the quantity of speech produced. With fluent speech, verbal output is preserved and rhythm, grammar, prosody, and articulation are normal. However, content is meaningless and paraphrases and neologisms are often used. In nonfluent speech, production is limited and speech is poorly articulated. Major types of aphasias are further described below.

Broca's Aphasia. Also known as motor or expressive aphasia, Broca's aphasia usually results from involvement of Broca's area or the precentral gyrus of the left frontal lobe. Speech is usually nonfluent and telegraphic, incorporating phrases or short sentences. In the most severe form of Broca's aphasia, mutism occurs. Paraphrasic errors and neologisms are common. Automatic speech appears to be intact. Auditory and reading comprehension appears intact, but subtle deficits are often present in these areas. Recurrent utterances may also occur and cursing is common. Writing ability is usually concurrently impaired (dysgraphia). Characteristically, the patient is aware of communication difficulties and makes attempts to correct speech but is unable to do so. This may lead to frustration, anger, and depression.

Wernicke's Aphasia. Also known as receptive or sensory aphasia, Wernicke's aphasia usually results from involvement of the left superior temporal gyrus. Speech is usually fluent but with inappropriate content. Auditory impairment and dyslexia occur. Anomia may be severe and circumlocution, paraphrases and neologisms may be used. The content of written expression may also be affected. Characteristically, the patient is unaware of language errors. Because of fluency of speech, the patient with Wernicke's aphasia may appear, on the surface, to be confused. Whole body commands, such as "sit down," may be understood better than those requiring fine motor coordination, such as "point to the picture". Behavioral changes (such as paranoia) are also common.

Global aphasia. Also known as sensory-motor or receptive-expressive or mixed aphasia, global aphasia results from extensive involvement of frontal-temporal areas and often has accompanying neurologic deficits that are fairly severe. Both language production and comprehension are impaired, rendering functional communication almost impossible. Often the patient is able to speak and understand only a few words. Remaining speech is nonfluent, and the patient is unable to write. Occasionally, global aphasia may improve to a Broca's, Wernicke's, or conductive aphasia.

Conductive aphasia. Also known as central aphasia, conductive aphasia occurs with involvement of the arcuate fasciculus, the connective pathway between Wernicke's and Broca's areas. Similar to Wernicke's aphasia, speech is fluent with literal paraphrasic errors. Although paraphrasic errors are noted in both verbal expression and writing, the errors are most marked in word repetition. In contrast, auditory and reading comprehension is relatively intact and the patient is aware of the language impairment.

Anomic aphasia. Also known as amnesic aphasia, anomic aphasia results from involvement of the parietal-temporal junction or the angular gyrus. Characterized primarily by difficulty with word retrieval (anomia), anomic aphasic speech is fluent, but generally vague because of frequent circumlocution. Patients are aware of what they want to say but cannot find the correct word; often they are able to describe it. Word repetition and auditory and reading comprehension are relatively intact.

Transcortical sensory aphasia (TCSA). An uncommon aphasia, TCSA occurs with damage in the "watershed" area—the border zone between the anterior, middle, and posterior cerebral arteries. This damage isolates unimpaired language centers from the motor-speech mechanism and ideation areas. Speech is fluent, but there is impaired auditory and reading comprehension. The patient is unable to write. Most striking is the use of paraphrasia and neologisms. The ability to repeat words is preserved, and the patient often echoes much of what she hears, a phenomenon known as *echolalia*.

Transcortical motor aphasia (TCMA). Also uncommon, TCMA results from damage to the periphery around Broca's area or deep within this area. Speech is nonfluent, and the patient has difficulty initiating speech and finding words. Auditory comprehension is usually intact, but reading comprehension may be mildly impaired. The ability to repeat words is usually preserved, but the ability to write is often impaired.

Apraxia

The motor-speech mechanism in the frontal lobe is responsible for converting the intended spoken word into the actual motor act of speech. Association fibers receive the appropriate motor-speech pattern from Broca's area, connecting it with the appropriate motor area in the precentral gyrus. Stroke in this area produces a speech disorder characterized by an inability to transform thoughts into meaningful language. The extent of apraxia ranges from mild to severe. Because of proximity to other language centers, aphasia may (but not always) accompany apraxia. Auditory and reading comprehension are intact with apraxia. Patients know what they intend to say but cannot and often become frustrated because of their errors. Speech is variable in fluency, with automatic speech being more clearly articulated. Word substitutions are common, and inconsistent language errors characterize this disorder.

Dysarthria

Speaking is a very complex motor function that involves the mouth, lips, tongue, palate, pharynx, larynx, and respiratory muscles. Muscle control of speaking occurs with input from corticobulbar tract via the vagus, hypoglossal, facial, and phrenic nerves. The basal ganglia and cerebellum (part of the extra-pyramidal system) also provide input into muscular control. Any disturbance in muscular con-

Table 11-2 Classification of Dysarthrias

Type	Involved anatomy	Characteristics*
Flaccid	Final common pathway (lower motor neuron)	Hypernasality, breathy voice, use of short phrases
Spastic	Corticobulbar tracts or extrapyramidal system	Slow muffled speech, hypernasality, pitch breaks, use of short phrases
Ataxic	Cerebellum	Slow, monotonous speech, explosive speech, scanning, hesitation
Hyperkinetic	Extrapyramidal system	Involuntary movement of speech musculature resulting in slow, twisted speech, pitch breaks, hesitation, use of short phrases
Hypokinetic	Extrapyramidal system	Short bursts of muffled speech, decay of loudness

*All dysarthrias characteristically include monopitch, monoloudness, slurring of consonants, and a harsh voice quality.

trol of speech is known as *dysarthria*. Characteristically, dysarthria results from damage to the central or peripheral nervous systems' muscular control of speech. Damage is manifested by weakness, incoordination, or altered tone of the speech musculature. Consonants are difficult to pronounce, giving speech a slurred and gutteral quality.

Dysarthrias, as classified here, are grouped by the specific type of muscular impairment rather than by an anatomic classification (Table 11-2).

Flaccid dysarthria. This type of dysarthria results from damage to the final common pathway (lower motor neuron damage). Speech is slurred and difficult to understand because of tongue weakness. Vibratory, lingual, and labial consonants (b,l,m,r,nk,ng,pt) are difficult for the patient to pronounce. A nasal quality (hypernasality) of speech exists along with a feeble or breathy voice because of weakness of the palate.

Spastic dysarthria. More common than flaccid dysarthria, spastic dysarthria results from damage to either the corticobulbar tracts or the extrapyramidal system (basal ganglia or cerebellum). Unilateral involvement produces mild impairment while bilateral involvement produces severe impairment. Speech is slow, muffled, and slurred with a harsh voice quality. Words may be spoken in short phrases with breaks in pitch.

Ataxic dysarthria. This type of dysarthria is associated with cerebellar hemorrhage or infarct. Slow, monotonous, and imprecise speech is characteristic. Explosive speech (speaking with too great a force) may be used because of incoordination between speech and respiration. Scanning, an unusual separation of spoken words with hesitation, is frequently seen. Ataxic dysarthria often sounds like speech associated with alcohol intoxication.

Hyperkinetic dysarthria. This type of dysarthria is related to extrapyramidal dysfunction, which leads to a decreased production of acetylcholine (ACh). Being the neurotransmitter at the myoneural junction, ACh is responsible for motor function. All motor speech functions are impaired. Characteristics include fast or slow involuntary movements of the speech musculature. Sounds may be expressed inappropriately, and words spoken may be delayed, drawn out, or twisted.

Hypokinetic dysarthria. Thought to be related to decreased production of dopamine (such as that seen with Parkinson's disease) hypokinetic dysarthria is characterized by marked limitation of speech muscle movement. Affect is flat, and short bursts of words are often used. Speech is muffled, and loudness of the voice decreases with continued effort.

Because of the interrelationships between pathways controlling the muscle speech effort, mixed dysarthrias are possible. For example, spastic and hyperkinetic dysarthrias may occur in combination. Multiple or extensive strokes may produce mixed dysarthrias.

Other Communication Deficits

Although not specifically an aphasia, *cognitive-linguistic impairment* deserves mention because it affects all language skills. With this type of impairment, language areas are intact, but cortical or subcortical damage affects language-related areas. Impairments include poor memory, inability to reason or concentrate, and decreased alertness. Damage may be right or left-sided or bilateral. Because of the diffuse nature of involvement, great variability is seen in speech-language deficits. Therefore, specific deficits are difficult to categorize. Aphasias, apraxia, and dysarthrias may all overlap. This type of impairment may be seen following stroke, but is more common following traumatic brain injury.

Although left hemisphere stroke is usually associated with communication impairment, language deficits may also occur with right hemisphere involvement. Aprosodia, the inability to comprehend or express meaning because of impaired speech prosody, may occur. Other difficulties originating from the right hemisphere include verbosity, difficulty understanding figurative language, flat affect, and visuospatial deficits that affect reading and writing (i.e., hemianopia). Because the many subtleties of right hemisphere functional integration are not well understood, the exact anatomic location and nature of these problems is still to be delineated. It appears that right hemispheric functions may be less focally organized than left hemispheric functions.

ASSESSMENT

The exact incidence of communication impairment following stroke is unknown. Estimates range from 20% to 60%, depending on the severity of the stroke and the location of the infarct. Because severe stroke may render the patient unresponsive, language and speech abilities cannot be evaluated. Although communication disorders are primarily related to left hemispheric involvement, evidence exists that infarction of the right hemisphere or in deeper structures affects speech and language. Therefore the communication abilities of every stroke patient should be assessed as early as possible in the course of the disease. Any deficits noted in this area warrant a comprehensive evaluation by a certified speech-language pathologist (SLP).

Nursing assessment for communication impairment is less formal than that conducted by the SLP. An assessment begins with an explanation to the patient of the purpose for the assessment. Any premorbid factors affecting language or speech are evaluated. Most important are the patient's ability to understand English, her level of education, and her ability to read and write. Visual or hearing impairments that may affect language should also be determined. Overall muscle strength should also be evaluated to determine the patient's ability to produce a motor response to a verbal command. Lastly, the patient's energy level and attention span and the presence of pain should be taken into consideration. Evaluation may need to be rescheduled or performed in short segments over a period of time.

Nursing assessment of language and speech skills is comprehensive and includes the following:

Automatic Speech

Automatic speech is often evaluated through simple observation. For example, the patient should respond to your "Good morning" greeting with a similar response. Note any slowness, word substitution, or unusual sounding speech.

Auditory Comprehension

Comprehension of sound should be evaluated on several levels. First, try simple commands that require a motor rather than verbal response, such as "stick out your tongue" or "squeeze my fingers." Next, try a complex command such as "pick up the comb and comb your hair." Also ask yes-no questions such as "are you in the hospital?" (yes) and "are you in church?" (no). Answers to questions must be known. For example, the patient's response to a question about his address can be verified with the patient's chart. It may be helpful to periodically intersperse a nonsensical question to validate comprehension. Avoid using gestures where possible because this gives the patient nonverbal cues. Note any inability to follow simple or complex commands or any inconsistency in responding to questions.

Written (Reading) Comprehension

Premorbid reading ability must be known before evaluating this area. Once established, ask the patient to read out loud a menu, card, headline, or short paragraph in the newspaper and then describe the content. For those with lower premorbid reading levels, write the names of objects in the room on a piece of paper. Then ask the patient to point out the object in the room. Note any word substitutions, difficulty describing content, neglect of any content (possibly indicative of hemianopia), or confabulation.

Expressive Ability

To evaluate expressive ability, ask the patient questions or engage in conversation with the patient. Ask about a program on television, what the patient ate for breakfast, or what color the patient's eyes are. Demonstrate a familiar object, such as a pen, key, or watch, and ask the patient to name it. Note any difficulty in naming the object (anomia) or inability to name an object but ability to describe it (circumlocution). Evaluate the rhythm of speech, noting any choppiness, halting (telegraphing), or monotony. Ask the patient to repeat words, then phrases, then sentences. Note any incorrectness or slowness in the response. Also, note any struggle in getting the words out. Evaluate the quantity of verbal output, noting a decrease in output ability (ability to answer questions with only one or two words) or an increase in output (rambling on). Listen for literal or verbal paraphrasias. Literal paraphrasias substitute similar sounds (i.e., "dake" for "cake"). Verbal paraphrasias substitute words with similar meanings (i.e., "knife" for "spoon"). Also, listen for any neologisms, or creation of new or nonsensical words. Examples of selected abnormalities are listed in Table 11-3.

Ability To Write

Since writing ability often parallels expressive abilities, similar deficits in writing ability may appear. If the patient is able to write (i.e., not hemiplegic), ask the patient to write down his name and address, what he had for breakfast, etc. Note any illegibility, spelling errors, inability to write, or nonsensical writing.

Formal evaluation by a certified SLP is necessary in any situation of impaired communication. The formal evaluation focuses on diagnosis of the type and extent of the communication disorder and identification of communication strengths and weaknesses. Information gained from the formal evaluation is used to develop a comprehensive treatment plan. Formal evaluation usually begins with a detailed speech-language history and includes hearing and vision screening. Standardized tests may be used to evaluate aphasias. Clinical and functional abilities are evaluated. More common standardized tests include the Boston Diagnostic Aphasia Examination, the Functional Communication Profile, and Communicative Abilities in Daily Living. Supplementary tests of other abilities may be incorporated as needed. Additional clinical evaluation may be undertaken to assess function in the aforementioned areas in a more detailed manner. There are currently no available standardized tests to evaluate affective language. However, a nonstandardized test, known as the RPC Evaluation of Communication Problems in Right Hemisphere Dysfunction (RICE), may be used. Abilities such as orientation, metaphoric meaning, memory, per-

Table 11-3 Types of language disturbances

Disturbance	Characteristics	Example
Verbal paraphrasia	Substitution of words with similar meaning	"I cut my meat with a spoon" (instead of knife)
Literal paraphrasia	Substitution of words with similar sounds	"I baked a dake" (instead of cake)
Perseveration	Continuous repetition of words, phrases, or sentences	"Don't know, don't know, don't know . . ."
Circumlocution	Ability to describe an object without being able to name it	When asked to name a watch, "It tells time and you wear it on your wrist"
Anomia	Inability to name an object or recall certain words	"I need . . . that" (points to object)
Neologism	Substitution of nonsensical word	"It's a pudgo"
Jargon speech	Extensive neologisms in speech making language incomprehensible	"Ta keo ep gob"
Telegraphic speech	Speech is halting, sentences are shortened to phrases with pauses in between but idea is still communicated	"Dinner . . . table . . . now"

ception, scanning and tracking, and others can be evaluated.

INTERVENTIONS

Once a communication impairment has been identified, it is generally accepted that a referral to a speech-language pathologist (SLP) is in order. In most circumstances, this requires a physician's order, but the nurse may be instrumental in relaying information regarding the need for therapy. The SLP may then institute a series of examinations of the patient to accurately diagnose the type and severity of deficit and begin to develop a comprehensive treatment plan. Before initiation of the treatment plan, the patient should be medically stable, aware of the immediate environment, and able to respond to auditory and tactile stimuli.

Treatment goals are based on the type of deficit and are individualized to the patient. General goals based on type of deficit are as follows:

Global Aphasia

The overall goal of therapy is to improve the patient's ability to communicate rather than to improve any one language area. Realizing that the patient with global aphasia may be sensitive to nonlanguage forms of communication, such as gestures and facial expression, this goal may be accomplished by emphasizing nonlanguage types of communication. Visual input is important to facilitate comprehension for these patients. One program that has shown some success with global aphasic patients is known as Visual Action Therapy (VAT). The VAT program teaches patients to associate visual ideas with objects and actions at various levels of communication. Communication boards have also been helpful to the global aphasic. However, coexisting hemiplegia and apraxia may make it difficult for the patient to use such a tool.

Broca's Aphasia

The major goal of therapy is to establish a reliable language output for self-expression. This may be accomplished by beginning to develop consistent yes-no responses through repeated drills. Repetition, reading out loud, sentence completion, and visual cueing (charts, diagrams, photos, etc.) may also be used. Two programs that have been useful in treating Broca's aphasia are (1) Melodic Intonation Therapy (MIT), in which the patient is asked to sing intonation of words, phrases, and sentences; and (2) Voluntary Control of Involuntary Utterances (VICU), in which involuntary words spoken by the patient are written down by the therapist and the patient is asked to read them out loud.

Wernicke's Aphasia

The major goals of therapy are to develop awareness of the language problem and to increase efficiency of the language output. This is generally accomplished by providing auditory stimuli, stressing comprehension, and providing feedback. This may initially require structuring the patient's environment to delete extraneous sounds, or the patient may be placed in a soundproof room and provided with selected auditory input. Directed reading and listening may also be used. Teaching the patient how to use nonverbal behavior to communicate may also be helpful. The therapist serves as a model for correct language rather than someone who points out errors. Repetition and other drills may reinforce learning.

Anomic Aphasia

The major goal of therapy is to assist the patient in rebuilding word associations and developing self-cueing strategies. This is accomplished by teaching the patient to personalize the unretrievable word, then to visualize it, thinking of its physical characteristics and function. Through the use of synonyms or homonyms, the word may be brought into speech. The patient may also be taught to use circumlocution more successfully. Role playing, i.e., putting the patient into an everyday scenario such as a trip to the bank, may also be helpful. Group interaction with other anomic aphasic patients allows for peer practice, learning new communication skills, and group support. The PACE program (Promoting Aphasic Communicative Effectiveness) has shown some benefit with anomia. This program focuses on ideas to be conveyed, rather than on linguistic accuracy.

Conductive Aphasia

The goals of therapy are similar to those for anomic aphasia. Additional emphasis is placed on decreasing frequency of paraphrasic errors.

Cognitive-Linguistic Impairment

The major goals of therapy focus on improving language-related areas of dysfunction. Therapy may be geared toward increasing attention and orientation, improving memory and visuospatial deficits, and facilitating integration skills, such as problem-solving and organization.

Dysarthria

The major goals of therapy focus on strengthening speech musculature and improving the patient's overall ability to communicate. Facial and oral exercises may be provided. Superficial stimulation of the peripheral portion of the facial nerve may be used when this nerve is affected. The patient may be instructed in alternative methods of communication, such as a communication board or a computerized talking board if the patient has severe dysarthria.

Right Hemisphere Language Deficits

The major goals of therapy focus on improving prosody and increased usage of language pragmatics. The patient is taught to focus on facial expressions, gestures, and voice tone, and is given the opportunity to practice turn-taking and voice inflections. Role playing and acting out to exaggerate language pragmatics are also helpful.

Other components of communication skills may need to be treated on an individual basis. Decreased visual acuity or hearing impairments may need attention. Impairments in ability to count or use money may need to be addressed. Since perseveration may be an underlying component to any aphasia, perseveration may need to be treated. The TAP program (Treatment of Aphasic Perseveration) has been used for various types of aphasia to teach the patient to control those factors that induce perseveration. However, long-term benefits of this program are yet to be determined because its use is still in the early stages.

Family involvement is essential to any successful therapy program. Family members provide not only support but also follow-through for the patient's therapy program at the bedside or in the home. Family members also need to learn how to cope with the altered relationship that the communication deficit produces. Counseling or a support group may help the family to cope.

One last point to remember is that although a communication impairment might be the sole deficit following stroke, it is far more common for other deficits to coexist. In that context, speech-language therapy is only one aspect of a multidisciplinary rehabilitation program. Aspects of the speech-language therapy program may be carried into other therapies.

Controversies exist about the actual efficacy of intensive speech-language therapy. There are a number of reasons for this. The natural course of recovery from communication impairment is unknown. As the patient experiences improvement with therapy, it is difficult to determine whether the improvement is due to therapy or to spontaneous recovery. Communication impairments are difficult to study for several reasons. To provide a definitive study, it would be necessary to randomize large numbers of patients into treatment and nontreatment groups. However, specific deficits are variable even with consistent lesions, and many other areas impact speech and language. Therefore, developing comparable study groups is a challenge. In addition, although the general principles of therapy may be agreed upon by clinicians, there is little agreement on how these principles are best accomplished. Therefore, standardized therapy is difficult to define. Finally, if the underlying assumption is that therapy does indeed make a difference, it is morally and ethically difficult to have a nontreatment group. Randomized studies have been conducted in spite of these difficulties, either comparing two types of treatment programs or comparing a treated group with an untreated group (usually patients who did not have physical or financial access to therapy). Results have been conflicting, with some studies demonstrating efficacy of therapy and others demonstrating no discernible differences between treated and nontreated groups. In spite of this, speech-language therapy continues to be an accepted treatment for communication deficits.

A recent development in the treatment of communication disorders is pharmacotherapy, based on the concept that stroke may decrease production of neurotransmitter substances necessary for speech-language function and replacement of these substances may improve language skills. In a case reported in the literature, bromocriptine was used successfully in a patient with transcortical motor asphasia to improve language performance (Albert and others, 1988). As more is learned about the effect of stroke on neurotransmitter function and pharmacotherapeutic treatment for such effects, this area may hold tremendous potential for the future.

The nurse may encounter a patient with a communication deficit in an acute care setting, hospital, rehabilitation facility, clinic, or in the home. Regardless of the setting or type of deficit, there are certain principles that guide nursing intervention:

- Approach and treat the patient as an adult. Treating the patient in a condescending or childish manner can negate the nurse-patient relationship. Conversation should be maintained at an adult level to stimulate interest in spontaneous conversation.
- Inform the patient of the nature of her impairment and the fact that treatment is available.
- Environmental control is important. To maximize communication efforts, provide a quiet, calm environment. Attempt to minimize distractions in the patient's environment. If the patient is easily distracted, a private room may be beneficial. Personalizing and arranging the patient's room to his wishes may convey caring, comfort, and encouragement.
- Be aware of the influence of your own behaviors on the patient. Nonverbal language, such as gestures, and voice intonation, may convey unintended meaning to the patient and should be controlled. Avoid raising or increasing the loudness of your voice unless the patient's hearing is impaired.

- Incorporate multimodal input. Pictures, photographs, drawings, and other visual cues may be used to supplement gestures and auditory input. Direct eye contact is also important; remember to stand in the patient's line of vision, especially if the patient has hemianopia.
- Don't assume the patient cannot comprehend simply because she may often appear to not understand. Conversations in the patient's proximity should be directed toward the patient. Avoid conversation about the patient within the patient's hearing.
- Simplify your communication with the patient. Use short, precise statements and familiar terminology. Use simple commands, pausing between steps when giving the patient directions that require his cooperation. If possible, structure questions to require yes-no answers rather than phrases.
- When reading comprehension is intact, written materials may be incorporated to supplement auditory input.
- Be honest when communicating with the patient. If you cannot understand the patient, say so; encourage the patient to try again. Point out to the patient progress she has made, giving realistic feedback.
- Allow adequate time for the patient to respond. Some patients may require as long as 30 seconds to process information and produce a response. Be patient when communicating with the patient who has a speech or language impairment.
- Provide opportunities for spontaneous or natural conversation. By determining the patient's interests, spontaneous conversation may be encouraged. Family should also be encouraged to engage the patient in conversation.
- Realize that frustration is a likely response for the patient. Instead of becoming involved in the frustration, reassure the patient that you understand her anger. If possible, eliminate frustrating factors.
- For patients with anomia, prompting may be beneficial. Offer clues rather than provide the word for the patient. Descriptive clues, phrase completion, functions, or even pantomime may facilitate the patient's recall of a particular word.
- Provide alternative methods for communication when necessary. Computerized talking boards, communication boards, an electronic voice, or other mechanical aids may be helpful. Specific suggestions in this realm may be obtained from the SLP.
- Family involvement is essential in any treatment plan. The family should be educated about the nature of the patient's problem and the family's role in treatment. The need for treatment and commitment to that treatment are also discussed. Interventions found to be successful can also be communicated to the patient.
- For patients with cognitive-linguistic impairment, interventions that promote orientation and facilitate attention are a priority. Frequent reorientation to the task at hand may be necessary.
- Ongoing assessment of the communication impairment is necessary to determine progress and the need for changes in the treatment plan.
- Communication with the SLP and other health care team members is vital. The treatment plan should be shared to promote follow-through and reinforcement wherever possible. The nurse can assist the patient in "homework" activities as well.
- Psychologic problems that warrant intervention (such as depression, withdrawal, rejection of therapy, or social isolation) may occur. Referrals to appropriate persons may be obtained. Information about support groups may also be offered.

Two nursing diagnoses may be incorporated into the plan of care for the stroke patient with a communication disorder.

Altered communication

Stroke involvement of the dominant left frontal, temporal, or parietal lobes may produce impairment in verbal and/or written language expression and in auditory or written comprehension. Stroke involvement of the cerebellum, brainstem, basal ganglia, or cranial nerves may impair articulation of speech. Specific deficits resulting are unique to the patient and depend on involved anatomy and severity of the insult. Assessment will reveal the specific type and severity of the patient's deficit, as mentioned in previous characteristics.

In providing intervention, the patient's needs are anticipated until an effective method of communication is developed. The patient may be questioned directly about needs, wishes, or discomforts. Necessary care may be offered, such as assistance with eating or a bedpan. Alternative means of communication are provided as necessary. Gestures, pictures, and written materials may be useful to enhance communication functions that remain intact. Assistive devices such as communication boards or talking boards may be utilized. Environmental control may also enhance patient communication efforts. Opportunities for spontaneous conversation may be provided to afford opportunities to practice functional communication. Minimizing extraneous distractions may also enhance efforts. Modulation of the nurse's own communication may be beneficial. Collaboration with the SLP is essential to implement a comprehensive treatment plan. Stimulation should be structured at a level appropriate to the patient, and aspects of the SLP treatment plan incorporated into nursing care activities.

Knowledge Deficit, Patient and Family, Regarding the Nature of Altered Communication and Measures to Enhance Communication Ability

Both the patient and family may be unaware of the existence or extent of communication impairment or unfamiliar with how the deficit relates to the stroke process. In addition, family members may be reluctant to attempt conversation with the communication-impaired family member because of lack of knowledge about the deficit. The nurse may be instrumental in explaining the nature of the deficit to the patient and family and providing information on the overall treatment plan and goals. Even though patients may not be able to comprehend the explanation, attempts should be made to provide information and reassurance. Family members may be encouraged to continue communication efforts with the patient, particularly spontaneous conversation. Family members and the patient may be involved in the development and implementation of the treatment plan. For example, the patient or family member may be asked to identify situations requiring communication that the patient is likely to encounter. Practice situations may then be structured around that information. Lack of knowledge may also contribute to patient frustration. Recognizing the frustration, attempting to minimize the frustration with patience, and demonstrating progress made may alleviate this problem.

FUNCTIONAL OUTCOME

Patients and families are naturally interested in prognosis for communication impairment. Prognosis is very individual and often difficult to predict. However, a number of factors have been related to outcome.

- The type of injury to the brain may relate to the outcome of communication impairment. Stroke patients have been noted to have lesser potential for language recovery as compared with head-injured patients. However, groups studied may not be comparable in terms of lesion site, age, and other factors. Therefore results must be viewed with caution.
- The type of aphasia appears to be related to outcome. Global aphasia appears to have the poorest prognosis for recovery, perhaps because of the diffuse nature of involvement. In contrast, patients with anomic or conductive aphasia often have complete or near-complete recoveries. Patients with Broca's or Wernicke's aphasia usually have incomplete recoveries, but their language skills can be expected to improve.
- The severity of aphasia may relate to outcome. Single, localized lesions are generally associated with more favorable recovery while recurrent, diffuse, or multiple lesions are generally associated with poor recovery of language skills.

- The time between onset of communication impairment and treatment may also affect outcome. Studies have shown the earlier the intervention, the greater the ability to promote spontaneous recovery. However, patients have received therapy as late as 2 years after stroke have been known to experience improvement. There is no agreement on the optimum time to begin therapy. One study recommended delaying treatment until 1 to 3 months after stroke because treatment before this time did not show any benefit.

Other factors related to outcome include error-awareness, age, handedness, and educational level. Those patients who are aware of their deficits and attempt to correct errors appear to have better recovery of language skills. Younger left-handed or ambidextrous persons also appear to have better recovery. Educational level and intelligence are difficult factors to measure and study prospectively, but both appear to have a positive relationship to recovery.

Since communication impairment has a psychological impact, psychological factors must also be taken into consideration. Psychological factors that appear to have a negative effect on recovery of language skills are depression, withdrawal, and social isolation. Therefore, interventions to promote psychological well-being are an important component of treatment.

NURSING CARE PLAN

Nursing Diagnosis	Interventions	Expected Outcomes
Communication, Impaired Verbal **Defining Characteristics** ■ Impaired verbal language expression ■ Impaired written language expression ■ Impaired auditory comprehension ■ Impaired comprehension of written language ■ Impaired articulation	**Ongoing Assessment** ■ Assess speech-language history A. Ability to read, write, and understand English B. Level of education ■ Assess speech-language function A. Automatic speech B. Auditory comprehension C. Comprehension of written language D. Expressive ability E. Ability to write ■ Assess the following additional factors A. Energy level B. Attention span C. Presence of pain **Therapeutic Interventions** ■ Approach the patient as an adult ■ Enhance the environment to facilitate communication, i.e., minimize distractions ■ Modulate personal communication, controlling body language and providing clear, simple directions ■ Incorporate multimodality input to enhance function in intact speech-language areas	■ Patient will be able to effectively communicate basic needs ■ Patient will be able to maximize remaining communication ability ■ Patient and family will be able to verbalize understanding of communication impairment ■ Patient and family will be involved in measures to promote communication

NURSING CARE PLAN — cont'd

Nursing Diagnosis	Interventions	Expected Outcomes
	■ Use written materials to supplement auditory input (when written comprehension is intact) ■ Use prompting clues ■ Allow adequate time for patient response ■ Provide opportunities for spontaneous conversation ■ Anticipate patient needs until alternative means of communication can be established ■ Provide reality orientation and focus attention ■ Collaborate with speech-language pathologist to implement a comprehensive plan of care	

Patient Education

- Inform patient and family of the nature of the communication impairment
- Inform patient and family of overall treatment plan and interventions they may use
- Encourage family to attempt communication with the patient
- Demonstrate to patient progress made

REFERENCES

Albert ML, Bachman DL, Morgan A, and others: Pharmacotherapy for aphasia, Neurology, 38:877, 1988.

Barnett HJ, Mohr JP, Stein BM, and others: Stroke: Pathophysiology, diagnosis, and management, New York, 1986, Churchill Livingstone, Inc.

Borenstein P, Linell S, and Wahrborg P: An innovative therapeutic program for aphasia patients and their relatives, Scand J Rehab Med, 19:51, 1987.

Boss BJ: Dysphasia, dyspraxia, and dysarthria: distinguishing features, part 1, J Neurosurg Nurs, 16:151, 1984a.

Boss BJ: Dysphasia, dyspraxia, and dysarthria: distinguishing features, part II, J Neurosurg Nurs, 16:211, 1984b.

Carriero MR, Faglia L, Vignolo LA: Resumption of gainful employment in aphasics: preliminary findings, Cortex, 26:667, 1987.

Gorelik PB, and Ross ED: The aprosodias: further functional-anatomical evidence for the organization of affective language in the right hemisphere, J Neurol Neurosurg Psychiatry, 50:553, 1987.

Halper AS, Mogil SI: Communication disorders: diagnosis and treatment, In: Kaplan PG and Cerullo LJ, editors: Stroke rehabilitation, Stoneham, Mass, 1986, Butterworth Publishers, Inc.

Hartman J and Landau WM: Comparison of formal language therapy with supportive counseling for aphasia due to acute vascular accident, Arch Neurol, 44:646, 1987.

Helm-Estabrooks N, Emery P, and Albert ML: Treatment of aphasic perseveration (TAP) program: a new approach to aphasia therapy, Arch Neurol, 44:1253, 1987.

Kaplan PE and Cerullo LJ: Stroke rehabilitation, Stoneham, Mass, 1986, Butterworth Publishers, Inc.

Kertesz A: What do we learn from recovery from aphasia? Adv Neurol, 47:277, 1988.

Koppel BS and Weinberger G: Pontine infarction producing dysarthria-clumsy hand syndrome and ataxic hemiparesis, Eur Neurol, 26:211, 1987.

Lebrun Y: Anosognosia in aphasics, Cortex, 23:251, 1987.

Legh-Smith JA, Denis R, Enderby PM, and others: Selection of aphasic stroke patients for intensive speech therapy, J Neurol Neurosurg Psychiatry, 50:1488, 1987.

MacKay S, Holmes DW, and Gersumky, AT: Methods to assess aphasic stroke patients, Geriatr Nurs, 9:177, 1988.

Mitchell PH, Hodges LC, Muwaswes M, and others: AANN's Neuroscience Nursing, New York, 1988, Appleton and Lange.

Nicolisi L, Harryman E, and Kresheck J: Terminology of communication disorders: speech, language, and hearing, Baltimore, 1978, Williams & Wilkins.

Ozaki I, Baba M, Narita S, and others: Pure dysarthria due to anterior internal capsule and/or corona radiata infarction: a report of five cases, J Neurol Neurosurg Psychiatry, 49:1435, 1986.

Pimental PA: Alterations in communication: biopsychosocial aspects of aphasia, dysarthria, and right hemisphere syndromes in the stroke patient, Nurs Clin North Am, 21:321, 1986.

Reedy DF: The client with aphasia—the assessment of language abilities, Top Clin Nurs, 8:67, 1986.

Ropper AH: Severe dysarthria with right hemisphere stroke, Neurology, 37:1061, 1987.

Sandson J, Albert ML, and Alexander MP: Confabulation in aphasia, Cortex, 22:621, 1986.

Scarpa M, Colombo A, Sorgato P, and others, The incidence of aphasic and global aphasia in left brain-damaged patients, Cortex, 23:331, 1987.

Tuszynski MH and Petito CK: Ischemic thalamic aphasia with pathologic confirmation, Neurology, 38:800, 1988.

Chapter 12

Alterations in Sexuality

Humans by their nature are sexual beings. Sexuality, a composite of sexual expression, is therefore basic to human existence throughout the life span. Yet sexuality is a very complex phenomenon with great variability in individual meaning. The physical and psychologic effects of stroke potentially affect the patient's sexuality, resulting in sexual dysfunction. Physical and psychologic disabilities associated with stroke alter body image and often impair sexual function. Disability also challenges the integrity of a relationship, ultimately affecting sexuality. To assist the nurse in approaching the multifaceted nature of sexual dysfunction in the stroke patient, this chapter will review human sexuality, describe sexual assessment and potential sexual dysfunctions, and provide suggested interventions.

HUMAN SEXUALITY

Major, and equally important, components of sexuality are sexual function, self-image, and interpersonal relationships. Sexual functioning, described as the "ability of an individual to give and receive sexual pleasure," (Renshaw, 1978) includes both the physical and psychologic components of the sex act. Body image and other related concepts comprise the sexual self-image and refer to the image an individual has of oneself as a sexual being. Because sexuality is expressed in an interpersonal relationship, the nature of the relationship is an important component of sexuality. Each of these components must be considered when evaluating sexual health.

Sexual Function

Sexual function is under neurogenic control. A total body response, sexual function is influenced by pathways involving the cerebral cortex, spinal cord reflex centers, autonomic nervous system, and peripheral nerves. Masters and Johnson originally conceptualized sexual functioning as the human sexual response. More recent work by Kaplan has identified three interrelated aspects of sexual response, based on distinct neurophysiologic mechanisms.

Sexual desire (libido). Described as the motivation for a person to seek out sexual activity, sexual desire occurs with activation of various cerebral systems. The exact areas of involvement are unknown, but the temporal lobe, limbic system, and preoptic nuclei of the hypothalamus are thought to be involved. It is postulated that these areas have chemical connections (most likely via endorphins) with pleasure areas of the brain. A variety of sensory stimuli are known to facilitate or inhibit sexual desire. Visual, auditory, olfactory, psychic, and tactile stimuli may facilitate or inhibit desire. Pain, stress, and fear are very effective inhibitors. Sexual desire may be enhanced by augmenting any of these stimuli. Certain neurotransmitters and hormones are also known to affect sex-

Table 12-1 Neurotransmitters and hormones affecting sexual desire

Substance	Effect
Endorphins	Stimulate pleasure centers
Serotonin	Inhibits sexual desire
Dopamine	Stimulates sexual desire
Testosterone	Mediates sexual desire
Luteinizing hormone	Mediates sexual desire

ual desire; these are described in Table 12-1.

Sexual excitement. Physical or psychic stimuli via sensory and corticospinal pathways are thought to be responsible for vasocongestion, the physiologic response characteristic of excitement. Reflex centers in the lower spinal cord produce arteriolar dilation, resulting in genital swelling. In males, parasympathetic impulses via the splanchnic nerve dilate penile arterioles while constricting penile veins, producing erection. Tactile stimuli via the sacral plexus (S2 to S4) and psychic stimuli via thoracolumbar pathways (T11 to L2) contribute to this response. In females, physical and psychic stimuli produce a similar response. Physical stimulation of the clitoris (analogous to the glans penis in the male) via the sacral plexus, or psychic stimuli via lumbar pathways, initiate a parasympathetic response via the splanchnic nerve. Arteriolar dilation occurs, causing swelling of the genitalia and vaginal lubrication. As excitement progresses, males secrete mucus from the bulbourethral glands, and females secrete mucus from the Bartholin's glands. Mucus secretion in both sexes is mediated by the parasympathetic system.

Orgasm. The peak of sexual response, orgasm is primarily controlled by spinal centers. Intensified stimuli transmitted via the sacral plexus activate a sympathetic response. In males, the bladder neck is occluded and rhythmic contractions of penile musculature occur. Parasympathetic stimulation of the vas deferens, prostate, and spermatic vessels causes a peristaltic movement known as ejaculation. A similar peristaltic movement of vaginal musculature, in addition to perineal musuclature, is noted in the orgasmic response in women. Orgasmic reflex centers in females are also located in the sacral cord and are under sympathetic control. Desire may exist without genital sensation or function, and genital ejaculation and orgasm may occur independent of the brain. Hence, sexual function is complex, and more is yet to be known. Because there are multiple levels of neurogenic control, sexual function may be preserved or facilitated by compensation in other areas when sexual dysfunction exists.

Self-concept

Sexual self-concept is an essential component of human sexuality and includes body image. How a person perceives his or her body and how the body is presented through grooming are important components of body image. The image a person holds of himself or herself as a sexual being is also important. This self-image may allow the person to seek out sexual activity or exhibit sexual behavior. Within self-concept are individual learned variations of what is perceived as pleasurable and what is not. Gender and role identity, sexual curiosity and fantasy, and sexual values are other aspects related to sexual self-concept. Changes in body image, denial of one's sexuality, or changes involving the related aspects may produce sexual dysfunction.

Relationships

Interpersonal relationships are the third component of sexuality. Sexuality is best expressed in relationships with others and is learned over time. Culture and societal values assist the person in a sexual relationship to define normal or acceptable sexual behavior. Frequency and techniques of sexual activity vary not only within the relationship but also among cultures. Intimacy is essential to any sexual relationship. When sexual function is not desired or possible, sexuality may be expressed primarily through intimacy. Dating, learning sexual roles, behavior and vocabulary, and commitment to and reciprocal involvement in a relationship are important related aspects. Social isolation produced by disability has an obvious impact on sexuality.

EFFECTS OF STROKE ON SEXUALITY

In spite of the hundreds of thousands of persons suffering stroke each year, little has been researched or written on sexual dysfunction in this population. Perhaps this is because other deficits, such as hemiplegia or aphasia, are more obvious. Or, perhaps stroke-related sexuality issues are just coming into perspective and little is really known on the topic. Whatever the reason, ongoing research is necessary to identify the nature of stroke-related sexual dysfunction and appropriate interventions. Material describing what is known about stroke-related sexual dysfunction will be presented in this section.

Several studies have been conducted in an attempt to identify sexual impairments in the stroke population.* These studies are largely descriptive and are not substantiated in a clinical setting. Results occasionally are contradictory but several strong themes are noted throughout.

In males affected by stroke, specific complaints relative to sexual function have been reported. These include decreased ability to achieve erection, decreased firmness of erection, inability to maintain erection, and decreased ability to achieve ejaculation or delayed ejaculation. Similar complaints have been reported by females affected by stroke, including decrease in vaginal lubrication and anorgasmia. Since these functions are mediated by the autonomic nervous system (ANS), and little is written about stroke effects on ANS function, these complaints need to be investigated.

Unless a stroke is very extensive or affects deeper structures (such as the limbic system), it is thought that higher cerebral areas responsible for sexual behavior are generally preserved following stroke. However, the magnitude of stroke-related sexuality issues suggests there are other cerebral mechanisms that play a role in sexual response that have not yet been determined. This idea is supported by a study that identified alterations in hormones unrelated to complaints of sexual dysfunction (Hawton, 1984).

Other changes noted in stroke couples include shorter duration of foreplay and intercourse and decreased frequency of intercourse. In addition, premenopausal women reported cessation or irregularity of menses. The exact mechanism for this problem is not understood. Difficulties imposed by disabilities may also impair sexual function. Hemiparesis or hemiplegia may make maneuvering during sexual activity difficult. Associated muscle spasms may become worse during sexual activity, frightening both partners. An aphasic person may become confused or frustrated in a sexual interaction and be unable to express sexual wishes or desires. In addition, during the intensity of sexual activity, the aphasic person may utter obscenities, which may inhibit stimulation for both partners. The patient with visual deficits may respond poorly to visual stimuli.

Interestingly, sexual dysfunctions have been reported to be more severe or disabling in persons with left hemispheric involvement. The reason for this is not clear. It may be that persons with right hemispheric lesions have a poorer perception of their problems rather than the problems actually being lesser with left hemispheric involvement.

Because sexual function should be anatomically and physiologically preserved following stroke, there must be other reasons for sexual dysfunction in this population. Decreased sensation is a common complaint of the stroke patient. Areas of the body (not just genitalia) that previously had been found to be stimulating no longer feel the same. Therefore sexual response is decreased or delayed. Medications commonly used by stroke patients, such as antihypertensive, anticholinergic, or antidepressant agents, may also contribute

*Bray and others, 1981; Griffith and others, 1975; Hawton, 1984; McIntyre and Elesha-Adams, 1990; Sjogren and others, 1983.

to a decrease in sexual response. Concomitant disease, such as diabetes, may also affect sexual function.

Some researchers and clinicians believe sexual dysfunction in stroke patients may be explained by coping deficits that alter sexual self-concept and relationships, indirectly affecting sexual function. Many patients or their partners have expressed fears that sexual activity may make their condition worse or cause another stroke. This may be a particularly important fear in patients whose stroke occurs in temporal proximity to sexual activity. Guidelines for resumption of sexual activity after stroke have not been delineated as they have for other disease states; however, there is no evidence to indicate that sexual activity after stroke can be harmful or cause additional neurologic damage. Another factor in the sexual relationship relates to other responsibilities of the partner. Often the patient's sexual partner is also the patient's caregiver. Caregiving activities may detract from sexual interest for both partners. In one study (Bray and others, 1981), couples with the greatest decline in sexual activity were those in which one partner was dependent on the other for activities of daily living. Both sexes have reported an overall decrease in sexual satisfaction, although there are some couples who reported increased sexual satisfaction following stroke. It may be that in these couples the threat to life and their relationship imposed by stroke actually brought the couples closer together, contributing to increased sexual satisfaction.

Depression has been shown to decrease libido and is associated with a decline in sexual response. Depression may occur in the stroke patient, contributing to sexual dysfunction. Changes in body image are also common, leaving the person feeling sexually unattractive or fearing inadequacy. The stroke patient experiences many losses, including loss of arm, leg, or speech function, employment, and independence. Each can contribute to altered sexuality. Additional psychosocial stressors affecting sexuality have been identified and are listed in the box above.

PSYCHOSOCIAL STRESSORS AFFECTING SEXUALITY

Grieving
Assumption of caretaker role
Social isolation
Loss of confidant relationship
Emotional fatigue
Anger
Guilt
Altered sleep patterns
Role confinement or overload
Fears or concerns about disability

Studies investigating sexual desire after stroke are contradictory. Although a few studies have found sexual interest to be decreased following stroke (Bray and others, 1981; Hawton, 1984; McIntyre and Elesha-Adams, 1990), a greater number of studies actually found no change in sexual desire after stroke. It appears that a temporary decline in sexual desire may occur acutely, possibly related to decreased production of neurotransmitter substances that play a role in desire. Desire has been found to return approximately 6 to 7 weeks after stroke. Interestingly, despite decreased sexual function following stroke, sexual desire remains unchanged, and sexual functioning is perceived to be an important part of life in both sexes. Rarely does sexual desire increase abnormally following stroke. Known as *hypersexuality,* this response is actually more common following head injury, but it may be seen with stroke involving frontal or temporal lobes. These areas are responsible for socially controlled behavior and when affected are no longer able to inhibit behavior. Hypersexuality is manifest in a variety of individual behaviors unique to the patient. Some of these behaviors include sexual aggression, frequent verbal innuendoes, genital exposure, public masturbation, confabulations with sexual overtones, or other sexual behaviors in inappropriate situations.

Table 12-2 Age-related sexual changes

Males	Females
Decreased size, firmness of testicles	Decreased vaginal lubrication
Longer time required to achieve erection	Thinning of vaginal walls
Decreased firmness of erection	Decreased elasticity of vaginal musculature
Less pronounced systemic response to arousal	Atrophy of clitoris
Decreased force of ejaculation	Less pronounced systemic response to arousal
Decreased amount of ejaculate (due to decreased amount of seminal fluid)	Shorter duration of orgasm

Sexuality changes throughout the life span. Since stroke is a disease that primarily affects the older population, age-related sexual changes (Table 12-2) may be superimposed upon those changes attributable to stroke. Changes in body image may occur with age-related physical changes. In addition, sexual relationships may change because of the death or illness of a spouse. Although sexual function changes with aging, it is important to remember that sexuality is important to a person's health throughout his life span.

Little information is available on outcome from sexual dysfunction following stroke. In one study involving only males (Hawton, 1984), sexual desire was found to return in 6.5 weeks and erectile capacity in 7 weeks following stroke. Over half of the stroke patients had resumed sexual activity within 6 months of the stroke, with a mean resumption time of 11 weeks. Persons with right brain lesions, who were younger and more physically independent, were also more likely to resume sexual activity. Persons with motor deficits were able to resume sexual activity, usually incorporating position changes into their relationship. Thus hemiparesis or hemiplegia does not prevent sexual activity. The most important indicator of potential for resumption of sexual activity after stroke was the level of prestroke activity. Those persons who were sexually active before the stroke were likely to resume sexual activity after the stroke. Those with altered sexuality before the stroke would be expected to continue with the same difficulties after the stroke.

ASSESSMENT

Sexuality may become an issue at various times during recovery from stroke. The early acute phase following stroke is probably not the ideal time to assess sexual health, because medical stability and, often, survival take precedence. However, basic information on interpersonal relationships can be gained during the initial history. Such information includes marital status and names of family members or other support persons.

When planning for discharge from the hospital to home, rehabilitation, or other setting, the nurse should perform a brief sexual assessment to facilitate later intervention if necessary. Questions are asked that focus on the three components of sexuality. Examples of questions are:

"Have you thought about how your stroke might affect your sexual function?"

"Do you feel your stroke has affected the way you think about yourself as a man/woman?"

"Do you feel your stroke might interfere with your role as a husband/wife?"

Depending on the response(s) obtained, the nurse may identify the need for additional assessment, intervention, or referral.

It is probably more common for sexuality to become an issue during rehabilitation or after return to the home. Physical or medical crises have passed, and maximizing remaining function becomes the emphasis of nursing care. A total rehabilitation approach demands that sexuality be addressed during stroke recovery, as any disability potentially affects this sensitive area.

Thus the nurse may become involved in a comprehensive assessment of a stroke patient's sexuality. Several tools or guidelines are available to the nurse in performing this assessment, each with distinct advantages and disadvantages. Components of a comprehensive assessment, regardless of the tool or guidelines used, include demographics, health history, sexual history, functional impairment, and effect on sexuality.

Demographic information includes age, marital status, identification of significant others (support systems), and number of children. In taking a health history, the nurse questions the patient about previous illnesses and surgery. Particular attention is paid to chronic illness other than stroke that may affect sexuality, e.g., diabetes or hypertension. Current medications should also be reviewed because certain medications may affect sexual function (Table 12-3).

Sexual history is obtained next. Elmassian and Wilson (1982) identify a format that can be used to obtain a brief sexual history:

- Are you currently sexually active? If so, what is the approximate frequency of sexual activity? Any changes in your (or your partner's) sexual desire or frequency?
- Are you satisfied with your sex life? If not, why not? (Are you dissatisfied with your or your partner's sexual functioning?)
- Is there anything about your (or your partner's) sexual activity (as individuals or as a couple) that you would like to change?
- For men: Do you have any difficulty obtaining an erection? Do you have difficulty controlling ejaculation?
- For women: Do you have any difficulties becoming sexually aroused? Do you experience any pain during intercourse? Do you have difficulty being orgasmic?
- Do you have any questions or problems related to sex that you would like to discuss?

A more detailed sexual history may be necessary to assist in the diagnosis of the exact type and severity of sexual dysfunction. A detailed sexual history usually begins with identification of the patient's perception of the problem. what it involves (severity, frequency), how long it has existed, and what it may be caused by. In addition, the patient is asked to identify any attempts to solve the problem and the results. Next, the patient is asked to identify goals for sexual counseling, focusing on expectations. The partner, if available, is asked the same questions. An in-depth sexual history format has been developed by Masters and Johnson. It takes several hours to complete and requires involvement of the partner. Such detailed history taking is usually beyound the realm of the nurse (unless specializing in sexual dysfunction). However, the nurse may be instrumental in explaining to the patient what such an assessment entails to alleviate concerns or fears.

Stroke may produce deficits that impair function in other areas related to sexuality. Functional impairments should be identified to minimize their effect on sexuality. Specific neurologic deficits may affect sexual function. Hand weakness or numbness may limit ability to provide physical pleasure. Leg weakness or numbness may prevent ambulation and subsequently limit social involvement. Aphasia may also limit socialization; in addition, verbal participation in a sexual relationship is limited. Face, mouth, or tongue weakness limits oral expression of sexuality. Bowel and bladder incontinence or the presence of an indwelling urinary catheter may detract from an environment conducive to a sexual relationship. Other related impairments that may affect sexuality and should be assessed include pain, fatigue, anorexia, nausea, sleep disorders, and behavioral changes (lability, withdrawal, depression, etc.). The patient should also be questioned about any other factors perceived to be problematic.

Physical examination may be necessary when the patient has complaints related to sexual function or when areas of the brain affected by stroke are those involved in sexuality. Touch or pain sensation is assessed in the genital or rectal areas. Reflex and volitional rectal control is assessed by inserting a lubricated gloved finger into the rectum and feeling for sphincter contraction. The patient is then asked

Table 12-3 Drug effects on human sexual behavior.

Drug or drug category	Effect	Probable mechanism of action
Oral contraceptives	Positive	Permits separation of sexual activity from concern about conception
Antihypertensives Clonidine (Catapres) Guanethidine (Ismelin) Methyldopa (Aldomet) Propranolol (Inderal) Reserpine (Serpasil) Trimethaphan (Arfonad)	Negative	Peripheral blockade of nervous innervation of sex glands
Antidepressants Amitriptyline (Elavil) Desipramine (Norpramin, Pertofrane) Imipramine (Tofranil) Nortriptyline (Aventyl) Pargyline (Eutonyl) Phenelzine sulfate (Nardil) Protriptyline (Vivactil) Tranylcypromine (Parnate)	Negative	Central depression; peripheral blockade of nervous innervation of sex glands
Antihistamines Chlorpheniramine (Chlor-Trimeton) Diphenydramine (Benadryl) Promethazine (Phenergan)	Negative	Blockade of parasympathetic nervous innervation of sex glands
Antispasmodics Glycopyrrolate methobromide (Robinul) Hexocyclium (Tral) Methantheline (Banthine) Poldine (Nacton)	Negative	Ganglionic blockade of nervous innervation of sex glands
Sedatives and tranquilizers Benperidol Chlordiazepoxide (Librium) Chlorpromazine (Thorazine, Megaphen) Chlorprothixene (Taractan)	Negative	Central sedation; blockade of autonomic innervation of sex glands; suppression of hypothalamic and pituitary function
Diazepam (Valium) Mesoridazine (Serentil) Methaqualone (Quaalude) Phenoxybenzamine (Dibenzyline) Prochlorperazine (Compazine) Thioridazine (Mellaril)	Positive	Tranquilization and relaxation
Ethyl alcohol	Negative	Central depression; suppression of motor activity; diuresis
	Transiently positive	Release of inhibitions; relaxation
Barbiturates	Negative	Central depression; suppression of motor activity; hypnosis

Continued.

Table 12-3 Drug effects on human sexual behavior.—cont'd

Drug or drug category	Effect	Probable mechanism of action
Diuretics Bendroflumethiazide (Naturetin) Chlorothiazide (Diuril) Spironolactone (Aldactone)	Negative	Diuresis
Sex hormone preparations Cyproterone acetate Methandrostenolone (Dianabol) Nandrolane phenpropionate (Durabolin) Norethandrolone (Nilevar)	Negative	Antiandrogenic effects on sexual function; loss of libido; decreased potency
Methadone	Negative	Suppressess secondary sex organ function in men
Potassium nitrate (saltpeter)	Questionable	Diuresis
Cantharis (Spanish fly)	Negative	Irritation and inflammation of genitourinary tract; systemic poisoning
Yohimbine	Questionable	Stimulation of lower spinal nerve centers
Strychnine	Questionable	Stimulation of neuraxis; priapism
Narcotics and psychoactive drugs Amphetamines Cocaine	Negative	Central depression; decreased libido and impaired potency
Heroin LSD Marijuana Methadone Morphine	Transiently positive	Release of inhibitions; increased suggestibility; relaxation
L-Dopa and *p*-chlorophenylalanine (PCPA)	Questionable	Improvement of well-being
Amyl nitrite	Questionable	Vasodilation of genitourinary tract; smooth muscle relaxation
Caffeine	Questionable	Central nervous system stimulant
Vitamin E	Questionable	Supports fertility in laboratory animals
Selenium	Questionable	Supports fertility in laboratory animals
Lithium carbonate	Questionable	
Produces broad endocrine changes; diuresis		
Clomiphene citrate (Clomid)	Questionable	Stimulates gonadotropic hormones; enhances expectations of achieving pregnancy
Bromocriptine (Parlodel)	Questionable	Stimulates gonadotropic hormones
Cimetidine (Tagamet)	Negative	Unknown
Clofibrate (Atromid S)	Questionable	Unknown
Disulfiram (Antabuse)	None by itself; negative with alcohol	Blocks alcohol metabolism; produces aldehyde syndrome

From Woods NF: Human sexuality in health and illness, ed 3, St Louis, 1984, The CV Mosby Co.

to contract the sphincter; contraction should again be felt. Further laboratory evaluation may be necessary to provide additional information. For example, a perinometer might be used to determine vaginal muscle strength. A penile tumescence monitor may be used to distinguish between organic and psychogenic impotence.

An environment appropriate to assessment should be considered when interviewing or examining the patient. Because of the sensitive nature of sexuality, privacy is essential. In addition, physical and psychologic comfort measures should be considered. Establishing a trusting interpersonal relationship with the patient is vital in gaining accurate and reliable information. Patient participation in the assessment may be declined at any time.

Because sexuality issues change or arise at different times during the course of stroke recovery, assessment of sexual health may be ongoing. In caring for stroke patients, the nurse should observe for certain behaviors that indicate the need for assessment. Sexual overtures or advances made to nurses usually indicate that the patient has sexual concerns. Indirect verbalizations regarding sexuality may also serve as cues for the nurse. For example, the patient might say, "I don't know why my wife even bothers to visit me." Direct verbalizations in the form of questions or complaints, although not as common, may also be noted.

Because nursing care involves an interpersonal relationship with the patient, the nurse should be aware of his or her own sexuality, even though the nature of the nurse-patient relationship is not sexual. The nurse brings certain sexual knowledge, values, and experience into the relationship. Awareness of one's own sexuality and the effect of this on the nurse-patient relationship is important in helping patients deal with sexuality issues. If a nurse is uncomfortable discussing sexual topics, then the patient should be provided the opportunity to discuss these issues with someone who is comfortable. Likewise, the nurse may not be educated in dealing with sexual dysfunction. Through continuing education, the nurse may become more knowledgeable in this area, or the patient may be referred to an appropriate health care professional for counseling.

Since a person's sexuality is usually expressed in the context of a relationship, the patient's partner should be included in the assessment. Questions asked of the patient may also be asked of the partner to determine a broader scope of any difficulties. For the patient with behavioral or cognitive problems, information from the partner may clarify information from the patient's perspective. When a partner is not available, as with the patient who is widowed or divorced and without a partner at present, it must *not* be assumed that sexuality isn't an issue. Such situations simply limit the scope of assessment.

INTERVENTIONS

Once assessment is completed, the nature of sexual dysfunction may be identified and appropriate interventions instituted. There are several general principles that guide nursing intervention. An *awareness of the problem* is important for both the nurse and the patient. Virtually every stroke patient is at risk for alteration in his or her sexuality, and sexual adjustment appears to be positively correlated with rehabilitation outcome. Patients should be informed of the potential sexual dysfunction and encouraged to ask for information or seek assistance if difficulties arise. It is important that a *trusting nurse-patient relationship* is established so that any problems may be openly discussed. *Privacy* is important. The environment in which sexual issues are discussed should be conducive to maintaining privacy. In addition, personal privacy is respected in giving the patient permission to not discuss sexual issues if she so wishes. *Early intervention* is important to reinforce self-esteem and facilitate recovery. Just as other deficits are treated as soon as possible, so should sexual dysfunction be. At times it can be difficult to identify patient readiness for sexuality information or rehabilitation. The nurse may be instrumental in initiating discussion even if readiness is not apparent. Patients often expect health care professionals to initiate such a discussion. Lastly, it is important to remember that preexisting sexual problems persist into the poststroke period. Although not specifically related to stroke, the stroke may exacerbate preexisting problems. Resolution of these problems may be necessary before new problems can be addressed.

Nursing interventions can be provided at various levels of involvement, depending on the nurse's comfort with intervening and the patient's specific needs. The PLISSIT model proposed by Annon (1974) allows for different levels of involvement as follows:

Permission—interventions at this level are directed toward providing the patient with permission to have sexual feelings and concerns, opening a relationship for discussion if necessary. The nurse may tell the patient and partner, "Your doctor feels it is acceptable for you to resume sexual activity."

Limited Information—interventions at this level are directed toward providing specific but not too detailed information related to the patient's sexuality. The nurse might say to the patient. "Many patients experience sexual problems following stroke. These problems can arise from physical disabilities that often occur. If you have specific questions or concerns, I would be happy to help you address them."

Specific suggestions—interventions at this level are directed toward solving specific problems identified through detailed history-taking. Specific suggestions are offered to the patient or partner, individualized to their unique situation. The nurse might say, "Some couples find morning is the best time for sexual relations, when both partners are well rested. You might want to see what time of day you feel you have the most energy."

Intensive Therapy—interventions at this level are provided by a health care professional with advanced training and expertise in sexuality and sexual dysfunction. Therapy may be indicated when interventions at previous levels have been unsuccessful. The nurse may be instrumental in referring the patient or couple for therapy.

Permission or limited information may be enough to help the patient or couple resolve or prevent sexual dysfuntion. Specific suggestions may be necessary; intensive therapy is often unnecessary unless preexisting problems are superimposed. The astute nurse who is comfortable in dealing with sexuality will know which level of intervention is required.

Several nursing diagnoses may be determined for the stroke patient with altered sexuality.

Altered Sexuality Related to the Physical Consequences of Stroke

Physical disabilities imposed by stroke have an impact on sexual function. While giving the sexual history, the patient may identify specific difficulties with maneuvering during sexual activity resulting from physical deficits. Physical examination may reveal deficits that potentially affect sexuality, such as hemiparesis or hemiplegia, spasticity, hemianopia, facial droop, oral weakness, or aphasia. Hemiparesis or hemiplegia may cause difficulty in coital positioning, particularly for the superior position if used by the affected partner. The unaffected partner could be encouraged to use the superior position (Fig. 12-1), which allows the stroke partner to lie down. The sidelying position may also be used with the stroke patient laying on the affected side. Males using a wheelchair may find the sitting position in the wheelchair most comfortable (Fig. 12-1). A trapeze, footboard, or handle on the headboard may also facilitate maneuvering. Pillows may be used to support spastic extremities for comfort. Some female patients with spasticity find the prone position minimizes the spastic response but it can make maneuvering difficult. Hemianopia may limit visual stimulation; therefore, the person should be approached from the visually intact side. Facial droop and oral weakness may make kissing or other oral contact difficult. Alternative forms of intimacy or stimulation, such as hugging, cuddling, or touching, may be encouraged. Aphasia may limit verbal exchange during sexual activity. Nonverbal communication should be encouraged. It may help the unaffected partner to know that an aphasic per-

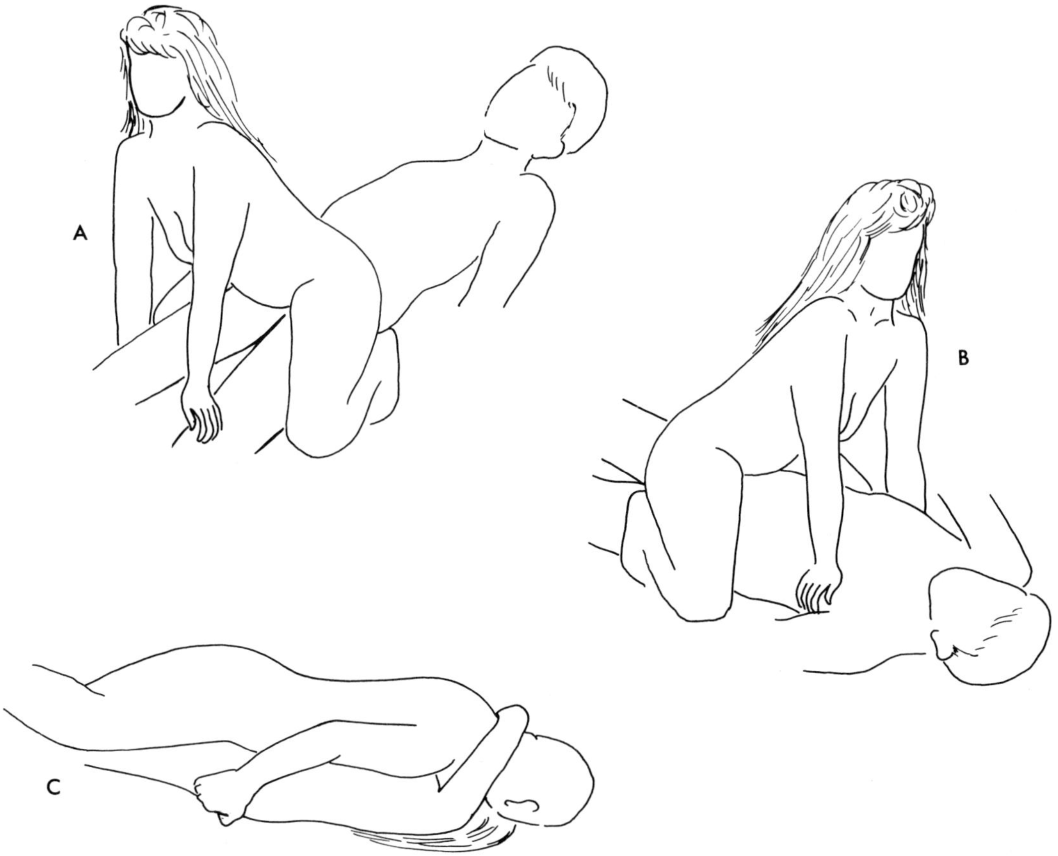

Fig. 12-1 **A** and **B**, The unaffected partner can use the superior position, allowing the stroke partner to lie down. **C**, The side lying position may be used with stroke partner on unaffected side.

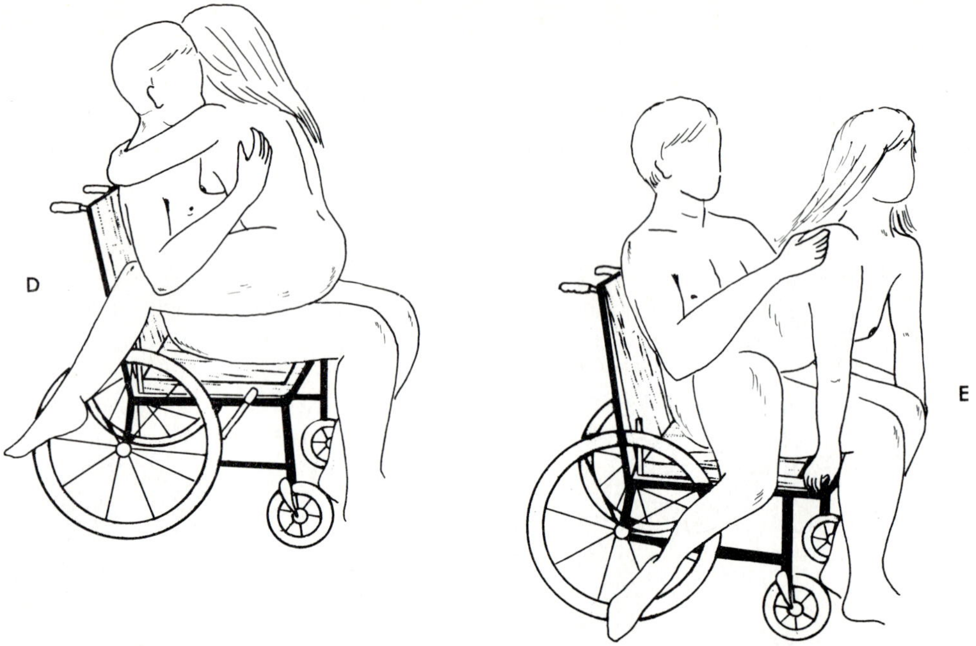

Fig. 12-1, cont'd D and E, Males may find the sitting position in the wheelchair most comfortable.

son may unintentionally use obscene language during the intensity of sexual activity. In addition, the nurse may individualize sexual history questions to focus on deficits commonly associated with right or left brain involvement. Persons with left brain involvement may be slow, hesitant, cautious, or disorganized, leading to difficulty in initiating or performing sexual activity and should be questioned about problems in these areas if the information is not offered directly. The unaffected partner should be encouraged to provide immediate feedback, reassurance, and encouragement. The unaffected partner may need to initiate sexual activity, even if this has not been a previous role. Individuals with right brain involvement may be impulsive, have a short attention span, and have difficulty sequencing activities, making it difficult to continue previous patterns of sexual activity. Foreplay may be forgotten or the partner's needs overlooked. The unaffected partner should be encouraged to provide simple directions; immediate feedback and encouragement are also helpful. In addition, the environment should be calm and free of distractions.

Altered Sexuality Related to Low Sexual Desire

Partners may directly identify decreased sexual desire as a problem or indirectly complain of decreased frequency of sexual activity during sexual history taking. Although sexual interest is thought to be preserved following stroke, an acute decline in desire may occur. It may be helpful to inform the patient that such a decline is normal and temporary. The patient should be questioned directly about fatigue, pain and discomfort, or depression because these may adversely affect sexual desire. Sexual activity may be planned when both partners are well-rested, in the morning or after a nap. Sexual positioning may incorporate comfort measures such as pillows. Depression may require medical attention and should be discussed with the patient's physician. Current medications should also be reviewed. Certain medications, such as antihypertensives, sedatives, narcotics, and testosterone antagonists may suppress sexual desire. Medications should be reviewed and discussed with the physician to determine whether changes in medication may enhance sexual desire. Alcohol has also been shown to suppress sexual desire and should be avoided. Concerns or fears about sexual activity may be voiced during sexual history taking. Patients or their partners may desire sexual activity less when fearful that sexual activity may cause another stroke or worsen their condition. The couple should be informed that sexual activity is permissible and will *not* cause another stroke or worsen the patient's condition (providing blood pressure is stable). In fact, sexual activity may enhance feelings of self-worth and facilitate overall rehabilitation. Support from couples in similar situations (such as through a stroke club) may also help to dissipate concern.

Altered Sexuality Related to Unrestrained Sexual Behavior

Often called hypersexuality, frontal lobe damage may cause unrestrained behavior, resulting in inappropriate sexual behavior. Characteristics to observe for during assessment include physical or verbal innuendos, frequent demands for sexual attention, exposure of genitalia, and sexual behavior in inappropriate situations. Because it is a behavioral problem, interventions to modify behavior are helpful. The patient should be informed about the inappropriateness of his behavior. When caring for patients with this problem, it is important to avoid becoming involved in their behavior by laughing or becoming offended. Removing the patient from the area where unacceptable behavior occurred may be helpful. Efforts at self-control should be praised. Group therapy may sometimes be helpful; patients may observe model behavior and attempt to imitate it.

Altered Sexuality Related to Decreased Sexual Arousal

From the sexual history specific complaints related to arousal may be obtained, including difficulty achieving or maintaining erection in males and decreased vaginal lubrication in females. In males, decreased arousal may be objectively measured by a penile tumescence monitor. Although objective measurement of arousal in females is difficult, it is possible to observe increased vaginal lubrication. More commonly, subjective reports provide information.

Physiologic mechanisms of arousal are thought to be preserved following stroke. However, subjective aspects of arousal may be impaired. These changes may be related to medications, other disease processes (e.g., diabetes), the aging process, or decreased sexual desire; therefore each of these aspects should be evaluated as previously discussed. Sensory loss is common following stroke, and it may be more difficult for the stroke person to become aroused. Partners may be encouraged to explore areas of the body with intact sensation to identify those that are stimulated. Information on areas involved in arousal (erogenous areas) may be provided. Both partners should be encouraged to verbalize feelings of what is pleasurable. In addition, alternative forms of stimulation, such as imagery, fantasy, or visual stimulation, may be encouraged. Vibrators may also be used. The physician may be consulted for change in medication to enhance sexual arousal. When medication cannot be changed, or when age-related changes are problematic, certain suggestions may be offered. Males may be counseled about the use of penile sheaths or prostheses. Females may be taught about substitutes for vaginal lubrication, such as hormonal cream, KY jelly, or saliva. Refer to the section on decreased sexual desire for interventions related to this problem.

Altered Sexuality Related to Anorgasmia

The identification of this diagnosis is based solely on complaints of anorgasmia elicited during the sexual history. Orgasm may be impaired in both males and females affected by stroke and is usually related to difficulty achieving adequate arousal. Generally, physiologic control of orgasm is preserved following stroke, but subjective aspects leading to orgasm may be impaired. Nursing interventions are the same as those in the section on decreased sexual arousal. However, the focus is on the type of stimulation that produces maximum pleasure. Often, arousal may improve over a period of time, and with selective attention toward this problem, the orgasmic ability will return.

Altered Sexuality Related to Altered Sexual Self-Concept

In obtaining the sexual history, the nurse may note specific feelings identified by the patient that are related to an altered body image or decreased self-worth. Disability from stroke potentially alters sexual self-concept, leaving the person feeling he or she is no longer a sexual being. Interventions are geared toward helping the patient to enhance body image and feelings of self-worth. Grooming and hygiene efforts are encouraged, with assistance provided as necessary. Concerns about bowel or bladder incontinence may need to be addressed. The patient is encouraged to attempt to fully empty the bladder before sexual activity. Intermittent self-catheterization may be performed before sexual activity. An indwelling catheter may be taped to the side of the leg or to the abdomen for females. Males may fold the catheter over the penis and apply a condom over both the catheter and penis. For both males and females, care should be taken to position the indwelling catheter to avoid traction and displacement of the inflated bulb into the urethra. A successful bowel program may enhance body image; sexual activity may be planned around the bowel routine. Otherwise it should be explained to both partners that incontinence may occur and a towel or disposable pad may be placed under the affected partner to minimize embarrassment. Other considerations include communication of feelings between partners. The affected partner should verbalize feelings about sexual self-worth. The unaffected partner could in turn express feelings of still finding the partner sexually attractive. Group interaction, through activities such as a stroke club, may also be helpful in enhancing self-worth and promoting sexual self-concept. Interventions to facilitate sexual desire may also be incorporated.

Altered Sexuality Related to Alteration in Sexual Relationship

A sexual assessment of both partners that reveals incongruities or dissatisfaction alerts the nurse to changes in the sexual relationship. Stroke is a phenomenon that affects not only the patient but close family and friends as well, potentially altering the sexual relationship. The unaffected partner may be confused about or fearful of changes in the stroke person. The nurse may be instrumental in explaining personality and behavior changes and other deficits to the partner. Illness, stress, or depression in the unaffected partner may decrease sexual desire and affect the sexual relationship. The unaffected partner should be encouraged to take time for himself or herself, strive to maintain health, and find creative outlets for stress. Changes in the way sexuality is expressed as a result of stroke affect the sexual relationship. Alternative forms of sexual expression may facilitate arousal, but one of the partners may find the alternative form of expression offensive. Couple communication is essential to resolving conflict and should be encouraged. Couple counseling might be beneficial. Caregiving responsibilities may make it difficult to maintain a sexual relationship. Caregiving and sexual activities should be kept as separate as possible. If possible, the unaffected partner could be relieved of caregiving responsibilities by obtaining outside help. Occasionally, caregiving responsibilities may actually enhance the relationship by assisting the unaffected partner in becoming accustomed to touching the affected partner. Finally, stroke may lead to social isolation for the couple. The couple should be encouraged to participate in social endeavors. A stroke club or similar group also provides opportunities for socialization.

Sexuality issues for the single person without a partner may be very difficult to address. Initial interventions may focus on assisting the disabled individual in socializing or dating. An exercise program may also be beneficial for the individual with altered sexuality. Exercise may improve energy level and enhance a feeling of self-worth. Group exercise also affords the opportunity for socialization. For the younger stroke patient birth control may need to be addressed. Although low-estrogen forms of oral contraceptives are available, many physicians are reluctant to prescribe this form of birth control for the female with a stroke history. Alternative forms of birth control may be recommended. Pregnancy is generally not contraindicated following stroke but should be discussed with the woman's physician.

Nursing research is limited in the area of sexuality following stroke. Reliable and valid instruments must be developed that assess sexuality in this population and determine readiness for sexual information. The effectiveness of recommended interventions also warrants further investigation, along with validity of proposed nursing diagnoses of altered sexuality.

NURSING CARE PLAN

Nursing Diagnosis	Interventions	Expected Outcomes
Sexuality Patterns, altered related to the physical consequences of stroke **Defining Characteristics:** ■ Difficulty in coital positioning due to hemiparesis, hemiplegia, and/or spasticity ■ Decreased arousal due to hemianopia, facial and/or oral weakness, or communication impairment ■ Changes in patterns of sexual activity due to cognitive-perceptual deficits	**Ongoing Assessment** ■ Conduct neurologic assessment for deficits affecting positioning A. Hemiparesis, hemiplegia, spasticity ■ Conduct neurologic assessment for deficits affecting arousal A. Hemianopia, facial droop, oral weakness, asphasia ■ Perform cognitive assessment for deficits affecting patterns of sexual activity A. Impulsivity, decreased attention span, difficulty sequencing activities **Therapeutic Interventions** (See Patient Teaching Section)	■ Patient will be able to maintain relationship with partner ■ Patient and partner will verbalize understanding of options for sexual satisfaction
Sexuality patterns, altered related to low sexual desire **Defining Charateristics:** ■ Verbalization of decreased sexual desire by patient and/or partner ■ Decreased frequency of sexual activity	**Ongoing Assessment** ■ Assess poststroke level of desire as compared with prestroke ■ Determine frequency of sexual activity ■ Assess related factors A. Pain, fatigue, fear, etc. **Therapeutic Interventions** ■ Review medications for effect on sexual desire	■ The patient and partner will be able to verbalize reasons for decreased sexual desire ■ The patient's sexual desire will improve

NURSING CARE PLAN — cont'd

Nursing Diagnosis	Interventions	Expected Outcomes
Sexuality patterns, altered related to unrestrained sexual behavior **Defining Characteristics** ■ Physical or verbal innuendos ■ Frequent demands for sexual attention	**Onging Assessment** ■ Assess A. Impulsivity B. Verbalization of sexual innuendos or attention demands C. Inappropriate sexual behavior **Therapeutic Interventions** ■ Reinforce appropriate behavior ■ Avoid becoming involved in inappropriate behavior ■ Remove patient from area where inappropriate behavior is exhibited ■ Allow patient to be exposed to situations of model behavior	■ Patient will be able to demonstrate appropriate sexual behavior

Continued.

NURSING CARE PLAN — cont'd

Nursing Diagnosis	Interventions	Expected Outcomes
Sexuality patterns, altered related to decreased sexual arousal **Defining Characteristics** ■ For males, difficulty achieving and/or maintaining erection ■ For females, decreased vaginal lubrication	**Ongoing Assessment** ■ Males—Ask about frequency and quality of erections ■ Females—Ask about vaginal lubrication with arousal ■ Conduct sensory assessment for areas of decreased tactile sensation ■ Assess factors patient and/or partner may perceive to negatively effect arousal **Therapeutic Interventions** ■ Review medications and medical history for factors that may decrease sexual arousal	■ Patient will achieve improved sexual arousal: A. Males: Ability to achieve/ maintain erection will improve B. Females: Increased vaginal lubrication
Sexuality Patterns, Altered related to anorgasmia **Defining Characteristics** ■ Subjective complaints of anorgasmia ■ Related complaints of difficulty achieving arousal	**Ongoing Assessment** ■ Ask about ability to achieve orgasm **Therapeutic Interventions** (See Patient Education selection)	■ Patient will be able to achieve orgasm

NURSING CARE PLAN — cont'd

Nursing Diagnosis	Interventions	Expected Outcomes
Sexuality Patterns, Altered related to alteration in sexual relationship **Defining Characteristics** ■ Expression of sexual dissatisfaction from patient and/or partner ■ Subjective reports of alteration in sexual relationship from patient and/ or partner A. Fear of sexual activity, confusion about sexual changes ■ Social isolation ■ Lack of sexual relationship	**Ongoing Assessment** ■ Conduct sexual assessment with both partners, noting any incongruencies ■ Identify primary caregiver ■ Identify extent of poststroke socialization **Therapeutic Interventions** ■ Encourage patient and partner to verbalize sexual concerns ■ Encourage couple communication, suggesting counseling where appropriate ■ Encourage socialization ■ Assist partner in obtaining outside help to gain relief from caregiving responsibilities	■ Patient's sexual relationship will be maintained.

Continued.

NURSING CARE PLAN — cont'd

Nursing Diagnosis	Interventions	Expected Outcomes
Sexuality Patterns, Altered related to altered sexual self-concept **Defining Characteristics** ■ Lack of interest in personal appearance, grooming, hygiene ■ Patient complaints of decreased self-worth, altered body image	**Ongoing Assessment** ■ Assess patient's physical appearance, grooming, and hygiene ■ Note verbal comments or complaints of decreased self-worth and/or altered body image ■ Ask about concerns related to sexual self-concept, e.g., incontinence **Therapeutic Interventions** ■ Encourage grooming and hygiene efforts, providing assistance as necessary ■ Encourage socialization ■ Encourage communication between partners ■ Incorporate interventions to facilitate sexual desire	■ Patient's sexual self-concept will improve

Patient Education

- Inform patient and family about potential alterations in sexuality following stroke
- Suggest alternative positions to facilitate comfort and activity
- Encourage partner to approach patient from visually intact side
- Encourage alternative forms of intimacy (e.g., hugging, cuddling, touching)
- Encourage both partners to use nonverbal forms of communication
- Encourage partner to provide feedback, assurance and encouragement
- Instruct patient and partner to minimize extraneous distractions during sexual activity
- Inform patient and partner about effects of stroke on sexual desire
- Instruct patient and partner to plan sexual activity when rested
- Encourage patient to seek medical attention for depression
- Instruct patient to discuss with physician change of medications that affect sexual desire
- Assure patient and partner that sexual activity is permissible following stroke
- Reassure patient and partner that sexual desire will improve

NURSING CARE PLAN — cont'd

Patient Education—cont'd

- Let patient know when sexual behavior is unacceptable and what is desired
- Encourage partner to explore areas of body with intact sensation to identify stimulating areas
- Provide information on erogenous areas
- Encourage patient to verbalize feelings of what is pleasurable
- Provide information on alternative forms of stimulation (e.g., imagery, fantasy, visual stimulation, mechanical stimulation [vibrator])
- Counsel males in use of penile prosthesis or sheath
- Counsel females in use of substitutes for vaginal lubrication (e.g., hormonal cream, KY jelly, saliva)
- Reassure patient and partner that problems relating to inability to achieve sexual satisfaction are common and usually resolve with time and selective attention
- Give permission to caregiver to relinquish some responsibilities and take some personal time
- Encourage partner to explore ways to improve self image
- Instruct patient to empty bladder or catheterize prior to sexual activity
- For males with an indwelling catheter, inform that it may be folded over penis and a condom applied. Care must be taken to avoid traction on or displacement of the catheter to avoid urethral damage
- For females with indwelling catheter, the catheter may be taped to the leg or abdomen
- Instruct patient to plan sexual activity around bowel program
- Explain to patient and partner that incontinence may occur
- Encourage partner to verbalize feelings of finding the patient sexually attractive

REFERENCES

Annon J: The behavioral treatment of sexual problems, Honolulu, 1974, Enabling System.

Bray GP, DeFrank RS, and Wolfe TL: Sexual functioning in stroke survivors, Arch Phys Med Rehabil, 62:286, 1981.

Bullard DG and Knight SE: Sexuality and physical disability, ed 1, St. Louis, 1981, The CV Mosby Co.

Elmassian BJ and Wilson RW: Assessment and diagnosis of sexual problems, Nurse Pract, 7:13, 1982.

Emick-Herring B: Sexual changes in patients and partners following stroke, Rehabil Nurs, 10:28, 1985.

Friedeman JS: Sexuality in older persons, Nurs Forum, 28:92, 1979.

Glover J: Human sexuality in nursing care, San Mateo, Calif., 1985, Appleton-Century-Crofts.

Griffith ER, Trieschmann RB, Hohmann GW, and others: Sexual dysfunction associated with physical disabilities, Arch Phys Med Rehabil, 56:8, 1975.

Hanson EI and Brouse SH: Assessing sexual implications of functional impairments associated with chronic illness, Sex Education and Therapy, 8:39, 1982.

Hawton K: Sexual adjustment of men who have had strokes, Psychosom Res, 28:243, 1984.

Kaplan HS: The new sex therapy, ed 1, New York, 1974, Brunner/Mazel Inc.

Katzin L: Chronic illness and sexuality, Am J Nurs, 90:55, 1990.

Lion EM: Human sexuality in the nursing process, New York, 1985, John Wiley & Sons.

Masters W and Johnson V: Human sexual response, Boston, 1966, Little, Brown & Co. Inc.

McCormick GP, Riffer DJ and Thompson MM: Coital positioning for stroke afflicted couples, Rehabil Nurs, 11:17, 1986.

McIntyre K and Elesha-Adams M: Sexual limitations caused by stroke, J Sex Education and Therapy, 16:57, 1990.

Monga TN, Lawson JS and Inglis J: Sexual dysfunction in stroke patients, Arch Phys Med Rehabil, 67:19, 1986.

Renshaw DC: Sexual problems in old age, illness, and disability, 22:975, 1981.

Renshaw DC: Stroke and sex. In Comfort A, editor: Sexual consequences of disability, ed 1, Philadelphia, 1978, George F. Stickley Co.

Sjogren K, Damber J and Liliequist B: Sexuality after stroke with hemiplegia, Scand J Rehab Med, 15:55, 1983.

Tilton C and Maloof M: Diagnosing the problems in stroke, Am J Nurs, 82:96, 1982.

White EJ: Appraising the need for altered sexuality information, Rehabil Nurs, 11:6, 1986.

Woods NF: Human sexuality in health and illness, ed 3, St. Louis, 1984,The CV Mosby Co.

Woods NF: Human sexuality: an overview, In Mitchell PH, Hodges LC, Muwaswes M, and others, editors: AANN's Neuroscience Nursing, New York, 1988, Appleton & Lange.

Woods NF: Alterations in human sexuality. In Mitchell PH, Hodges LC, Muwaswes M, and others, editors: AANN'S Neuroscience Nursing, New York, 1988, Appleton & Lange.

Chapter 13

Alterations in Coping

One's health is disrupted by a stroke; this can result in unparalleled physical and emotional losses producing substantial psychological disability (Goodstein, 1983). Thus the effects of a stroke, and subsequent adaptation, consist of physiological, psychological and social dimensions. Stroke-related deficits may affect how individuals perceive and interpret their situation, their hopes for recovery and how they cope. If persons accurately appraise their situation and mobilize resources then they will be able to cope with the stress of a stroke. By identifying how stroke patients cope, nurses can better facilitate adaptive coping in this population and play a crucial role in assisting the patient to cope (Roy, 1970).

Coping is often neglected in discussions about stroke. Frequently, the emphasis on stroke outcomes is on physical improvement, as indicated by level of functional abilities, health status, discharge placement and employment status. Despite the growing interest in stroke care, relatively little attention has been given to the psychological effects of stroke, particularly how patients and their families cope. Coping should concern clinicians in light of research findings regarding mood disturbances and the frequent cognitive and perceptual deficits that one potentially may experience after a stroke. It is almost certain that the concomitant cognitive and mood changes will interfere with one's ability to cope. One of the goals of the nurse is to facilitate patient coping and to help the family understand changes they may see in the patient. By assisting the patient and family to cope, the nurse is giving the patient and family every possible chance to understand and to live with their stroke.

This chapter will discuss general coping as it has been studied in a variety of populations; then, specifically, coping with stroke. A model for coping with stroke will be presented. Tools for nurses to subjectively and objectively assess coping will be described; and, nursing interventions to facilitate coping after stroke will be discussed.

GENERAL COPING

This section will examine four areas in the general coping literature: an overview of the coping process, the nature of the stressful event, the coping response to a stressful event, and personal and situational variables affecting coping.

Overview

Definitions of coping found in the literature are diverse. In its broadest sense, coping is the way in which humans react and respond to the environment. Coping consists of psychosocial processes aimed at establishing balance in the person-environment interaction (Carlson, 1981) in response to a fairly drastic change or problem (White, 1976). More specifically, coping is defined as dynamic cognitive and behavioral efforts to manage specific external and/or internal demands that are appraised as taxing or exceeding the resources of the person (Lazarus and Folkman, 1984).

Coping has many facets and is influenced by many factors. Coping is a process involving cognitive, emotional and behavioral components, and includes efforts a person makes to master conditions of harm, threat or challenge (Lazarus and others 1974). Coping occurs across the life span to manage transitions that accompany each developmental stage. The coping response is also elicited by unusual and extreme stressors such as illness. The nature of the stressful event may affect how a person copes.

Nature of the Stressful Event

The stressful event (such as illness) has many dimensions, including the nature of onset, the course of the illness, and the duration of the illness. Each of these dimensions of the stressful event will be discussed.

The nature of the onset of illness has a major effect on how patients cope. Sudden illness can put a person in a crisis state, which has implications for the person's capability for action and for the type of adaptive tasks he perceives as important. For example, when a person suddenly becomes ill or injured, the changes in body image or functioning, the separation from family, and the feelings of anxiety, uncertainty, and helplessness are also sudden (Moos & Tsu, 1977). If the person is in a crisis, adaptive tasks and coping stategies will be directed toward resolving the crisis.

A major adaptive task in sudden physical illness is dealing with uncertainty (Moos and Tsu, 1977; Cohen and Lazarus, 1979). Event uncertainty has great potential for creating psychologic stress because it immobilizes anticipatory coping (Lazarus and Folkman, 1984) and makes it difficult for the person to choose appropriate coping strategies. For example, a stroke patient may have to cope with the threat of a permanent loss of hand function while still maintaining hope that function will be restored. The uncertainty of the event outcome causes the individual to frequently appraise and reappraise what is happening; this process can induce conflicting thoughts, emotions, and behaviors and mental confusion (Lazarus and Folkman, 1984). Thus the suddenness of the event will influence the person's coping responses.

In contrast to a sudden illness, a gradual onset of illness warns the person and provides her with opportunities to use a greater variety of coping mechanisms (Lazarus and Folkman, 1984). Event imminence refers to how much time there is before the event occurs. Although simulated studies suggested that the longer the interval of time before the event, the greater the threat (Nomikos and others, 1968), more anticipation time was associated with less stress because the person had time to mobilize coping strategies to minimize the threat (Lazarus and Folkman, 1984). Thus the nature of the onset of illness may affect how the person copes.

Another dimension of the stressful event that must be considered is whether the course of the event is static or changing. If the nature of the stress changes over time, the nature of the coping response may also change over time. Coping responses over time have been explained by stage theory, which Cobb (1962) derived from her early studies with dying patients.

Stage theory proposes five stages of psychologic adjustment to physical trauma and disability: shock, denial, depression, reaction against independence, and adaptation (Krueger, 1984). Patients usually move through all stages but may oscillate between them. Shock is characterized by the person not comprehending the magnitude or consequences of what has occurred. Denial, a necessary defense against depression, enables the person to deny severity or irreversibility and maintain hope. Depression occurs when the person recognizes the loss. Reaction against independence may be expressed by ambivalence or deliberate behavior to interfere with progress. Adaptation is characterized by coping behaviors that reduce stress and result in effective problem-solving. Some studies have investigated stages of adaptation and coping after disability, but few of these are conclusive (Hamburg and others, 1953; Visotsky and others, 1961). Future studies should incorporate qualitative and quantitative measures to investigate the validity of stage theory in long-term recovery.

One concern with stage theory is that it suggests that patients progress through stages at a certain pace and in a prescribed sequence. The danger with this interpretation of stage theory is that health care providers may expect patients to feel and act a certain way at different times in recovery; if patients fail to meet these expectations, they may be labeled as not well-adjusted. Though advocates of stage theory acknowledge individual differences in the coping response, they do not emphasize differences among individual patients. In contrast, recent research in the area of coping demonstrates that coping responses may be more variable than was initially thought because coping varies with the person and the situation (Billings and Moos, 1981; Lazarus and Folkman, 1984; Pearlin and Schooler, 1978).

The final dimension to be considered is the duration of the illness, i.e., whether an illness is short-term or chronic. While interviewing chronically ill patients, Strauss and others (1984) documented extensively the work involved in managing a chronic illness and the related coping responses. Problems that chronically ill persons face include preventing and managing medical crises, controlling symptoms, managing health regimens, and dealing with social isolation. The extent of these problems, of course, will depend on the type and severity of the illness and the available resources. However, daily management of a chronic illness may deplete coping resources and interfere with overall coping effectiveness. One study found that prolonged stress on coping style reduced a person's tendency to use active coping processes (Shanan and other, 1976). The presence of prolonged stress may be physically and psychologically exhausting, resulting in a decrease of overall coping effectiveness. The effects of chronic illness on coping responses, however, are not all negative.

While some studies have pointed out the negative effects of chronic stressors (Selye, 1977; Shanan and others, 1976), none have investigated how the negative effects might be controlled by individual factors. Lazarus and Folkman (1984) suggest that chronic stressors give the person a chance to learn how to deal with demands, develop new skills, and identify realistic goals. Thus the chronicity of the stressor may be an advantage in that patients have opportunities for appraisal and reappraisal of their situation.

Although patients appraise and reappraise some chronic-illness stressors, stressors related to the duration of an illness are not always predictable. For example, uncertainty as an influencing factor in coping response is an issue for people with terminal illness. In a longitudinal study of adults with leukemia in remission, patients reported using anticipatory grief and denial as the most common coping strategies to deal with the uncertainty of their own outcome (Sanders and Kardinal, 1977). Thus uncertainty is an issue faced by terminally ill people; similarly, people with chronic illness face uncertainty of different types.

In summary, the duration of an illness has implications for coping. Coping is influenced by whether the stressor is short-term or chronic. Chronic illness imposes different adaptive tasks on the individual; these adaptive tasks may require using different coping strategies or using strategies similar to those used for persons with short-term illness but at different times. Although the stressors of chronic illness may afford the individual opportunities for identifying coping strategies, the net effects of chronic illness may also deplete coping resources. Whether coping resources are depleted or not will depend on additional personal and situational variables and the effectiveness of the coping response.

Coping Response to the Stressful Event

Responding to a stressful event is a complex process. Four dimensions of this process must be considered: selection, use, and effectiveness of coping stategies, and the change of coping strategies over time.

First, in response to a stressor, patients will select coping strategies. *Coping strategies* have been defined as techniques used to deal with a particular stress (Carlson, 1981); using coping strategies may involve learning new skills and techniques to manage the stressors (Moos and Tsu, 1977; Wright, 1983). Strategies have been categorized into several evolving taxonomies. In one taxonomy, those strategies that manage the problem are called *problem-focused,* and those strategies that regulate the emotional response evoked by the situation are called *emotion-focused* (Folkman and Lazarus, 1980). A third type, *palliative coping,* is suggested as tension-modulating, with components of both emotion-focused and problem-solving strategies (Jalowiec, 1986). Recent attempts to describe coping strategies suggest even greater variety and may include evasive, optimistic, fatalistic, supportant and self-reliant strategies (Jalowiec, 1987). Second, the individual uses coping strategies to problem-solve, to modify the stressor, to control the emotional stress arising from the stressful situation itself (Cohen and Lazarus, 1979), and to control the meaning of the stressor so as not to be overwhelmed by it (Pearlin and Schooler, 1978). Using a variety of coping strategies may promote healthy coping.

Another dimension of the coping process is coping effectiveness. Researchers have investigated coping strategy types (coping dispositions) to determine if certain strategies are more effective than others. Coping dispositions were investigated in preoperative stress and recovery in surgical patients (Cohen and Lazarus, 1973). Results suggested that avoidant copers did better after surgery than vigilant copers. In contrast, Roberts and others (1987) found that adult burn patients who scored higher on adjustment ratings used less avoidance coping and more problem-solving coping. Additional support for the effectiveness of problem-solving strategies can be found in a study of coping strategy types of middle-aged and elderly adults with hypertension, diabetes, cancer, or arthritis (Felton and others, 1984). Positive affective states were associated with cognitive strategies, while negative affect and lowered self-esteem were linked to use of emotional expression, avoidance, and blaming strategies and poorer adjustment. Thus these studies imply that certain types and combinations of coping strategies may be more effective than others.

Given the finding that certain coping strategies may be more effective than others, one must ask what is meant by coping effectiveness. Some researchers consider coping is effective if there is a good match between the way a person actually copes and his or her preferred coping style, which encompasses values, goals, commitments, and beliefs (Lazarus and Folkman, 1984). Also, two other dimensions of coping effectiveness can be measured: the effectiveness of individual coping strategies and overall coping effectiveness. In addition, coping effectiveness can be evaluated by the patient and/or by others. Thus coping effectiveness is both subjective and objective, and it is contextual.

One difficulty in measuring coping effectiveness is defining and measuring it consistently. In the previously mentioned studies that correlate coping strategies with adjustment, it is notable that none measure coping effectiveness. Although there are studies that focus on single and group indicators of adjustment, such as psychosocial adjustment (Roberts and others, 1987), self-esteem (Felton and others, 1984; Mitchell and Hodson, 1983), acceptance of illness (Felton and others, 1984), and depression and mastery in a person's life (Mitchell and Hodson, 1983), the relationship between coping effectiveness and adjustment is implied. Therefore there is a need to evaluate how the patient evaluates each coping strategy and her overall coping effectiveness.

Finally, how coping strategies change over time must be considered. Logically, since coping is dynamic, one might assume that coping changes over time. However, few studies have investigated the complex effect of time on coping. Typically, studies of how people cope measure coping at one point in time. An exception to this is a study by Coyne and others (1981) that investigated coping in depressed and nondepressed middle-age people during a 1- year period. Findings supported that depressed and nondepressed people differed in how they coped and that coping was different in different situations. Thus, because coping is dynamic and changes from one stressful situation to another, one can assume that coping may change during the course of a stressful event. Therefore it is important that coping strategies be measured longitudinally to get an accurate picture of coping throughout the course of a stressful event.

PERSONAL AND SITUATIONAL FACTORS MEDIATING COPING

The coping process is mediated by personal variables and situational variables. Personal variables include the demographic variables of age, race, sex, marital status, education, employment, socioeconomic status, and occupation. Situational variables that may affect coping include illness-related and environmental variables. Demographic variables often measured in stroke patients include age, sex, and educational level, when investigating depression and functional outcomes (Sinyor and others, 1986); social psychologic determinants of performance in rehabilitation (Hyman, 1972); and coping strategies and poststroke adaptation (Bronstein, 1986).

Personal Variables

Age. Though age has not been shown to affect functional gains after stroke (Heinemann and others, 1987), older persons tend to have more severe strokes, making it important to collect data on age of the subjects (Lind, 1982). While age did not seem to make a difference on coping efficacy (Pearlin and Schooler, 1978) in general, older persons may have to cope with more losses and may have access to fewer resources that may enhance coping than younger persons. On the other hand, having a stroke at a young age may be more difficult to accept because it happens out of sequence in a person's life. While health is desired at any age, younger people expect to be healthy; older people may have had experience with some chronic illness and so may have different expectations for health. Thus age should be considered when assessing and evaluating coping.

Race. Though little has been investigated on coping and race, transcultural studies in health care suggest that cultural beliefs and norms may influence a patient's appraisal of the illness situation and the treatment sought and that these may influence the coping process.

Sex. Differences between females and males have been noted in a study of psychologic variables and physical functioning (Rosillo and Fogel, 1971). However, other studies of stroke patients showed sex was not a predictor of functional outcomes (Lehmann and others, 1975, Heinemann and others, 1987). In addition, coping patterns were found to be different based on sex (Kleinke and others, 1982), and women were socialized to use less effective coping patterns than men (Pearlin and Schooler, 1978).

Marital status. Being married exposes people to different types of stressors and has complex implications for the quantity and quality of social support. Thus coping effectiveness may be influenced by marital status (Pearlin and Schooler, 1978).

Education. It is suggested that greater intellectual capacity may be positively correlated with higher functional gains (Lind, 1982). Also, educational background may have an effect on the coping process by affecting cognitive appraisal and identification and use of different types of coping strategies.

Socioeconomic status, employment, and occupation. Socioeconomic status was found to be correlated positively with improvement after stroke (Feldman, 1962; and Katz, 1966). More recently, a high correlation was found between socioeconomic status and family involvement; in turn, family involvement was highly correlated with stroke recovery (Lehmann and others 1975). In relation to coping, more affluent people may have access to more effective coping techniques and a stronger sense of mastery and optimism (Pearlin and Schooler, 1978). Occupational status may affect coping as it relates to education and socioeconomic status. Higher levels of education and higher income are achieved statuses that are closely associated with higher self-esteem and mastery (Pearlin and Schooler, 1978).

Illness-related Variables

Illness-related variables of interest include location and extent of stroke lesion, time since stroke, cause of stroke, and past medical history.

Location and extent of stroke lesion. Many studies have investigated the importance of the location and the extent of the stroke lesion on outcomes after stroke. Lesion location accounted for significant differences in performance (Novack and others, 1987) and in the severity of poststroke depression (Sinyor and others, 1986; Robinson and others, 1984; Robinson and Szetela, 1981), which could affect coping. Depressed patients were found to be significantly more likely to use emotive coping strategies (Foster and Gallagher, 1986). Also, coping has been studied in relation to event seriousness. That is, patients who perceived their illness as serious used different types of coping strategies and had a poorer adjustment to illness than persons not perceiving the illness as serious (Roberts and others, 1987).

Time. In clinical interviews with stroke patients, time since stroke appeared to have some effect on the coping process; that is, individuals who relied heavily on certain coping strategies soon after stroke did not necessarily use the same strategies later in their recovery (Popovich, 1987). Another dimension of time of illness is the length of time the person is sick. In a study of renal patients, Shanan and others (1976) found that prolonged stress reduced the tendency to cope actively.

Past medical history. It is expected that patients with several chronic illnesses may have different coping strategies and have different stroke outcomes than patients with fewer chronic illnesses. In addition, stroke patients with other chronic illnesses may have different and more illness-related stressors than patients with no chronic illnesses. More research is needed in this area.

Environmental variables. One environmental variable is whether or not the patient receives rehabilitative care, and the type and extent of that care. This is an important variable because patients learn problem-solving activities in rehabilitation that might predispose them to using certain types of coping strategies.

A MODEL FOR COPING WITH STROKE

A conceptual model describes the complex factors involved in the process of coping after stroke (Popovich, 1987) (Fig. 13-1). Based on clinical interviews with stroke patients (n = 36), previously reviewed models were adapted to produce the Coping After Stroke Model (Popovich, 1987). The Coping After Stroke Model combines the concepts of loss, cognitive appraisal, adaptive tasks, coping strategies, coping effectiveness, hope, and rehabilitation outcomes to describe a dynamic process that is influenced by feedback from variables in the model. Because this process is dynamic, stroke patients' use of coping strategies, coping effectiveness, hopes, and rehabilitation outcomes may change over time during their recovery.

Loss

At the time of the stroke, a person's response will be influenced by personal factors that include the state of balance or imbalance the person has in life before the stroke. According to the Coping After Stroke Model, when experiencing a stroke, a person perceives an actual or potential loss or change in functioning. *Loss* or *change* is defined as perceived and actual alterations in physical, psychologic and/or social functioning that are directly or indirectly related to the physiologic changes from the stroke. Whether or not the patient perceives them, loss or changes in functioning act as stressors by disrupting his previous functioning and previous relationships in the environment. Alterations can result in complete or partial loss of functioning; if the loss is complete, the patient may be unable to perform an activity. With partial loss of functioning, the patient can still perform the activity but must change the manner in which he does it. Stroke patients identify a broad range of physical, psychologic, and social loss or changes after a stroke. Some of these include loss of independence in ADLs, feelings of vulnerability, and loss of employment. Loss or change in functioning interferes with the person's ability for simple and complex tasks, resulting in a partial or complete dependence on others.

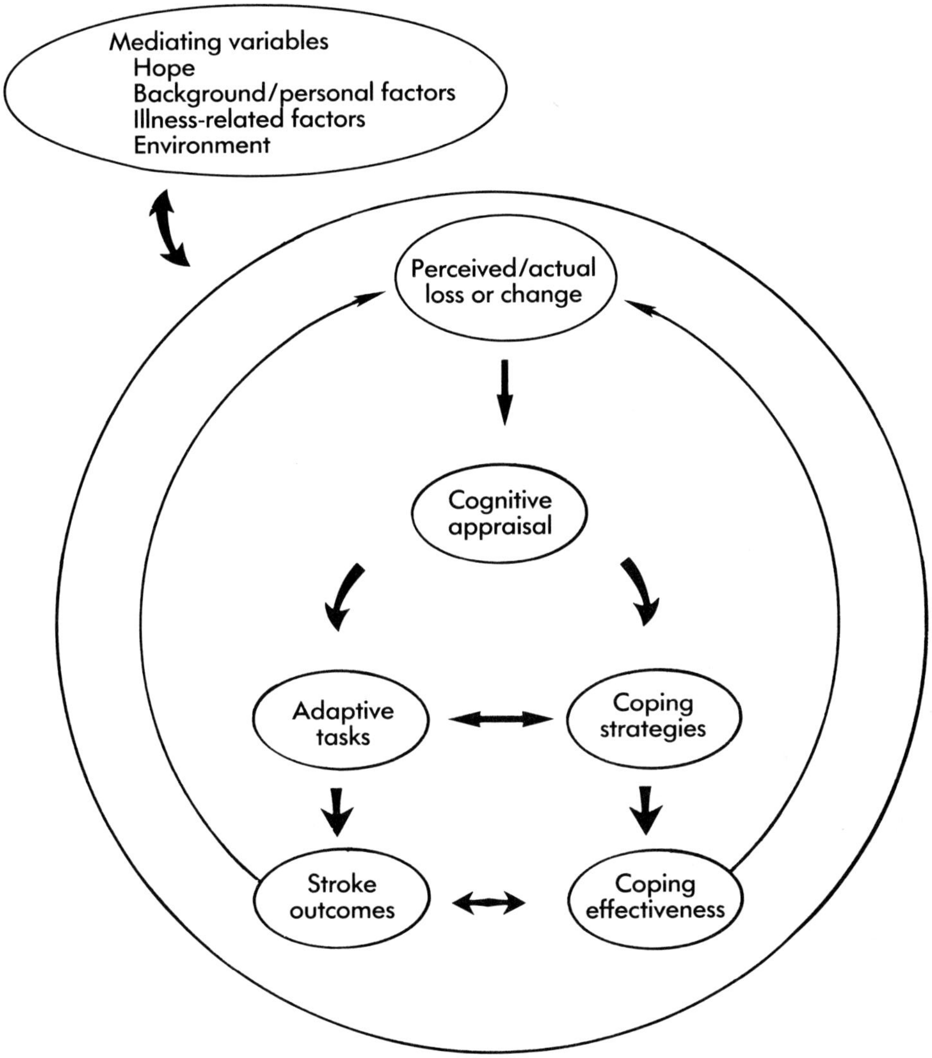

Fig. 13-1 A conceptual model of coping after stroke. © 1990 by Judith M. Popovich.

Cognitive Appraisal

After perceiving or experiencing the loss or change in functioning, the patient interprets and evaluates the stressor. This process is called *cognitive appraisal* (Lazarus and Folkman, 1984). Appraisal is a cognitive process because the patient interprets what the stroke means for her. This cognitive process underlies the ebb and flow of emotional responses and their quality and intensity (Lazarus, 1976). When the person cognitively appraises the situation, this appraisal elicits emotional responses and the person thinks and acts to respond to the stressor. Appraisal is both primary and secondary. That is, primary appraisal is the initial interpretation of the event; secondary appraisal is ongoing, during which the person evaluates her initial interpretation and coping strategies and the effectiveness of the coping strategies (Lazarus and Folkman, 1984). In other words, appraisal and reappraisal influence the coping process continuously.

Cognitive appraisal is a significant component in coping with stroke because of the stroke-related deficits that can interfere with accurate appraisal of the situation. An extreme example of this is a patient with anosognosia (complete denial of illness) secondary to a parietal lobe lesion. This person would be unable to accurately interpret his stroke experience, thus affecting his emotional responses and his ability to identify coping strategies. Other persons may demonstrate less severe cognitive and perceptual deficits, which may also alter their individual appraisal. Two people experiencing a stroke may appraise their situation in very different ways. For example, when asked about the problems he was having since his stroke, a man said:

> Look at my right side and my speech! I lost my job and my responsibilities. I used to teach. Now I stay in my room a lot. I don't want to see anyone. I need help for the simplest things.

This patient expresses how the stroke has threatened his very existence. His life has significantly changed; he is unable to do most of his previous activities. His emotional response is almost desperate as he describes how he feels about being dependent on others. Yet, another patient when asked about the problems she was having since the stroke replied:

> I have weakness in my right hand, arm, and leg, which causes me to have to wear this leg brace. I also have shoulder pain a lot. But I get out into my flower garden and I like to see my friends. I have to learn new ways to do things but I figure it out.

This patient describes the changes brought about by her stroke more as a challenge that she is determined to overcome. Thus, as a result of different appraisals, individuals interpret the meaning of the stroke differently, have different degrees and types of emotional responses, and perceive different options for coping. Once the patient appraises the situation, she then determines both the necessary adaptive tasks and coping strategies to manage the stroke-related stressors.

Adaptive tasks are new psychologic and physical work the patient must accomplish to achieve optimum potential during recovery from stroke. These tasks build on each other, are goal-oriented, and are directly related to stroke outcomes. For example, if a stroke patient's expected stroke outcome is to walk, her tasks will include actively participating in therapy and practicing what she learns in therapy on the nursing unit. Other tasks the patient may need to accomplish include developing self-confidence to walk with a cane, conquering the fear of falling, and knowing when to ask for help.

Adaptive tasks are especially relevant in the study of coping with stroke. Patients identify many stroke-related adaptive tasks, including relearning self-care activities, being patient with themselves, and dealing with the reactions of others (Popovich, 1987). Because a stroke causes temporary and/or permanent changes in body functioning the stroke survivor must learn new ways of doing things, such as moving, taking care of himself, and relating to others. Stroke-related adaptive tasks are physical, psychologic, and social and require a range of complex skills. Additionally, adaptive tasks are dynamic; i.e., the tasks change as the patient's perception and actual health status change; and adaptive tasks directly affect stroke outcomes.

Rehabilitation Outcomes

Stroke outcomes are the direct result of the patient's accomplishing a series of physical, psychologic, and social adaptive tasks. *Stroke outcomes* are the patient's optimum functional gains in the physical, psychologic, and social domains. Stroke outcomes are usually evaluated in these three domains by measuring functional ability, the presence or absence of depression, and some dimension of social functioning. Stroke outcomes are related to other variables in the model (Fig. 13-1) by the relationship to coping effectiveness and the feedback loop to perceived or actual loss or change. Stroke outcomes may positively or negatively influence coping effectiveness. For example, if outcomes exceed what the patient perceives he should accomplish, this may enhance coping effectiveness. If outcomes do not meet the patient's expectations for recovery, outcomes may function as a stressor that may interfere with coping effectiveness. Finally, outcomes change over time and may influence the overall coping process. This influence on the overall coping process is illustrated by the feedback loop between stroke outcomes and perceived or actual loss of change.

Coping Strategies

In addition to identifying adaptive tasks, the stroke survivor employs certain coping strategies. Coping strategies are dynamic; they are influenced by how effective the patient perceives the strategies to be in managing the stressors and by her capabilities and resources at different times during recovery. And, because they are part of the larger process of coping, coping strategies are influenced by other variables in the model.

Coping strategies can be distinguished from adaptive tasks in that coping strategies reflect previous coping efforts and newly learned ways to manage the stressful situation. However, adaptive tasks are new and represent something with which the patient is likely to have had no prior experience. Both adaptive tasks and coping strategies must be learned and both have affective and behavioral components. Coping strategies help to identify and accomplish the necessary adaptive tasks to achieve outcomes.

Stroke patients identify a variety of coping strategies, including talking with other patients, praying, and thinking positively (Popovich, 1987). Coping strategies that stroke patients use may be internal (self-directed) or external (other-directed). Both internal and external strategies reflect a wide range of emotions and behaviors that patients use to manage stroke-related stressors. Some are familiar to the patient in that they have used these strategies in other stressful situations in their lives (for instance, praying or being with family), while other strategies, such as seeing their progress and comparing themselves with others, may be newly learned.

Coping Effectiveness

Coping effectiveness is directly related to coping strategies. *Coping effectiveness* is how productive or useful individual strategies are in helping the patient manage the stroke-related stressors. Coping effectiveness may be perceived and/or actual. One's coping effectiveness may be measured by evaluating how effective the individual or others perceive the coping strategies to be and by evaluating overall coping effectiveness as it is perceived by the stroke survivor and others in the stroke survivor's environment.

Coping effectiveness is related to both stroke outcomes and the overall coping process. If coping effectiveness is high, this may enhance outcomes because the patient will be able to manage stroke-related stressors as they arise. If coping effectiveness is low, this may inhibit rehabilitation outcomes because the individual will have difficulty managing stroke-related stressors when they occur. Coping effectiveness influences the overall process as indicated by the feedback loop from coping effectiveness to perceived or actual loss or change. The level of coping effectiveness will affect how the patient perceives the stroke-related loss or change, the appraisal and reappraisal process, the identification of new adaptive tasks, and the selection of new coping strategies. These relationships further emphasize that this model represents a dynamic and interactive process that changes during stroke recovery.

Four variables mediate the adjustment after stroke process: hope, background and personal factors, illness-related factors, and environmental factors. These mediating variables may facilitate or inhibit coping at different steps in the coping process and/or at different points during recovery.

Hope

In the model, hope is conceptualized as a mediating variable in the coping process. The mechanisms by which hope is believed to work have been discussed earlier. The literature supports the inclusion of hope as an important variable in the Coping After Stroke Model. Further support for including hope in the model can be drawn from interviews with stroke patients (Popovich, 1987). Patients describe three major sources or experiences that strengthened their hope: self (internal feelings or behaviors), others (support from other people), and religion (spiritual attitudes or religious activities). These data support three of the four attributes of hope identified by Farran (1985). The "rational" attribute includes the patient's thinking and feelings about herself and about the future. The "relational" attribute includes references to other people, who either fostered or strengthened hope in the patient. The attribute of "transcendence and faith" includes all spiritual thoughts and behaviors. The fourth attribute, hope inspired by captivity or suffering is not supported by these data, probably because the sample was limited and patients had difficulty in answering this question.

Other findings from the interviews were that stroke patients had both global (generalized) and specific (particularized) hopes. This is congruent with hope spheres identified by Dufault and Martochhio (1985). Generalized hope is broad and casts a positive glow on life; particularized hope is concerned with a valued outcome or state of being and clarifies a specific goal important to the person. Patients reported global hopes that included hopes for full recovery and to not get worse. Some specific hopes that stroke patients in this sample reported included hopes for movement to return, to be independent, and to resume all prestroke activities (Popovich 1987).

In this model, hope may positively influence coping at any point in the process. Hope may influence how the patient perceives the loss or change in function, and hope may enable the patient to appraise the situation as challenging rather than threatening. In addition, hope may help the patient to identify adaptive tasks and coping strategies that would facilitate stroke outcomes and effective coping.

Hope may also be influenced by other variables in the model and by different stages of recovery. For instance, a patient who experiences more functional gains may be more hopeful than a patient who sees little return in function. An environmental variable, such as a strong social support network, may facilitate hopefulness. And hope may be directly or indirectly influenced by coping strategies; patients who find coping strategies that are effective in managing the stroke-related stressors may be more hopeful than patients who use fewer effective coping strategies.

Three remaining external variables in the model are *background and personal factors, illness-related factors,* and *environmental factors* (Moos and Tsu, 1977). These factors represent a broad scope of possible influences on the coping process. The importance of these factors for individual coping will vary from person to person. For instance, illness-related factors may have a major influence on coping for one person, while environmental factors may be a stronger influence on coping for another person. In addition, the effect of these factors on the coping process is not static throughout a person's stroke experience; i.e., some variables may play a stronger role in the coping process than others at different points in poststroke recovery. For example, coping in the patient with medical complications may be influenced strongly by illness-related factors during the development and resolution of the complications; however, later during recovery, illness-related factors may have a smaller influence on the person's attempts to cope.

The patient's background and personal factors (such as personality type, culture, education, age, race, sex, occupation, religion, attitudes, self-esteem, prior coping experiences, and the premorbid state of balance and imbalance) may affect how he copes. Therefore, background and personal factors are included in the model as mediating variables of the coping process.

Illness-related factors are those situations or conditions brought about directly or indirectly by the illness that affect the patient's ability to cope. Some of these factors include pain, life stage of illness, illness-severity, presence of complications, resulting physical and psychologic deficits, and change in body image. Illness-related variables of interest in stroke studies include location of lesion (Folstein and others, 1977; Robinson and others, 1984; and Sinyor and others, 1986), cognitive and emotional deficits (Charatan and Fisk, 1978), and functional outcome after stroke (Bourestrom, 1967; Lehmann and others, 1975). Thus illness-related factors are included in the model because of their key role as mediating factors in coping with stroke.

The environment is considered an important mediating factor in the Coping After Stroke Model. *Environmental factors* are conditions in the patient's physical and social environment that may affect the patient after a stroke at any point throughout the coping process. Environmental factors include problems and/or resources in the physical surroundings, nursing care, social support, and amount and type of rehabilitative care the patient receives. Studies on the effects of environmental variables on patients with chronic illness, including stroke patients, have evaluated family adjustment to illness (Derogatis, 1986), family functioning (Bishop and others, 1986), social support (Dimond, 1979; and Mahoney, 1985), and rehabilitative care (Heinemann and others, 1987). Therefore the environment is considered an important mediating factor in the Coping After Stroke Model.

DEPRESSION AFTER STROKE

When compared with other patient populations, stroke patients are frequently more depressed (Folstein and others, 1977; Finklestein and others, 1987). Significant depression after stroke has been reported between 40% and 60% (Morris and Raphael, 1987), especially during the time period from 6 months to 2 years after stroke (Robinson and Price, 1982). While most researchers agree that stroke patients are more depressed than other patients with comparable physical disabilities, there is less agreement on what clinical indicators predict poststroke depression.

Over the past 10 years, there has been much research on the relationship of laterality and lesion location to depression in stroke patients (Robinson, Starr, and Price, 1984; Lipsey and others, 1983). The incidence of depression was higher in patients with left-anterior brain lesions, and among these patients, the severity of depression increased the closer the lesion was to the frontal pole. These findings are thought to be due to neurochemical brain processes and the effects of damage on catecholamine-containing pathways as they pass through the frontal cortex.

Recently, some researchers have questioned the strong emphasis on lesion location and depression and suggest that depression may be due to a complex interaction of variables. Variables that have also been investigated in relation to depression include loss of functional independence (Wade and others, 1987; Sinyor and others, 1986), coping strategies, and stroke outcome (Sinyor and others, 1986).

Assessing the patient for depression in the clinical setting should be done both objectively and subjectively. Objective measures of depression include paper-pencil tests that the patient may be asked to complete or that the nurse can read to the patient and record the responses. One example of an instrument used to measure depression is the Center for Epidemiologic Studies of Depression (CES-D) Scale. This is a 20-item scale that includes short questions that ask the patient how she has been feeling in the past week. The patient answers using a 4-point Likert-type scale, indicating how frequently she has been feeling a certain way. The CES-D has frequently been used with stroke patients and has been demonstrated to be reliable and valid in screening for depression in stroke patients (Shinar and others, 1986).

Another objective measure that is used for diagnosing depression is the Dexamethasone Suppression Test (DST). The test is performed by drawing a baseline serum cortisol and administering 1 mg of dexamethasone to the patient on the evening before the test. The next day serum cortisol levels are drawn at 8 AM and 4 PM. Normally, both cortisol levels should be less than 5 μg/ml If one or both cortisol levels exceed 5 μg/ml, the test is abnormal. However, specificity of the test is only 70% because patients with large lesions may have abnormal results and not be depressed (Price, 1987).

The nurse can subjectively evaluate the patient for depression by interviewing and observing the patient. The nurse should ask the patient how he feels, if he has had appetite or sleep disturbances, loss of energy, anxiety, difficulty concentrating, and feelings of hopelessness. She should also observe the patient's affect, her interaction with family and friends, and her active participation in her care.

ASSESSING COPING

Assessing coping is the first step in the nursing process to determine if patients are coping with the stroke adequately and what nursing interventions may facilitate coping. Whitney (1987) suggests seven characteristics of adequate coping. These include the ability to (1) contain distress within personally tolerable limits, (2) maintain self-esteem and identify one's role, (3) preserve interpersonal relationships, (4) convert unfamiliar to familiar, (5) meet the conditions of new circumstances, (6) control and predict situations, and (7) maintain meaningful human attachments. Determining the adequacy of coping can be accomplished only by combining nursing observations with subjective and objective data collected from the patient and family.

Subjective data the nurse collects include observing the patient and family and interviewing them about how they are managing their concerns about the stroke. Things to consider in assessing how patient and family are coping with a stroke include background and personal, illness-related, and environmental factors. Questions the nurse should consider in her assessment of coping are listed in the box on p. 251. Subjective information the nurse collects will facilitate an accurate assessment of how patient and family are coping. In addition, the nurse should observe the patient's affect and participation in his care, the interaction between patient and family, and the interaction among patient, family and the health care team.

In addition to subjective data, objective data enhance the nursing data base and helps the nurse to make the most accurate assessment possible. Objective measures to assess coping include paper-pencil tools that the nurse may administer to the patient. If the patient is able, he may complete the tool independently, or the nurse can read the questions to the patient and record his responses. One example of an instrument used to measure coping is the Ways of Coping (Revised) (Lazarus and Folkman, 1984). This is a 67-item scale that asks the patient to identify the coping strategies she uses and how often she uses them. An example of questions on the Ways of Coping (Revised) is given in the box on p. 252. The items represent eight coping subscales catergorized as (1) confrontive, (2) distancing, (3) self-controlling, (4) seeking social support, (5) accepting responsibility, (6) escape-avoidance, (7) planful problem-solving, and (8) positive reappraisal. Reliability and validity are being determined by repeated use of the tool in healthy

FACTORS TO CONSIDER WHEN ASSESSING COPING IN STROKE PATIENTS

What losses has the patient experienced due to the stroke?
Has the patient experienced other recent losses in his life?
How does the patient and family appraise their situation (primary, secondary)?
Does the patient have deficits that interfere with appraisal of her situation?
What adaptive tasks does the patient have to accomplish?
What goals do the patient and family have?
Are goals of the patient and family consistent with one another?
How did the patient cope before the stroke?
How did the family cope before the stroke?
Are the patient's coping strategies enabling him to manage his stressors effectively?
Are the family's coping strategies effective?
What are the sources of hope for the patient and family?

BACKGROUND/PERSONAL

What was the patient's premorbid lifestyle?
What strengths do the patient and family exhibit?
What weaknesses do the patient and family exhibit?
What are the patient's and family's values and beliefs?
What is the control orientation of the patient and family?
What are the patient's demographic characteristics (age, sex, cultural background, education level, employment status, socioeconomic status, and occupation)?
What is the likelihood that the patient will resume prestroke roles in family, school, and employment?

ILLNESS-RELATED FACTORS

Was the stroke onset sudden or gradual?
How recently did the stroke occur?
In what part of the brain is the lesion located?
How extensive is the stroke lesion?
What was the cause of the stroke?
Is the patient at high risk for recurrence?
Does the patient have concomitant acute or chronic illnesses?
What cognitive/perceptual deficits are present that may impair coping?
What are the type and severity of the patient's functional limitations?

ENVIRONMENTAL FACTORS

Does/will the patient receive rehabilitative care?
What is the extent and level of social support from family and friends?
What material resources are available (money, equipment, place for discharge)?
Will the patient require a caregiver? If so, who?

SAMPLE ITEMS ON THE WAYS OF COPING

	Not Used	Used Somewhat	Used quite a bit	Used a great deal
1. I tried to analyze the problem to understand it better.	0	1	2	3
2. I was inspired to do something creative.	0	1	2	3
3. I made light of the situation; refused to get too serious about it.	0	1	2	3

From Lazarus RS and Folkman S: Stress, appraisal, and coping, New York, 1984, Springer-Verlag.

SAMPLE ITEMS ON THE JALOWIEC COPING SCALE

	Never Used	Seldom Used	Sometimes Used	Often Used	Not Helpful	Slightly Helpful	Fairly Helpful	Very Helpful
1. Worry about the problem	0	1	2	3	0	1	2	3
2. Exercise or do some physical activity	0	1	2	3	0	1	2	3
3. Get mad and let off steam	0	1	2	3	0	1	2	3

From Jalowiec: Jalowiec Coping Scale, 1987.

populations. Because the Ways of Coping (Revised) has been used primarily on healthy people, its usefulness with hospitalized patients requires further evaluation.

Another tool to objectively measure coping is the Revised Jalowiec Coping Scale (Jalowiec, 1987). This is a 63-item scale that lists coping strategies and asks the patient to identify how frequently she uses the strategy and if it is helpful. Sample items of the Jalowiec Coping Scale are listed in the box above. The items represent eight subscales identified as (1) confrontive, (2) evasive, (3) optimistic, (4) fatalistic, (5) emotive, (6) palliative, (7) supportant, and (8) self-reliant. Reliability and validity of this scale will be determined when sufficient data are collected using the revised scale.

With use of the Jalowiec Coping Scale, the coping strategies of stroke patients were investigated in 46 patients to determine the type of strategy used and the relationship between strategy and degree of poststroke adaptation (Bronstein, 1986). Problem-oriented coping behaviors showed a significant positive correlation to total adaptation scores ($p < 0.05$). Emotion-focused coping behaviors were positively correlated to depression ($p < 0.07$). Findings demonstrated that stroke patients used a wide variety of coping strategies and that problem-solving stategies may facilitate adaptation.

Though the Ways of Coping scale and the Jalowiec Coping Scale both have similar items and are designed to measure the coping process in a particular stressful encounter, the Jalowiec Coping Scale also asks the patient to rate perceived helpfulness of the coping strategies used. In addition, the Jalowiec Scale has been used in patient populations. Both scales are lengthy and require that the patient have good physical endurance to participate.

One of the difficulties of assessing coping with both subjective and objective measures is that the coping process is dynamic and changes over time. For example, how a patient copes may be affected by her recovery, how she appraises her situation, and by changing available resources. For example, the patient may employ a greater number of coping strategies and/or use different types of coping strategies in response to change in her situation over time. Considering this, it is crucial that the nurse's assessment of coping be ongoing.

INTERVENTIONS

The goal of nursing interventions to facilitate coping is to maximize the patient's and family's resources to enable them to manage their situation. To accomplish this goal, the nurse must accurately assess what the patient and family need and then implement the appropriate interventions.

Following are nursing diagnoses relevant to the stroke patient with a altered coping.

Coping, Ineffective Individual Related to Lack of Information

The goal in resolving ineffective individual coping related to a lack of information is to make sure that the patient has accurate information about his situation. Common concerns of patients include the possibility of a recurrent stroke, the time period of and the extent to which they can expect recovery, and what life-style changes they should make to maintain their current level of health.

Nursing interventions might include giving the patient this information, considering the learning style of the patient. Having access to information helps the patient to feel some control over her situation; information regarding recovery and life-style changes enables the patient to do anticipatory coping in preparation for discharge.

Another important nursing intervention is to find out how the patient and family appraise the situation; the nurse must reevaluate these appraisals regularly. Because of the complexity of information delivered to patients and families by many members of the health care team, misunderstandings are common. In addition, the stress of the hospital experience may interfere with information that patients and families are able to process. Repetition and feedback from the patient enable the nurse to evaluate the patient's understanding as well as the nursing interventions.

Coping, Ineffective Individual Related to Inability to Mobilize Effective Coping Strategies

In resolving ineffective individual coping related to the patient's inability to mobilize effective coping strategies, the goal of nursing interventions is to identify the types of coping strategies the patient is currently using, help her to evaluate the effectiveness of familiar strategies, and assist her in finding ways to cope effectively. Common difficulties that hospitalized stroke patients experience include limited activities related to the hospital environment and/or their unstable physical condition. These limitations keep patients from using as many familiar coping strategies as they are used to and sometimes create feelings of powerlessness.

Appropriate nursing interventions might include educating the patient about alternate coping strategies that are either easier to use in the hospital and/or may be more effective than familiar ones. Coping strategies such as finding ways to relax, thinking about the good things in one's life, talking with professionals and other patients, and finding activities to take one's mind off the stroke may be useful for some hospitalized stroke patients.

In the case of teaching a patient new coping strategies to enhance her overall coping effectiveness in the present and after discharge, the nurse can discuss new coping strategies with the patient, demonstrate their use, and provide opportunities for the patient to practice these in the hospital setting. As patients implement new strategies, the nurse should point out any changes in the patient's ability to manage the situation. Feedback will enable the patient to have insights about how she copes, and practicing new strategies in the hospital may facilitate the patient's mastery in learning.

Coping, Ineffective Individual, Related to Change in Physical Functioning

The loss of physical functioning may affect coping in situations in which the stroke patient has significant functional deficits in the areas of speech, perception, cognition, and mobility or in which his physical condition is deteriorating. The goal of nursing interventions is to minimize the stress on the patient and to maximize how the patient is able to compensate for these deficits. Ultimately, the outcome should be that the patient continues to cope by using as many effective and familiar coping strategies as possible. In complex situations that demand more coping efforts than the patient has to give, the nurse must minimize the stress on the patient and provide support.

Nursing interventions to facilitate effective coping in the previous situations include providing support to the patient, promoting relaxation, providing alternate ways for communicating when necessary, and fostering realistic hope in the patient. The nurse can minimize stress by keeping the environment as routine and relaxed as possible and by explaining activities and procedures to the patient when appropriate. The nurse also acts as a patient advocate to other members of the health care team and facilitates family understanding of the patient's needs when the patient is unable to express his own needs.

Coping, Ineffective Individual, Related to Fear (of Dying, of New Procedures, of Getting Worse)

Fear is not an uncommon feeling in the hospital. Stroke patients may fear further loss of function and fear having another stroke. Unstable patients with severe strokes may fear dying. The goal of nursing interventions is to diffuse the fear as much as possible by allowing the patient to express her feelings and to provide the support the patient needs. For some patients, support may mean providing information to them about procedures; however, for other patients, receiving information in advance may intensify their fear. It is the nurse's responsibility to assess the patient's needs and determine the appropriate interventions.

Coping, Ineffective Family

Family coping will be determined by a constellation of factors, some of which include previous coping styles in the family, the patient's condition, and concomitant stresses. The goal of nursing interventions is to make an accurate assessment and implement ways for the family to mobilize the coping resources that they have available to them.

Nursing interventions include developing a professional relationship with the patient's significant others, engaging them in the patient's care when appropriate, and addressing their concerns. It is important for the nurse to determine the extent to which family members are able to be involved in the patient's care so that appropriate arrangements are made if the patient should need a caregiver.

Hopelessness

Patients and family members may feel hopeless when they think there is nothing that they can do to make the situation better. Some of the situations when patients and family may feel hopeless include when the patient's deficits impair his ability to communicate, when his condition is deteriorating, and if he is not seeing recovery as expected. Because the patient and family may not be able to express their feelings, the nurse must pay careful attention to nonverbal cues.

Nursing interventions to foster hope include identifying sources of hope to the patient and, whenever possible, supporting those things that provide hope. For example, the nurse might support the patient's relationships with significant others (friends, spouse, children, grandchildren); also important is encouraging the patient's belief in herself and the spiritual beliefs and activities that are important to her.

Other coping-related nursing diagnoses the nurse should consider when caring for the stroke patient and family are given in the care plan on p. 256.

NURSING CARE PLAN

Nursing Diagnosis	Intervention	Expected Outcomes
Coping, Ineffective Individual related to lack of information **Defining Characteristics** ■ Anxiety ■ Difficulty problem solving ■ Patient/family may or may not express need for information ■ Change in communication patterns ■ Patient and family verbalize inability to cope ■ Inappropriate use of defense mechanisms ■ Reluctance to participate in self-care activities and/or health regimen ■ Change in patterns of social interaction with staff, other patients, and/or family ■ Verbal manipulation ■ Frequent accidents and/or illnesses	**Ongoing Assessment** ■ Determine immediate concerns of patient and family ■ Identify any impending change (i.e., routine, procedure) requiring explanation ■ Determine current level of patient and family understanding ■ Find out how patient and family appraise their situation ■ Assess patient and family learning needs ■ Determine preferred learning style for patient and family ■ Assess stroke-related deficits that may impair learning (i.e., aphasia, alterations in cognition, sensation, and/or mood ■ Determine long-range concerns of patient and family ■ Assess ways patient and family communicate with staff and with one another ■ Assess ways patient and family interact with others ■ Determine whether patient is participating in self-care activities appropriately ■ Assess accidents and complaints of stress-related symptoms ■ Evaluate the quality of the patient's and family's support system	■ The patient and family will describe factors that influence coping ■ The patient and family will understand the relationship between stress and physical and psychologic functioning ■ The patient and family will identify effective coping strategies to manage stress ■ The patient and family will communicate concerns or needs for information to the nurse ■ The patient and family will understand the mechanisms of stroke, course of recovery, and expected outcomes

NURSING CARE PLAN — cont'd

Nursing Diagnosis	Intervention	Expected Outcomes
	Therapeutic Interventions ■ Discuss immediate concerns; provide information as appropriate ■ Provide reassurance and emotional support ■ Collaborate with patient, family, and team members regarding learning needs ■ Implement patient and family education program, considering learning styles and needs ■ Assist patient and family in identifying own personal effective and ineffective coping strategies ■ Provide opportunities for patient and family to implement effective coping strategies; give positive reinforcement ■ Make ongoing evaluation of program effectiveness; increase patient and family involvement at a pace appropriate to meet their needs, considering external constraints ■ Model open communication with the patient and family; encourage them to express feelings; be a good listener ■ Help patient to understand relationship between difficulty coping and stress-related symptoms and accidents ■ Encourage patient and family to ask questions	

Continued.

NURSING CARE PLAN — cont'd

Nursing Diagnosis	Intervention	Expected Outcomes
Coping, Ineffective Individual related to inability to mobilize effective coping strategies **Defining Characteristics** ■ Anxiety ■ Difficulty problem solving ■ Difficulty managing changes in routine ■ Difficulty participating in self-care activities and/or health regimen ■ Change in communication patterns ■ Patient and family verbalizes inability to cope ■ Inappropriate use of defense mechanisms ■ Change in patterns of social interaction with staff, other patients, and/or family ■ Verbal manipulation ■ Frequent accidents and/or illnesses ■ Self-destructive behaviors	**Ongoing Assessment** ■ Determine coping strategies used by the patient and family ■ Ask about previous coping style of family ■ Assess personal, illness-related, and environmental variables that interfere with patient and family implementing familiar coping strategies ■ Assess stroke-related deficits that may impair coping (i.e., aphasia, alterations in cognition, sensation, and/or mood) ■ Find out how patient and family appraise the stroke and the illness experience ■ Determine patient and family learning needs ■ Determine preferred learning style for patient and family ■ Determine whether patient is participating in self-care activities appropriately ■ Assess accidents and complaints of stress-related symptoms ■ Assess self-destructive behaviors ■ Evaluate quality of patient and family support system	■ The patient and family will replace self-destructive behaviors with constructive, self-nurturing behaviors ■ The patient and family will describe factors that influence coping ■ The patient and family will understand obstacles to implementing familiar coping strategies ■ The patient and family will identify alternative coping strategies to manage stress ■ The patient and family will implement alternative coping strategies during stroke recovery as appropriate ■ The patient and family will understand long-range consequences of ineffective coping

NURSING CARE PLAN — cont'd

Nursing Diagnosis	Intervention	Expected Outcomes
	Therapeutic Inventions ■ Assist patient and family in identifying their own personal effective and ineffective coping strategies ■ Assist patient and family to identify obstacles to implementing familiar strategies ■ Collaborate with patient, family, and team members regarding learning needs ■ Implement patient and family education considering learning styles and needs ■ Provide opportunities for patient and family to implement alternative coping strategies; give positive reinforcement ■ Make ongoing evaluation of effectiveness of patient and family coping ■ Model open communication with the patient and family; encourage them to express feelings; be a good listener ■ Help patient to understand relationship between difficulty coping and stress-related symptoms, accidents, self-destructive behaviors ■ Promote and support constructive and self-nurturing behaviors ■ Provide reassurance and emotional support	
Coping, Ineffective Individual related to change in physical functioning **Defining Characteristics** ■ Anxiety ■ Difficulty participating in self-care	**Ongoing Assessment** ■ Assess stability of patient's physical condition ■ Determine whether patient has uncontrollable pain ■ Assess side effects of medications that may impair functioning (e.g., causing drowsiness, incontinence, weakness etc.)	■ The patient and family will understand the mechanisms of stroke, reasons for change in functioning, and course of recovery ■ The patient and

Continued.

NURSING CARE PLAN — cont'd

Nursing Diagnosis	Intervention	Expected Outcomes
activities and/or health regimen ■ Difficulty problem-solving ■ Exhibiting behaviors or feelings of low self esteem ■ Change in communication patterns ■ Patient and family verbalize inability to cope ■ Inappropriate use of defense mechanisms ■ Change in patterns of social interaction with staff, other patients, and/or family ■ Verbal manipulation ■ Frequent accidents and/or illnesses ■ Self-destructive behaviors	■ Determine coping strategies typically used by patient and family ■ Ask about previous coping style of patient and family ■ Assess personal, illness-related and environmental variables that interfere with patient and family implementing familiar coping strategies ■ Assess stroke-related deficits that may impair coping (i.e., aphasia, alterations in cognition, sensation, and/or mood) ■ Determine how patient and family appraise the stroke and illness experience ■ Assess patient and family learning needs, learning style ■ Determine whether patient is participating in self-care activities at the expected level ■ Assess accidents and complaints of stress-related symptoms ■ Assess self-destructive behaviors ■ Evaluate quality of patient and family support system	family will understand the side effects of medications ■ The patient and family will understand obstacles to coping in familiar ways ■ The patient and family will identify alternative coping strategies to manage stress ■ The patient and family will implement alternative coping strategies during stroke recovery as appropriate ■ The patient and family will understand long-range consequences of ineffective coping ■ The patient will replace self-destructive behaviors with ones that are constructive and self-nurturing

NURSING CARE PLAN — cont'd

Nursing Diagnosis	Intervention	Expected Outcomes
	Therapeutic Interventions ■ Provide information as needed regarding change in patient physical functioning ■ Get feedback from patient and family on their understanding of the situation ■ Assist patient and family in identifying own personal effective and ineffective coping strategies ■ Provide opportunities for patient and family to implement alternative coping strategies; give positive reinforcement ■ Collaborate with patient, family, and team regarding learning needs; implement program that considers learning styles ■ Make ongoing evaluation of effectiveness of coping ■ Model open communication; encourage patient and family to express feelings; be a good listener ■ Help patient to understand relationship between difficulty coping and stress-related symptoms, accidents or self-destructive behaviors ■ Promote and support constructive and self-nurturing behaviors ■ Provide reassurance and emotional support ■ Facilitate patient self-esteen by providing opportunities for patient to function at optimum level of independence ■ Foster realistic hopes and expectations for recovery	

Continued.

NURSING CARE PLAN — cont'd

Nursing Diagnosis	Intervention	Expected Outcomes
Coping, Ineffective Individual related to fear (of dying, of new procedures, of getting worse) **Defining Characteristics** ■ Fear ■ Anxiety ■ Difficulty participating in self-care activities and/or health regimen ■ Difficulty problem-solving ■ Change in communication patterns ■ Patient and family verbalize inability to cope ■ Inappropriate use of defense mechanisms ■ Change in patterns of social interaction with staff, other patients, and/or family ■ Verbal manipulation ■ Frequent accidents and/or illnesses ■ Self-destructive behaviors	**Ongoing Assessment** ■ Assess patient and family fears ■ Determine whether fears represent a realistic understanding of the situation ■ Determine appropriate level of information needed to minimize fear (For other assessment parameters, see previous nursing diagnosis) **Therapeutic Interventions** ■ Identify interventions that will minimize patient and family fears (i.e., providing accurate information, keeping everyone informed appropriately, facilitating coping strategies to promote relaxation) (For additional therapeutic interventions, see previous nursing diagnosis)	■ The patient and family will be less fearful, based on realistic understanding of situation ■ The patient and family will express fears and accept support and encouragement as needed ■ The patient and family will implement coping strategies that help to minimize fear (See Outcomes accompanying previous nursing diagnosis)

NURSING CARE PLAN — cont'd

Nursing Diagnosis	Intervention	Expected Outcomes
Coping, Ineffective Family: Compromised related to inability to mobilize coping resources **Defining Characteristics** ■ Anxiety ■ Family or significant other not involved appropriately in patient activities and/or health regimen ■ Difficulty in problem-solving ■ Change in communication patterns ■ Family verbalizes inability to cope ■ Inappropriate use of defense mechanisms ■ Change in patterns of social interaction with staff, patient, and/or other family members ■ Verbal manipulation ■ Frequent accidents and/or illnesses ■ Self-destructive behaviors	**Ongoing Assessment** ■ Assess whether patient's condition is stable, deteriorating, or improving ■ Determine family's current use of coping strategies ■ Ask about family's previous coping style ■ Assess factors that interfere with family implementing familiar coping strategies ■ Assess stroke-related deficits that may impair patient and family interaction (i.e., aphasia, alterations in cognition, sensation and/or mood) ■ Determine how family appraises the stroke and illness experience ■ Assess family learning needs, learning style ■ Determine whether family is participating in patient's program at the appropriate level (underinvolved, overinvolved) ■ Assess accidents and complaints of stress-related symptoms ■ Assess self-destructive behaviors ■ Determine quality of family's support system **Therapeutic Interventions** ■ Provide information as needed regarding change in patient's physical functioning ■ Get feedback from family on their understanding of the situation ■ Assist family in identifying own personal effective and ineffective coping strategies	■ The family or significant other will be involved at an appropriate level in the stroke victim's care ■ The family or significant other will understand the mechanisms of stroke, course of recovery, and expected outcomes ■ The family or significant other will understand obstacles to coping in familiar ways ■ The family or significant other will identify alternative coping strategies to manage stress ■ The family or significant other will implement alternative coping strategies during stroke recovery as appropriate ■ The family or significant other will understand long-range conse-

Continued.

NURSING CARE PLAN — cont'd

Nursing Diagnosis	Intervention	Expected Outcomes
	■ Provide opportunities for family to implement alternative coping strategies; give positive reinforcement ■ Collaborate with patient, family, and team regarding learning needs; implement program that considers learning styles ■ Make ongoing evaluation of effectiveness of coping ■ Model open communication; encourage family to express feelings; be a good listener ■ Help family to understand relationship between difficulty coping and stress-related symptoms, accidents, or self-destructive behaviors ■ Promote and support constructive and self-nurturing behaviors ■ Provide reassurance and emotional support ■ Foster realistic hopes and expectations for recovery	quences of ineffective coping ■ The family or significant other will replace self-destructive behaviors with behaviors that are constructive and self-nurturing
Hopelessness related to feeling of loss of control **Defining Characteristics** ■ Feeling that life has no meaning or purpose ■ Feeling of emptiness and/or a sense of loss or deprivation	**Ongoing Assessment** ■ Assess role illness plays in patient's hopelessness (i.e., level of physical functioning, endurance, duration and course of illness, prognosis) ■ Assess physical appearance (i.e., grooming, posture, hygiene) ■ Assess appetite, exercise, sleep patterns ■ Determine patient's ability to set and accomplish goals ■ Note whether patient emphasizes failures over accomplishments ■ Assess feelings of hopelessness, lack of	■ The patient will recognize and implement alternative coping strategies ■ The patient will identify potential sources of hope ■ The patient will express feelings, and accept support and encouragement as needed

NURSING CARE PLAN — cont'd

Nursing Diagnosis	Intervention	Expected Outcomes
■ Expression of sustained apathy in response to a situation perceived as impossible with no solutions ■ Lack of ambition, initiative, interest; passivity with decreased verbalization ■ Difficulty problem-solving ■ Difficulty making decisions ■ Difficulty integrating information ■ Difficulty identifying and accomplishing goals ■ Inability to recognize sources of hope ■ Weight changes, anorexia, sleep disturbances ■ Feelings of incompetence, vulnerability, discouragement with self, others ■ Social withdrawal, poor eye contact ■ Lack of involvement with self-care	self-worth, suicidal ideas ■ Identify potential sources of hopes (i.e., self, others, religion) ■ Evaluate patient's expectations for the future ■ Assess patient and family appraisal of stroke experience ■ Assess patient's perception of and need for control ■ Determine current coping strategies and level of effectiveness ■ Assess patient's belief in self **Therapeutic Interventions** ■ In a manner that communicates warmth, respect, and acceptance, provide physical care the patient is unable to perform ■ Implement individualized strategies to resolve difficulties with diet, sleep, activity endurance ■ Implement physical care routine that enables patient to function at optimum level and is compatible with patient and family resources ■ Encourage the patient to express feelings ■ Express hope for the patient ■ Encourage hopes that are active and reality-based ■ Help the patient set realistic goals; identify short-term goals and revise as needed ■ Help patient to evaluate situations and accomplishments	■ The patient will appraise his situation accurately ■ The patient will recognize accomplishments and set realistic goals ■ The patient will implement self-nurturing behaviors

Continued.

NURSING CARE PLAN — cont'd

Nursing Diagnosis	Interventions	Expected Outcomes
▪ Resignation, depression, anger, destructive behavior ▪ Lessened ability to recall the past and to perceive time accurately ▪ Distorted thought perceptions and associations ▪ Impaired judgment ▪ Confusion ▪ Overall sense of sadness	▪ Recognize patient accomplishments no matter how small ▪ Support patient's relationships with significant others ▪ Provide opportunities for patient to control own care ▪ Promote ego integrity by encouraging patient to reminisce about his life (self-validation) ▪ Facilitate patient's problem-solving ▪ Provide support and encouragement	

Patient Education

- Educate patient and family about effective coping strategies
- Educate patient and family about signs and symptoms of stress
- Educate about effect of stress on physical and psychological functioning
- Educate patient and family about stroke, course of recovery, and expected outcomes
- Educate patient and family how to evaluate effectiveness of their own personal coping strategies
- Educate patient and family about alternative coping strategies if current strategies are not effective
- Educate about signs and symptoms of stress and ineffective coping
- Educate patient in constructive problem-solving and setting realistic goals
- Educate patient and family about coping strategies to promote relaxation when fearful
- Educate about sources of hope and ways of sustaining hopefulness

Other Relevant Nursing Diagnoses

Adjustment, impaired
Coping, defensive
Denial, ineffective
Coping, ineffective family: disabling
Decisional conflict (specify)
Family processes, altered

REFERENCES

Billings AG and Moos RH: The role of coping responses and social resources in attenuating the stress of life events, J Behav Med 4:139, 1981.

Bishop DS, Epstein MB, Keitner GI, and others: Stroke: morale, family functioning, health status, and functional capacity, Arch Phys Med Rehabil 67:84, 1986.

Bourestom NC: Predictors of long-term recovery in cerebrovascular disease, Arch Phys Med Rehabil 48:415, 1967.

Bronstein K: Coping strategies and adaptation poststroke, unpublished doctoral dissertation, Chicago, 1986, University of Illinois.

Carlson CE: Methods of coping. In Martin N, Holt NB, and Hicks D, editors: Comprehensive rehabilitation nursing, New York, 1981, McGraw-Hill, Inc.

Charatan FB and Fisk A: Mental and emotional results of stroke, New York State J of Med 78:1403, 1978.

Cobb B: Cancer. In Garrett JF and Levine ES, editors: Psychological practices with the physically disabled, New York, 1962, Columbia University Press.

Cohen F and Lazarus RS: Active coping processes, coping dispositions, and recovery from surgery, Psychosom Med 35:375, 1973.

Cohen F and Lazarus RS: Coping with the stresses of illness. In Stone GC, Cohen F, and Adler NE, editors: Health psychology, San Francisco, 1979, Jossey-Bass Inc, Publishers.

Coyne JC, Aldwin C, and Lazarus RS: Depression and coping in stressful episodes, J Abnorm Psychol 90:439, 1981.

Derogatis LR: The psychosocial adjustment to illness scale (PAIS), J Psychosom Res 30:77, 1986.

Dimond M: Social support and adaptation to chronic illness: the case of maintenance hemodialysis, Res Nurs Health 2:101, 1979.

Dufault K and Martocchio BC: Hope: its spheres and dimensions, Nurs Clin North Am 20:379, 1985.

Farran CJ: A survey of community-based older adults: stressful life events, mediating variables, hope and health, unpublished doctoral dissertation, Chicago, 1985, Rush University.

Feldman DJ, Lee PR, Unterecker J, and others: Comparison of functionally oriented medical care and formal rehabilitation in management of patients with hemiplegia due to cerebrovascular disease, J Chronic Dis 15:297, 1962.

Felton BJ, Revenson TA, and Hinrichsen G: Stress and coping in the explanation of psychological adjustment among chronically ill adults, Soc Sci Med 18:889, 1984.

Finklestein SP, Weintraub RJ, Karmouz N, and others: Antidepressant drug treatment for poststroke depression: retrospective study, Arch Phys Med Rehabil 68:772, 1987.

Folstein MF, Maiberger R, and McHugh PR: Mood disorder as a specific complication of stroke, J Neurol Neurosurg Psychiatry 40:1018, 1977.

Foster JM and Gallagher D: An exploratory study comparing depressed and nondepressed elders' coping strategies, J Gerontol 41:91, 1986.

Goodstein RK: Overview: cerebrovascular accident and the hospitalized elderly—a multidimensional clinical problem, Am J Psychiatry 140:141, 1983.

Hamburg DA, Hamburg B, and deGoza S: Adaptive problems and mechanisms in severely burned patients, Psychiatry 16:1, 1953.

Heinemann AW, Roth EJ, Cochowski K, and others: Multivariate analysis of improvement and outcome following stroke rehabilitation, Arch Neurol 44:1167, 1987.

Hyman MD: Social psychological determinants of patients' performance in stroke rehabilitation, Arch Phys Med Rehabil 53:217, 1972.

Jalowiec A: Construct validity of the Jalowiec coping scale. Paper presented at Rush University College of Nursing, Chicago, July, 1986.

Jalowiec A: Personal communication, Winter 1987.

Katz S, Ford AB, Chinn AB, and others: Progrosis after strokes, part II: long-term course of 159 patients, Medicine (Baltimore) 45:236, 1966.

Kleinke CL, Staneski RA, and Mason JK: Sex differences in coping with depression, Sex Roles 8:877, 1982.

Krueger DW: Psychological rehabilitation of physical trauma and disability. In Krueger DW, editor: Rehabilitation psychology. Rockville, Md, 1984, Aspen Systems.

Lazarus RS: Patterns of adjustment, ed 3, New York, 1976, McGraw-Hill Inc.

Lazarus RS, Averill JR, and Opton EM: The psychology of coping: issues of research and assessment. In Coehlo GV, Hamburg DA, and Adams JE, editors: Coping and adaptation. New York, 1974, Basic Books Inc, Publishers.

Lazarus RS and Folkman S: Stress, appraisal, and coping, New York, 1984, Springer Publishing Co Inc.

Lehmann JF, Delateur BJ, Fowler RS, and others: Stroke rehabilitation: outcome and prediction, Arch Phys Med Rehabil 56:383, 1975.

Lind K: A synthesis of studies on stroke rehabilitation, J Chronic Dis 35:133, 1982.

Lipsey JR, Robinson RG, Pearlson GD, and others: Mood change following bilateral hemisphere brain injury, Br J Psychiatry 143:266, 1983.

Mahoney EK: The interaction of physical illness, coping focus, and perceived social support and their relationship to recovery from stroke, unpublished doctoral dissertation, San Francisco, 1985, University of California.

Mitchell RE and Hodson CA: Coping with domestic violence: social support and psychological health among battered women, Am J Community Psychol 11:629, 1983.

Morris PL and Raphael B: Depressive disorder associated with physical illness, Gen Hosp Psychiatry 9:324, 1987.

Moos RH and Tsu VD: The crisis of physical illness: an overview. In Moos RH, editor: Coping with chronic illness, New York, 1977, Plenum Medical Book.

Nomikos MS, Opton EM, Averill JR, and others: Surprise versus suspense in the production of stress reaction, J Pers Soc Psychol 8:204, 1968.

Novack TA, Haban G, Graham K, and others: Prediction of stroke rehabilitation outcome from psychologic screening, Arch Phys Med Rehabil 68:729, 1987.

Pearlin LI and Schooler C: The structure of coping, J Health Social Behav 19:2, 1978.

Price TR: Depression and stroke. In Dunkle RE and Schmidley JW, editors: Stroke in the elderly, New York, 1987, Springer Publishing Co Inc.

Popovich J: A study of hope and coping in stroke patients, Unpublished manuscript, 1987.

Roberts JG, Browne G, Streiner D, and others: Analyses of coping responses and adjustment: stability of conclusions, Nurs Res 36:94, 1987.

Robinson RG, Kubos KL, Starr BK, and others: Mood disorders in stroke patients, Brain 107:81, 1984

Robinson RG and Price TR: Poststroke depressive disorders: a followup study of 103 patients, Stroke 13:635, 1982.

Robinson RG, Starr LB, and Price TR: A two year longitudinal study of mood disorders following stroke, Br J Psychiatry 144:256, 1984.

Robinson RG and Szetela B: Mood change following left hemispheric brain injury, Ann Neurol 9:447, 1981.

Rosillo RH and Fogel ML: Correlation of psychologic variables and progress in physical rehabilitation: the relation of body image to success in physical rehabilitation, Arch Phys Med Rehabil 52:182, 1971.

Roy SR: Adaptation: a conceptual framework for nursing, Nurs Outlook 18:42, 1970.

Sanders JB and Kardinal CG: Adaptive coping mechanisms in adult acute leukemia patients in remission, J Am Med Assoc 238:952, 1977.

Selye H: The stress of life, New York, 1977, McGraw-Hill Inc.

Shanan J, De-Nour AK, and Garty I: Effects of prolonged stress on coping styles in terminal renal failure patients, J Human Stress 12:19, 1976.

Shinar D, Gross CR, Price TR, and others: Screening for depression in stroke patients: the reliability and validity of the center for epidemiologic studies depression scale, Stroke 17:241, 1986.

Sinyor D, Amato P, Kaloupek DG, and others: Poststroke depression: relationships to functional impairment, coping strategies and rehabilitation outcome, Stroke 17:1102, 1986.

Strauss AL: Chronic illness and the quality of life, St. Louis, 1984, The CV Mosby Co.

Visotsky HM, Hamburg DA, Goss ME, and others: Coping behavior under extreme stress, Arch General Psychiatry 5:27, 1961.

Wade DT, Legh-Smith J, and Hewer RA: Depressed mood after stroke: a community study of its frequency, Br J Psychiatry 151:200, 1987.

White RW: Strategies of adaptation, In Moos RH, editor: Human adaptation, Lexington, Ma, 1976, DC Heath & Co.

Whitney FW: Using physical and neuropsychological assessment in the nursing care of the acute stroke patient, In Dunkle RE and Schmidley JW, editors: Stroke in the elderly, New York, 1987, Springer Publishing Co.

Wright BA: Physical disability—a psychosocial approach, ed 2, New York, 1983, Harper & Row, Publisher's Inc.

Section III

Community Transition

Chapter 14

Discharge Planning and Home Assessment

Discharge planning is the key link in the continuum of care for the stroke patient and family. Depending on the nature and extent of deficits, the stroke patient and family may require support as minimal as instruction before discharge and a follow-up phone call, or as much as home health care and referrals for additional community services. To meet the individual needs of each patient, the nurse must activate the discharge plan upon admission to the inpatient setting, view discharge planning as a process, and understand factors affecting this process. Well-coordinated discharge planning by the nurse enables the patient and family to begin anticipating their own needs, learn problem-solving skills, and use resources available to them in the community.

This chapter will describe the process of discharge planning and discuss factors affecting this process in the inpatient setting. Practice models to promote efficient and timely discharge planning will be critiqued, and adjuncts to facilitate the stroke patient's transition from inpatient setting to the community will be described. Finally, recommendations will be made for assessing the stroke patient and family or caregiver needs (including home assessment) and for nursing interventions to assist in community transition.

Discharge planning is defined as a process during which planned activities in the inpatient setting are coordinated to promote continuity of care and a smooth transition of the patient and family into the next setting (i.e. another institution or the community) (Povse & Keenan, 1981). According to the American Hospital Association (AHA) (1984), discharge planning is essential to maintain high quality patient care. The AHA further states that discharge planning serves important functions by helping patients and families to make appropriate decisions and by helping to reduce length of stay and the rate of increase of health care costs. Thus, discharge planning benefits patients and families as well as health care providers.

The immediate goal of discharge planning is to ensure uninterrupted health care and to meet both actual and anticipated patient needs. Additional patient-centered goals of discharge planning have been delineated by the National League for Nursing (1984). Patient-centered goals include:

- patient and family actively participate in discharge planning
- high risk patients or patients with potential discharge planning problems are identified soon after admission
- solid collaboration and communication exist among all individuals involved in discharge planning
- the most economical and appropriate options are selected
- current knowledge of available health care

providers, programs and resources is maintained.

Thus, the benefits of discharge planning for the stroke patient and her family are obvious and will facilitate the patient's transition from one setting to another.

Ideally the nurse is the key person to initiate and coordinate a discharge plan because of her or his global view of the stroke patient's performance and needs, the nurse's constant contact with patient and family, and the nurse's ongoing interaction with all members of the health care team (Povse and Keenan, 1981). The discharge plan is best formulated with input from all disciplines involved in the patient's care. Thus, although the title or role of the nurse responsible for discharge planning may differ from one institution to another, an assumption underlying this chapter is that the process of discharge planning is implemented and coordinated by a nurse.

Discharge planning is a process that begins the day the patient is admitted to the hospital and continues through the day of discharge. Little information is available on outcomes and evaluation of discharge planning; however, discharge planning is believed to facilitate the continuum of care in the following ways: it lowers the hospital readmission rate for previously treated illnesses; maintains the patient's level of functioning after discharge; assists the patient and family to plan appropriate and continuing follow-up care; and improves the ability of the patient and family to identify and use available resources (Shine, 1983).

Although most health care professionals would agree that discharge planning is an ongoing process, the reality is that the plan often is not initiated until near the time of discharge, creating the potential for incomplete planning and referral. Mechanisms for discharge planning vary from institution to institution; however, guidelines to promote consistency and quality among institutions are available from the Joint Commission on Accreditation of Hospitals (1984), the American Hospital Association (1984), and the National League for Nursing (1984). Six essential elements of discharge planning are identified (American Hospital Association, 1984):

- early identification of patients needing complex posthospital care
- patient/family education
- patient/family assessment and counseling
- develop the plan
- coordinate and implement the plan
- follow-up after discharge

These components are the core of every discharge plan regardless of the institution or who facilitates the process. If the discharge planning process does not include these components, there may be negative consequences for the patient and family. Possible deleterious effects on the stroke patient and family include lack of follow-up medical care, increased stress on the caregivers because of lack of knowledge of support services, and an unsafe home environment if the family does not understand subtle deficits that the patient may have. Early involvement of the patient's family or significant other can facilitate a more complete and timely discharge plan.

Discharge planning is affected by various factors. First, the patient is in the hospital for shorter hospital stays. Since the federal government implemented a prospective payment system (PPS) known as diagnostic related groups (DRGs), Medicare reimburses a preestablished payment amount to the hospital based on the diagnosis of the patient. This predetermined payment provides incentives for acute care hospitals to reduce costs by shortening the length of stay. Since the development of DRGs, patients spend fewer days in the hospital. For example, the average length of stay per PPS discharge in fiscal year 1984 was 7.5 days, compared with 9.5 days (pre-PPS) in 1983 (Balinsky and Starkman, 1987). Specifically, Medicare patients with a diagnosis of cerebral vascular accident and no complications are allowed a mean length of stay of 7.5 days in the acute care setting (Jones and LeBlond, 1989). Because time spent in the hospital is so short, it is crucial that patient discharge needs be evaluated on admission.

A second factor affecting discharge planning is

that hospitalized patients may be sicker at the time of discharge than they used to be. A U.S. General Accounting Office preliminary study on the effect of DRGs on posthospital long-term care services noted that patients were being discharged "in a poorer state of health than prior to PPS. . .and in need of more extensive services" (Chelimsky, 1985). The fact that patients are in a poorer state of health at the time of discharge is of great concern because the majority of stroke patients are discharged into the community. In addition, the increased need for services requires a more comprehensive assessment and increased coordination between agencies. Elderly stroke patients and those with functional impairments could benefit greatly if transferred to a rehabilitation unit to assist them in learning how to care for themselves and return to an optimum level of functioning.

Another factor affecting discharge planning is whether the patient is going home or to a rehabilitation facility from acute care. The stroke patient who is discharged with minimal deficits to home from acute care will have different needs than the moderately or severely impaired patient who is discharged from the rehabilitation unit to home. Studies investigating the care of stroke patients report that only 10% to 18% of stroke patients are transferred from acute care to rehabilitation facilities (Gibson, 1974; Herman and others, 1984; Mayo and others, 1989; Dombovy and others, 1987). For stroke patients transferred from acute care to other units or facilities, communication about the plan of care not only provides essential information to the new care providers but also facilitates the transition of the patient and family into the new setting.

Of those stroke patients who do receive inpatient rehabilitative care, one study reports that 70% were discharged from rehabilitation facilities into the community, 17% were discharged to long-term care facilities, and 8% were transferred back to an acute care hospital (Granger and others, 1988). Although stroke patients who are discharged from rehabilitation facilities into the community may have additional skills for self-care and knowledge about community resources, each patient must be evaluated individually to determine the need for supportive services after discharge.

Considering that the survival rate for stroke is roughly two thirds and that for strokes due to atherothrombotic brain infarctions the survival rate is as high as 85% during the initial 30 days after stroke (Goldberg and Berger, 1988), a significant number of stroke patients are discharged from acute care into the community. These patients may need supportive services such as home nursing care, physical or occupational therapy, and information about preventing a recurrent stroke. Stroke caregivers need to know how to care for their loved ones and what resources are available to them in the form of services, information, support groups, and follow-up care.

A fourth factor influencing discharge planning is the patient's status at the time of discharge. Patient status after stroke is influenced by intrinsic and extrinsic variables (see the box on p. 274); these variables will affect subsequent discharge needs of the patient and his prognosis for recovery. Many stroke survivors sustain considerable physical deficits as a result of the stroke. For example, of stroke survivors in the Framingham study 31% were dependent in self-care and 20% were dependent in mobility (Gresham and others, 1975). Patients with these residual deficits may require discharge planning to assess things such as equipment needs, caregiver's needs, safety in the home and home modifications, and community services. The nurse must evaluate the effect of the stroke on the patient by assessing these intrinsic and extrinsic factors and determining patient needs for a smooth transition into the community.

Thus many factors affect the discharge planning process. For stroke patients, their often complex needs and short hospital stays present a serious challenge to nurses to coordinate comprehensive and timely discharge planning.

APPROACHES TO DISCHARGE PLANNING

Although the concept of discharge planning is accepted as an integral part of quality patient care, there is a fair amount of variability among institutions in how this is operationalized and who is responsible. Three approaches to facilitate discharge planning will be discussed: case management, the interdisciplinary team, and primary nursing.

VARIABLES CONSIDERED DETERMINANTS OF FUNCTIONAL OUTCOME IN STROKE SURVIVORS

Intrinsic Characteristics of the Patient

- Demographic: age, sex, race, and marital status
- Precise neurologic deficit:
  - Motor (hemiparesis, bilateral motor deficit, no motor deficit); degree of spasticity
  - Sensory (hemisensory deficit or other)
  - Hemianopia
  - Speech problems (dysphasia, dysarthria)
  - Organic cognitive deficits
  - Other (i.e., cerebellar ataxia, cranial nerve palsies)
- Etiology of stroke (atherothrombotic brain infarct, hemorrhage)
- Comorbid processes (concurrent medical conditions that may affect survival or functional abilities)
- Psychosocial factors (premorbid personality, usual socialization patterns, affective state, and others)
- Educational level and other skills
- Vocational status
- Financial assets

Extrinsic Characteristics of the Patient's Environment

- Family constellation or significant others
- Physical environment of home
- Type of community (physical environment, resources, attitudes)
- Services available (medical, rehabilitative, ongoing)

From Barnett HJ, Mohr JP, Stein BM, and Yatsu FM: Stroke: pathophysiology, diagnosis, and management, New York, 1986, Churchill Livingstone, Inc, p. 1260.

Case management is a coordinated approach to continuous patient care, spanning from preadmission, to discharge and postdischarge (Olivas and others, 1989) and involving an agreement between the patient and case manager regarding problems, outcomes, and services needed. The case manager's role in the institutional setting is to integrate services and facilitate activities, tasks, and procedures for the duration of the patient's illness. The case manager, then, is the coordinator whose focus is to help bring about the best patient outcome in the most effective and efficient manner. Although the overreaching goals of case management are the same for the patient in the community, aspects of the case manager's role may be different. For example, the case manager working with patients after discharge functions as an advocate, interpreter, and advisor, linking patients and their families to necessary services and helping them to negotiate their way through bureaucracy (Perlman and others, 1985).

Although the concept of case management is growing in popularity, a major problem is a lack of operational clarity. The main source of controversy regarding the role of case managers is whether the case manager functions primarily as a coordinator and expediter of services or if the case manager will also provide therapeutic services (Johnson and Rubin, 1983). As this model of practice evolves and is implemented to meet the needs of specific patient populations, the concept of case management should become more clear.

Case management has evolved as a model of practice to meet the complex needs of select patient populations, including patients with complex disabilities. Though no studies have evaluated this model specifically in the coordination of care for stroke patients, it is a promising alternative that may facilitate efficient and comprehensive care, throughout the course of an illness such as stroke.

The interdisciplinary team approach is common in rehabilitation settings and typically consists of a nurse, a physician, occupational, physical, and speech therapists, a social worker, and a psychologist. A dietician and chaplain may also be part of the team. Each team member evaluates the patient's abilities, provides therapeutic interventions, and educates the patient and family, within their domain of expertise. Team members usually meet weekly as a group to present their findings and interventions, to evaluate patient progress, and to set goals for continuing treatment. The team discusses issues such as variation in patient performance between therapy department and nursing unit, concerns or obstacles impeding the patient's progress, and plans and needs for discharge. In addition to weekly team meetings, family conferences may be set up any time during the course of hospitalization to address patient and family concerns, facilitate mutual goal setting, and to provide information and support. The team approach is valuable because the interdisciplinary involvement provides comprehensive assessment and interventions for patient and family. The goals of the team are to accurately assess patient functioning, use therapeutic interventions to help the patient achieve a maximum level of functioning in all domains, assist the patient and family in adjusting, and promote a smooth transition to home. While all members of the team work together to facilitate quality discharge planning, the nurse and social worker closely collaborate to facilitate this process. Stroke patients in particular benefit from an interdisciplinary approach because of the broad range of potential stroke-related deficits (Bukowski and others, 1986). The sometimes complex but subtle presentation of these deficits can interfere significantly with self-care activities, interpersonal relationships, and family functioning. Members of the team provide education and support to the patient and family to facilitate a quality transition into the community.

Though primary nursing is not distinct from the interdisciplinary team concept, it is presented here as a model of nursing practice regarded as a superior way to promote continuity of nursing care throughout the patient's hospitalization. The primary nurse is a registered nurse who takes responsibility for a patient for the duration of her hospitalization and assumes 24-hour accountability for the nursing plan of care. Although the primary nurse does not always provide the care for the patient, he or she is responsible for ongoing assessment, planning, implementation, and evaluation of nursing interventions; the primary nurse also assumes responsibility for coordinating all discharge needs of the patient and family.

Some institutions have nurses whose primary role is discharge planning. In these situations, the discharge planner collaborates with the primary nurse for essential information to facilitate discharge. The multiplicity of factors affecting the health care climate and the patient's hospitalization (i.e., length of stay, whether or not he goes to a rehabilitation facility, cost-containment, and staffing issues in health care environments) demands that nurses find innovative ways to meet the discharge planning needs of their patients. Additionally, current nursing shortages make it difficult in some settings for primary nurses to coordinate all aspects of patient care. An alternative, such as a discharge planning nurse, may facilitate a quality transition into the community for the patient and family.

ADJUNCTS TO DISCHARGE PLANNING

Three adjuncts to discharge planning have been used in the rehabilitation setting: self-medication programs, therapeutic passes, and rehabilitation home visits. Each of these programs facilitates discharge planning by providing opportunities for the patient to practice self-care behaviors and to develop problem-solving skills so she is better prepared to manage her care after discharge.

A *self-medication program* refers to patients being in charge of managing their own medications, including administering the medications themselves and getting the medications refilled as needed. The goals of self-medication are threefold: to help the patient to learn about her medications, including dosage, actions, and side effects; to provide a supervised trial to evaluate the patient's knowledge and compliance before discharge; and to enable the patient to increase her responsibility for her own care (Thompson and Ellenberg, 1987).

To begin a self-medication program, the nurse must ascertain that the patient is able to reliably participate and to identify modifications that might be necessary to help herself be successful. The nurse instructs the patient on the types of medications she is taking, the dosage, and the potential side effects, using whatever visual aids are appropriate. When the patient begins the program, the nurse checks with the patient at each dose to make sure that she took her medication. As the patient gets into the routine of taking her own medications, gradually she will not need to be checked on for each dose. However, the pharmacist usually monitors the frequency at which the patient requests a refill and notes if the patient is taking the medication in the prescribed amount and frequency. The stroke patient may need modifications to participate in the program, such as medication lids that can be opened with one hand and medication cards to remind her of the purpose of the medication. Color-coding medication bottles to correspond to time taken may be beneficial for some stroke patients with vision or memory problems. Thus self-medication programs are customized to meet individual needs and represent the interdisciplinary efforts of the nurse, physician, pharmacist, and sometimes an occupational therapist. The major benefit is that patients learn about their medications and get into the habit of taking their pills correctly; both of these are thought to increase patient compliance after discharge (Anderson and Poole, 1983).

Therapeutic passes are another adjunct therapy that is believed to facilitate discharge planning and the patient's transition into the community. *Therapeutic passes* are defined as the process of allowing the patient to return to the home or family environment for short stays (Rao and others, 1986). For the patients, the goals are to help the stroke survivor adjust to the home environment, to allow the patient to practice self-care activities and transfers, and sometimes to evaluate home accessibility. For the family, the goals are to help family members or significant others to adjust to living with the stroke survivor with alterations in physical, cognitive, and emotional functioning, and in some cases to experience the caregiving role for a short time to promote problem-solving and identify their own needs for further education. Patients usually are candidates for therapeutic passes as discharge approaches and when patients and families learn the necessary skills to be safe at home for short periods of time. Much effort goes into preparing the patient and family for a therapeutic pass, including educating them in all domains of care that the patient will need during that time at home, practicing skills, and demonstrating safe transfers, wheelchair management, ambulation, and self-care activities to the nurse and therapists. Once the patient and family are ready, the patient usually starts by going out on an 8-hour pass. If the 8-hour pass goes well, the patient then goes out on a weekend pass to allow him more opportunity for acclimating to the home environment. Upon returning from the pass, the patient and family discuss any difficulties they had during the pass, and team members provide additional information, suggestions for problem-solving, and in some cases, additional adaptive equipment. Researchers suggest that therapeutic passes are especially valuable for patients with brain injury (such as after a stroke) to help families prepare for any social and cognitive changes the patient may have (Rao and others, 1986). Therapeutic passes are useful in anticipating discharge needs and helping the stroke patient and family be as prepared as possible for leaving the institutional setting.

Finally, rehabilitation home visits are another adjunct to facilitate discharge planning. A *rehabilitation home visit* is a visit to the patient's home by members of the health care team together with the patient. Members of the team who might participate include the nurse, the social worker, and the physical therapist and/or the occupational therapist. The purpose of the visit is to evaluate accessibility of the environment and the patient's ability to safely maneuver in that environment. Specific things to be evaluated include the patient's ability to get in and out of the house, to perform specific tasks in each room, to transfer onto and off the commode, bed, and chair, and to move about from room to room. The patient's ability to safely use appliances and to use the phone are also evaluated. Based on findings during the home visit, the rehabilitation team makes further recommendations regarding self-care activities, adaptive equipment, and home modifications. The rehabilitation home visit was useful in a study evaluating the ability of forty elderly hip fracture patients to function at home prior to discharge from rehabilitation (Rosenblatt and others, 1986). This therapeutic adjunct is believed to promote patient satisfaction with discharge planning by fostering the patient's confidence and motivation, decreasing the anxiety present for some patients about discharge, and ultimately facilitating a safe transition into the home environment.

ASSESSMENT

Assessing the stroke patient's needs during hospitalization as they relate to discharge planning falls into several categories: educational needs, equipment needs, assessment of home environment, and psychosocial needs. Assessment in all categories is ongoing throughout hospitalization; and changing needs of the client will be reflected in this ongoing assessment. Guidelines for nursing assessment are listed in the box on p. 278. It is only through a thorough and constant assessment that the nurse can identify relevant and effective interventions to facilitate discharge.

Patient and family education is ongoing throughout hospitalization. To meet the individualized needs of each patient, the nurse must assess the patient's and family's knowledge about stroke, self-care activities, possibility for recurrent stroke, and their educational background and learning style. The nurse gathers objective and subjective information to formulate the plan. Two very important points about patient and family education are that patient and family priorities must be identified, and that adequate time must be allowed for learning. Before deciding what educational content to provide the patient and family, the nurse must assess their needs and find out what their priorities are. Once knowing their priorities, the nurse can incorporate this into the overall educational process. Finally, adequate time for learning offers the patient the best chance to absorb new information. This is especially important with stroke patients who may be elderly or have cognitive deficits or with patients who have decreased endurance from prolonged inactivity.

Often the equipment the stroke patient uses is provided by occupational and physical therapists. It is important for the nurse to assess the patient's use of this equipment to determine if the patient is using it properly and regularly, and how she feels about using adaptive equipment. Sometimes a patient feels uncomfortable using adaptive equipment and would prefer performing a task without it even if it is more difficult. Ongoing assessment of the patient's use of equipment provides valuable information to the nurse and other members of the team. Finally, the nurse assesses the patient's need for additional equipment and collaborates with therapists as appropriate. Equipment commonly used by stroke patients is described in Fig. 14-1.

An integral part of planning the patient's discharge is to assess the environment in which he will live. Once the location of discharge is known, it is important to determine what modifications are needed to make the environment accessible, convenient, and safe for the stroke patient. This may be done by asking the family to make a home assessment and bring this back to the team for evaluation. However, if the patient is severely impaired or the patient or family have special needs, it may be more appropriate for members of the health care team to make a home visit for the assessment. It may be beneficial for the patient to participate in the home visit.

Although home visits by members of the health care team can be time consuming, a visit may provide valuable information, for example, about family functioning, safety of the environment (in and outside the home), and availability of resources that was not readily apparent from interviewing and observing the patient and family in the inpatient

GUIDELINES FOR NURSING ASSESSMENT IN PREPARATION FOR DISCHARGE

EDUCATION

Is the patient knowledgeable about all aspects of his or her own care? (i.e., secondary stroke prevention, activities of daily living (ADL), functions of eliminations, sexual functioning, compensatory behaviors for sensory, perceptual, and cognitive deficits, medications, importance of health care follow-up)

Is the family or caregiver knowledgeable in all of these?

Does the patient, family, and/or caregiver demonstrate reasonable problem-solving skills when making decisions about health care?

Is the patient participating in prescribed health care behaviors in the institutional setting? Is this supported by the family?

Does the patient, family, and/or caregiver demonstrate a readiness for learning?

What learning style does the patient, family, or caregiver exhibit?

Does the patient, family, and/or caregiver participate in available group activities?

EQUIPMENT

Does the patient have the necessary equipment to function at an optimum level at home (i.e. equipment for dressing, toileting, grooming, bathing, and to facilitate social and vocational interests)?

Can the patient safely use all equipment?

Is the equipment well-maintained?

Is currently used equipment compatible with the home environment?

Has the family been instructed in the proper use of equipment?

If the patient needs to purchase new equipment from community sources after discharge, has he or she been instructed in ordering instructions and possible vendors?

HOME ENVIRONMENT

Is the home environment accessible for using the equipment the patient needs? (Fig. 14-2)

Can the patient maneuver around the home safely?

Has the patient gone on a therapeutic pass or rehabilitation home visit?

What are the anticipated needs for services in the community?

PSYCHOSOCIAL

What is the patient, family, and/or caregiver response (behavioral and emotional) to the patient's impending discharge?

What are the expressed needs for support from the patient, family, and/or caregiver?

What are the unexpressed needs for support from the patient, family, and/or caregiver?

setting. In situations in which discharge needs are complex, information obtained by a home visit may enable the health care team to better provide the understanding, support, and information that a patient and family need to make a more successful transition to home.

The home environment is assessed for accessibility. Accessibility means that the environment is free of physical barriers that interfere with the patient's convenience and her ability to move about and function independently and safely (Goldman, 1987). Guidelines for determining home accessibility are provided in Fig. 14-2.

INTERVENTIONS

Nursing interventions to prepare the stroke patient for discharge include educating the patient and

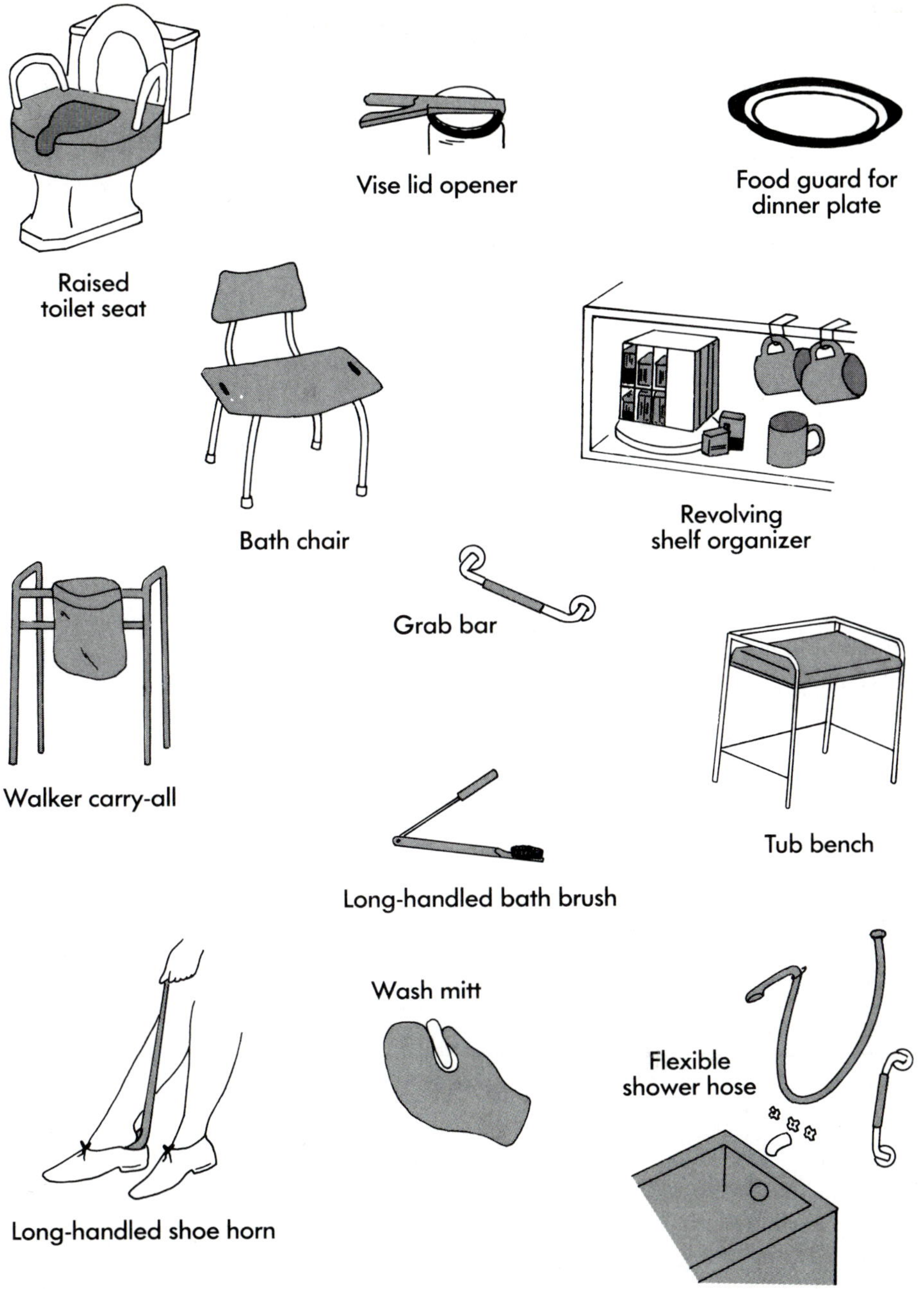

Fig. 14-1 Equipment commonly used by stroke patients.

Accessibility checklist for the home

Area	Yes/no	Length	Width	Height
Outside/approach slope at entrance				
parking near entrance				
dimensions of walkway				
connection of walkway to other surfaces (platforms, ramps)				
surface nonskid				
Ramps/stairs slope				
dimensions				
surface nonskid				
handrails (height, side)				
clearance at bottom				
landing dimensions				
edge protection (ramps)				
Entrances number				
dimensions				
Kitchen doorway				
door swings out/in to kitchen				
counters				
cupboards				
sink				
adequate lighting				
outlets				
controls for stove (front, back)				
hot water pipes covered				
water temperature regulated				

Fig. 14-2 Accessibility checklist for the home.

Accessibility checklist for the home (continued)

Area	Yes/no	Length	Width	Height
Bathroom				
doorway				
door swings out/in to bathroom				
commode				
grab bars				
space next to commode for w/c				
bathtub				
space next to tub for w/c				
shower/tub faucets				
shower				
threshold into shower				
sink				
hot water pipes covered				
water temperature regulated				
Miscellaneous				
telephones (location, number)				
smoke detectors (location)				
fire extinguisher (location)				
flooring (type)				
extension cords				
throw rugs				

Fig. 14-2, cont'd

family, providing support, making appropriate referrals, giving suggestions for home modifications, and ensuring health maintenance by arranging follow-up care.

Education about stroke is important to facilitate the patient's and family's understanding of what occurred, the treatment, and what they need to do once the patient is home. Stroke patients must learn about what a stroke is and its causes. Many patients are anxious about having another stroke. Because recurrent stroke is a possibility, it is crucial that the patient and family be able to recognize signs and symptoms of stroke. In addition, education about prestroke health problems and their management may enable families and patients to recognize symptoms and seek help for problems when they are detected. In addition to learning skills for self-care and behaviors to compensate for the deficits, the stroke patient must learn problem-solving skills to deal with unexpected situations and be able to recognize signs and symptoms of another stroke. The nurse must identify patient readiness for learning and the patient's individual learning style to design the most effective approach with the patient and family.

Support is another important intervention that nurses provide to stroke patients and their families. Patients and families may need support concerning many issues of the stroke, including frustration resulting from loss of mobility and frustration at not being able to do things as quickly as before. If the patient has had a particularly unstable medical course after stroke, he may be fearful of dying and afraid to exert himself for fear of damaging his health. Another potential area of support is the case of a family with unrealistic expectations for the patient. Sometimes families may believe that the stroke patient can do things if he really wanted to; these unrealistic expectations are further complicated when stroke-related deficits are subtle and not always visible to the family, such as sensory and perceptual difficulties. Nursing interventions include providing opportunities for the patient to verbalize his feelings and express fears, anxieties, and frustration in appropriate ways.

The nurse provides support to the family by involving them in the patient's care as appropriate and keeping them informed about the patient's progress. Often families need clarification about why things happen and what they can do to be supportive of their family member. The nurse also provides support to caregivers by encouraging them to allow time for themselves and to take breaks from caregiving as needed. Sometimes caregivers need permission to not be caregivers or reminders to take care of themselves. Thus providing support to patients and families is an important nursing intervention in the care of the stroke patient.

Another common intervention is for the nurse to collaborate and make appropriate referrals to meet the needs of the stroke patient. These referrals might be to a psychologist, a vocational counselor, a chaplain, or a peer visitor. Depending on the needs of the patient and family, referrals for information or services may facilitate problem-solving and educating the patient and family about potential places to get help after discharge.

Another nursing intervention to facilitate discharge planning is for the nurse to make suggestions for home modifications. When discussing with the patient how she will continue her routine of self-care at home, the nurse can suggest ways to organize supplies to promote convenient access at home and energy conservation techniques to promote the patient's endurance throughout her daily activities. Stroke patients with altered mobility and sensory and perceptual deficits may require specific home modifications to function safely at home.

Finally, the nurse facilitates health maintenance by helping the patient to set up clinic appointments for a time and place convenient for the patient, and provides this information to the patient and family in writing. Special transportation services may be needed if the family is working during the time of the appointment. The nurse should discuss this with the patient and give him the information needed to arrange his own transport. It is important for the nurse to explain the rationale for follow-up care and what will occur at the follow-up visit. Patients and families should be encouraged to write down any questions to ask the nurse or the doctor and to take them with them when they come back for follow-up care. In addition, patients should have someone they can call if they have questions about their medications or about any new symptoms they may be experiencing. On some stroke units, nurses make a follow-up phone call at 1 month after discharge to check on how the stroke patient is doing and to evaluate how well their hospital care prepared them for home. Contact with patients after discharge may facilitate their satisfaction with their hospital care and provide some continuity in the community.

Now, nursing diagnoses relevant to stroke patient and family discharge needs will be discussed. One pertinent nursing diagnosis for the stroke patient is:

Translocation Syndrome Related to Impending Discharge After Stroke

As discharge approaches, the stroke patient may experience feelings of anxiety, insecurity, loss of control, and separation from staff. These feelings are precipitated by plans for discharge and change in the environment and caregivers. The goals of nursing interventions are to help the patient prepare for change, provide a supportive environment for the patient and family to express their feelings, and to promote the patient's self-confidence by providing every opportunity for the patient to function at his or her optimum level of independence.

Interventions include making an ongoing assessment of patient and family skills for care, assessing feelings about impending discharge, supporting open communication between patient and family, and making referrals to community agencies as appropriate. Throughout these interventions, the nurse must promote balance between allowing the patient to do as much for himself as he is able, while supporting the family's involvement as they develop their skills in caregiving. Education about the transition home, problem-solving in the new environment, and all aspects of stroke recovery will help the patient and family to feel less anxious about change and more confident about their abilities. Nurses play a crucial role in facilitating this transition for both the patient and family.

Potential for Altered Health Maintenance Related to Stroke Related Deficits

Upon leaving the institutional setting, patients have the potential for altered health maintenance if they are not knowledgeable about their needs and if they do not have the resources (i.e., equipment, caregiver, support services) necessary to enable them to follow their health care routine at home. Patients may not follow through with clinic appointments and with aspects of their self care if they lack resources and/or they do not understand the importance of these activities. Some problems stroke patients may encounter after discharge include injury to their affected side, falls, difficulties taking their medications, not being able to identify an emergent problem (such as a transient ischemic attack or medication side effects), and accessing transportation to keep clinic appointments.

The goal of nursing interventions is to prepare the patient and family for discharge so that the potential for altered health maintenance is minimal. Nursing interventions include openly communicating with patient and family during the discharge process to address their concerns and answer questions; helping them to develop problem-solving skills; and providing information regarding dietary restrictions, signs and symptoms of stroke, side effects of medications, and the importance of keeping follow-up appointments even when one feels good. Also, by promoting appropriate and increasing levels of responsibility for self-care throughout hospitalization, the nurse enables the patient and family to develop levels of competence with skills necessary to function in the home environment. A care plan of nursing diagnoses and additional interventions can be found on p. 284.

NURSING CARE PLAN

Nursing Diagnosis	Interventions	Expected Outcomes
Translocation Syndrome* related to impending discharge after stroke **Defining Characteristics** ■ Temporary loss (or change) of: decision making control of own life and environment support systems trust in family and new caregivers familiarity with environment feelings of security ■ Anxiety ■ Withdrawal ■ Confusion ■ Anger ■ Fear of independence ■ Noncompliance ■ Change in eating or sleeping habits ■ Change in bowel and bladder functions ■ Change in level of participation of self-care activities	**Ongoing Assessment** ■ Assess feelings of anxiety, anger, withdrawal, fear of independence ■ Assess areas of noncompliance or nonparticipation in self-care ■ Evaluate physical symptoms (i.e., confusion, changes in sleeping or eating habits) ■ Assess loss of change as perceived by the patient and family ■ Assess needs for reassurance, support, and services to promote a smooth transition **Therapeutic Interventions** ■ Plan strategies to facilitate client participation in self-care ■ Determine cause of physical symptoms and strategies to alleviate these ■ Discuss plans for impending discharge (estimated time, transportation, immediate needs for care and equipment in new environment) ■ Instruct caregiver on necessary skills, procedures ■ Facilitate home assessment for accessibility ■ Encourage patient and family to express feelings (fears, anxiety, anger, anticipation) ■ Facilitate discussion of concerns between patient and family ■ Provide support ■ Make referrals to community agencies as appropriate ■ Emphasize change as positive	■ The patient and family will prepare for discharge physically and emotionally ■ The patient and family will have the knowledge and/or skills to foster safe care in the new environment ■ The patient and family will express concerns and fears about impending discharge ■ The patient and family will be comfortable with the new environment ■ The patient and family will describe ways to make decisions and problem-solve after discharge ■ Identify available support systems

*Currently, there is no NANDA nursing diagnosis that describes this clinical problem. This nursing diagnosis is taken from Mumma, CM, editor: Rehabilitation nursing: concepts and practice, a core curriculum, ed 2, Evanston, Ill., 1987, Rehabilitation Nursing Foundation.

NURSING CARE PLAN — cont'd

Nursing Diagnosis	Interventions	Expected Outcomes
Potential for altered health maintenance related to stroke deficits **Defining Characteristics** ■ Difficulties managing health routine ■ Difficulties asking for help ■ Lack of knowledge of basic health practices ■ Demonstrated lack of adpative behaviors ■ History of lack of health-seeking behaviors ■ Expressed interest in improving health behaviors ■ Reported or observed lack of equipment, financial or resources ■ Reported or observed difficulty with personal support systems	**Ongoing Assessment** Assess patient and family's ability to ask for help ■ Assess knowledge of stroke and preventive behaviors ■ Assess patient and family's ability to manage health routine (via return demonstration of skills, procedures, performing ADLs). ■ Assess adaptive behaviors ■ Assess concerns expressed about improving health behaviors ■ Assess need for resources (i.e., equipment, financial, or others) ■ Assess personal support available to patient, family, caregiver **Therapeutic Interventions** ■ Promote health behaviors by modeling quality nursing care ■ Instruct patient and/or caregiver in skills, procedures, and assistance with ADLs ■ Explain rationale for care provided ■ Provide opportunity for patient and/or caregiver to demonstrate skills ■ Determine patient and family readiness for learning and involve them as soon as appropriate ■ Discuss importance of preventive health behaviors (diet, exercise, rest, monitoring medication effects, health care follow-up after discharge, etc.) ■ Assist patient and family to access resources when appropriate	■ The patient and family will have the knowledge and/or skills to follow health maintenance routine in the new environment ■ The patient and family will understand the potential consequences of not following health maintenance routine in the new environment ■ The patient and family will state signs and symptoms of potential health care problems ■ The patient and family will demonstrate use of effective coping mechanisms to manage stress ■ The patient and family will demonstrate knowledge and responsibility for behaviors necessary to maintain health after discharge

NURSING CARE PLAN — cont'd

Patient Education

- Educate patient and family about health maintenance routine at home
- Educate patient and family about stroke recovery and prevention
- Educate patient and family about constructive problem-solving
- Educate patient and family about signs and symptoms of potential health care problems
- Educate patient and family about community resources and ways to access them

Other Relevant Nursing Diagnoses

- Injury, potential for, related to knowledge deficit
- Injury, potential for, related to sensory or motor deficits
- Injury, potential for related to lack of awareness of environmental hazards
- Family processes, altered
- Role performance, altered

REFERENCES

American Hospital Association: Guidelines for discharge planning, Chicago, 1984, The Association.

Anderson K and Poole C: Self-administered medications on a post-partum unit, Am J of Nurs 83:1178, 1983.

Balinsky W and Starkman JL: The impact of DRGs on the health care industry, Health Care Manage Rev 21:61, 1987.

Bukowski L, Bonavolonta M, Keehn MT, and others: Interdisciplinary roles in stroke care, Nurs Clin North Am 21:359, 1986.

Chelimsky E: Information requirements for evaluating the impacts of medicare prospective payment on post-hospital long-term care services: preliminary report, US General Accounting Office Pub No GAO/PEMD-85-5, 1985, Washington, DC, US Government Printing Office.

Dombovy ML, Bamford JF, Whisnant, JP, and others: Disability and use of rehabilitation services following stroke in Rochester, Minnesota, 1975-1979, Stroke 18:830, 1987.

Gibson CJ: Epidemiology and patterns of care of stroke patients, Arch Phys Med Rehabil 55:398, 1974.

Goldman C: Disability rights guide: practical solutions to problems affecting people with disabilities, Lincoln, Neb., 1987, Media.

Gresham GE: The rehabilitation of the stroke survivor. In Barnett HJ, Mohr JP, Stein BM, and others, editors: Stroke: pathophysiology, diagnosis, and management, vol 2, New York, 1986, Churchill Livingstone.

Gresham GE, Fitzpatrick TE, Wolf PA, and others: Residual disability in survivors of stroke: the Framingham study, New England J Med 293:954, 1975.

Hartigan EG and Brown DJ, editors: Discharge planning for continuity of care (revised edition), New York 1984, National League for Nursing.

Herman JM, Culpepper L, and Franks P: Patterns of utilization, disposition, and length of stay among stroke patients in a community hospital setting, J Am Geriatr Soc 2:421, 1984.

Johnson PJ and Rubin A: Case management in mental health: a social work domain? Social Work 25:49, 1983.

Joint Commission on Accreditation of Hospitals: Accreditation manual for hospitals, Chicago, 1984, The Commission.

Jones MK and LeBlond J: St. Anthony's 1989 DRG Optimizing Card System, Washington, D.C., 1989, St. Anthony's Hospital Publications.

Mayo NE, Hindlisz J, Goldberg MS, and others: Destinations of stroke patients discharged from the Montreal area acute-care hospitals, Stroke 20:351, 1989.

Mumma, CM, editor: Rehabilitation nursing: concepts and practice, a core curriculum, ed 2, Evanston, Ill., 1987, Rehabilitation Nursing Foundation.

Olivas GS, Togno-Armanasco VD, Erickson JR, and others: Case management: a bottom-line care delivery model, J Nurs Adm 19:16, 1989.

Perlman BB, Meinick G, and Kentera A: Assessing the effectiveness of a case management program, Hosp Community Psychiatry 36:405, 1985.

Povse SM and Keenan ME: Discharge planning for the transition from a health care facility to the community. In Martin N, Holt NB, and Hicks D, editors: Comprehensive Rehabilitation Nursing, New York, 1981, McGraw Hill Book Co.

Rao N, Sulton L, Young CL, and others: Rehabilitation team and family assessment of the initial home pass, Arch Phys Med Rehabil 67, 759-761, 1976.

Rosenblatt DE, Campion EW, and Mason M: Rehabilitation home visits, J Am Geriatr Soc 34:441, 1986.

Shine MS: Discharge planning for the elderly patient in the acute care setting, Nurs Clin North Am 18:403, 1983.

Thompson TC and Ellenberg M: A self-medication program in a rehabilitation setting, Rehabil Nurs 12:316, 1987.

Chapter 15

Community Reintegration

One of the challenges in discussing the needs of stroke patients in the community is that this population is such a diverse group. Stroke survivors may be young or old, minimally or severely impaired, employed or unemployed, and have many or few family and community resources upon which to draw. These factors will have a major influence on the type and amount of assistance needed in the community. Regardless of how minimal the assistance needed by the patient and/or family, that assistance may be the crucial link to the patient's successful immediate transition and long-term adjustment to her stroke. This chapter will define community reintegration and resources, describe types of assistance available, and discuss factors affecting the survivor's and family's use of resources. Additionally, guidelines will be presented for the nurse to assess patient and family community needs; nursing interventions to promote appropriate and independent use of resources; and recommendations for priorities in stroke care and research for the 1990s.

Traditionally, successful recovery from stroke has been measured in terms of physical functioning. Stroke patients were judged as successfully recovering if, within a few months after the stroke, they could physically care for themselves and return to work. Rehabilitation health care specialists are beginning to identify the problems with valuing physical function alone and are making efforts to evaluate stroke-related effects on psychologic and social functioning.

Three observations in particular justify a more holistic approach to evaluating stroke survivors in the community. First, stroke patients may experience subtle problems such as mood disorders, altered sexual functioning, problem-solving difficulties, and sensory changes that may interfere with psychologic and social functioning. In spite of visible independence in physical care, these subtle difficulties may result in life changes that ultimately affect the quality of life of the stroke survivor and his family. Second, because the population is aging, more stroke survivors will be older, have more severe strokes, and potentially have concomitant chronic illnesses that limit their physical independence. The question then becomes, how can one lead a productive and satisfying life in spite of physical limitations? Third, as advances in technology enable more people to survive, the possibility of surviving a stroke with significant deficits, increases. Thus the emphasis must shift from measuring physical function alone to a broader view of evaluating this along with other dimensions of functioning that affect the quality of the patient's life after stroke.

Outcomes after stroke are beginning to be defined in terms of overall quality of life, which includes subjective well-being, satisfaction with one's life, and reintegration to normal living. These domains encompass dimensions of mental and physical health, interpersonal relationships, employment, personal development and fulfillment, and community and recreational activities (Freed, 1984; Anderson, 1982; Flanagan, 1982; Kottke, 1982).

REINTEGRATION TO NORMAL LIVING

Reintegration is the reorganization of physical, psychologic, and social characteristics of a person into a harmonious whole so that she can resume well-adjusted living after an incapacitating illness or trauma (Wood-Dauphinee and Williams, 1987). Three characteristics of reintegration that distinguish it from medical outcomes are: (1) it considers issues of living that are centrally important to the individual, (2) it extends to months and years after the stroke, and (3) the focus is the subjective perceptions of the patient rather than the objective perceptions of the health care provider. Reintegration to normal living is relevant for patients for whom a cure and a return to normal is not expected (Wood-Dauphinee and Williams, 1987), such as after a stroke. Regardless of how minimal stroke-related deficits are, survivors have to compensate for any impairments and resulting disability. Thus reintegration is relevant to the discussion of stroke survivors in the community, a diverse group.

A portrait of stroke survivors in the community can be drawn from studies evaluating outcomes over time from 3 months to 10 years after stroke in the United States, Canada, the Soviet Union, Finland, and Sweden. Among stroke survivors, approximately two-thirds are 65 years old or older (Mayo and others, 1989), and two-thirds have residual disabilities (Schmidt and others, 1986; Gresham and others, 1979). Older survivors have more disabilities and increasing numbers of chronic illnesses (Dombovy and others, 1987), and the stroke recurrence rate was 4.9% over 5 years in one study (Dombovy and others, 1987). Fewer than 1% in one sample of 367 community-dwelling survivors experienced medical complications, including cardiac problems, extending the stroke, and renal decompensation (Granger and others, 1988). Although women have a higher survival rate than men at 5 years (Dombovy and others, 1987), women are more often institutionalized than men despite marital status (Kelly-Hayes and others, 1988).

A multisite study of stroke patients at 6 months after discharge from inpatient medical rehabilitation units found that approximately 70% of stroke survivors return to the community, living either at home or in long-term care facilities (Granger and others, 1988). Of the survivors living at home, 15% live alone and 65% live with others. About 20% of stroke survivors are institutionalized (Granger and others, 1988). Community-dwelling stroke survivors were homemakers (24%), employed (5%), unemployed (15%), and many were retired (56%). While 5% of stroke survivors were employed in this sample, a study in Sweden reports that one third of stroke survivors return to work (Fugel-Meyer and others, 1975), with an even higher rate of employment (42%) in the Soviet Union 1 year after stroke among survivors who were working at the time of their stroke (Vladimirovitc and others, 1988). Thus the majority of stroke patients sustain some residual disability and live at home. The type of assistance stroke survivors need can vary from minimal help to much help to remain in their homes. The nurse can facilitate the patient's reintegration into the community by assessing the patient and family resources and needs before discharge and by determining learning needs and necessary support services.

COMMUNITY RESOURCES

Community resources are supportive services that meet the health, psychologic, and/or social needs of the stroke survivor and family. Resources are tools that facilitate the stroke survivor's reintegration to normal living after the stroke. The resource may be needed for a brief period and may be as simple as an organization for information, a support group, or a provider of equipment and supplies. On the other hand, resources may be more complex, such as services to provide skilled nursing care, delivered meals, or respite care for a family caregiver. The type of assistance needed will vary greatly and depend on the stroke survivor and family needs, their values, and their currently existing skills and resources.

For example, in a study of how patients adjust in the first 3 months, stroke survivors (n = 60) and family members needed help with a wide range of stroke-related problems, including obtaining acute and chronic medical treatment, getting medical clearance to return to work, managing activities of home health aides, completing insurance forms, and interpreting and managing residual effects from the stroke (Popovich, 1990). In most cases, problems were detected by routine follow-up phone calls, patients or families either did not perceive the need for help or did not know how to get assistance, and interventions facilitated stroke survivor and family problem-solving. Thus a broad scope of services address the needs of this population living in the community.

Possible community resources for survivors living at home fall into two major categories: those that provide support for survivors returning to their prestroke living arrangements and those that provide alternative living arrangements.

Many services are available that provide support to stroke survivors living at home. These include home health care services of a nurse, therapist, or home health aide; outpatient medical care; emergency alerting services; meals and transportation; equipment and supplies; homemakers; adult day care; respite care; stroke clubs and stroke support groups; and organizations providing information and referral.

Home Health Care

Home health care may be provided by a registered nurse, a licensed practical nurse, a nurse's aide, or a therapist, depending on the type of care needed. Home care provided by a nurse or therapist is available from home health agencies, visiting nurses associations, and private registries. Though this type of care can be quite expensive, Medicare will subsidize visits for skilled care ordered by a physician, for a limited time. Skilled care may include physical therapy and nursing care required to administer intravenous feedings, to assess a significant change in health status, to manage tubes and catheters, and to educate patient and family about equipment, medications, or procedures. In some cases, help is needed to perform ADL such as bathing, dressing, feeding, and monitoring blood pressure and medications. These activities can be performed by a home health aide and may not be subsidized by Medicare. During hospitalization, the nurse should assess the type of home health care the patient and family need; needs for education, equipment, and some services that are detected early may be met before discharge from the hospital or rehabilitation unit.

Outpatient Medical Care

After discharge, stroke patients may have their health monitored by a family physician, a health maintenance organization (HMO), or an ambulatory care clinic at a medical center. Services may be provided on a fee-per-visit basis or, in the case of HMOs, services are prepaid and the patient participates in regularly scheduled health visits. Although HMOs intend to provide regular supervision and health promotion, it is sometimes difficult for a client to gain timely and efficient access to the needed services. Barriers to accessing such care develop if the client does not know whom to call, how to communicate that a health problem is emergent, and if the client is not seen by the same physician each time. Nurses can facilitate this process before discharge by making sure that the patient and family understand which physician they will be seeing after discharge, where the office is, and whom to contact to make an appointment.

Emergency Alerting Services

Emergency alerting services are set up to send an alert, via an electronic device or other signal, to someone outside the home that the stroke survivor needs help. This alert sets into motion a preplanned system that ensures an emergency response. These services are especially useful for people with impaired mobility who spend a lot of time at home alone and find security in knowing they can get help in an emergency. Services are usually operated around the clock, 24-hours a day, and may be operated by a variety of companies, agencies, and hospitals. The signal may be initiated by an electronic device worn by the patient who is alone. When the patient is in trouble, a signal is transmitted to a switchboard operator, who then seeks help. Another alerting service, the Postal Alert, was developed by the US Postal Service and alerts the carrier by a red sticker on the mailbox. If mail is not picked up, the carrier will notify an appropriate agency or service to intervene (National Stroke Association, 1989).

Meals and Transportation

Meals and transportation may be provided to assist stroke survivors whose nutritional status may be compromised or for those who need transportation for health care or community events. These services may be arranged on a regular or sporadic basis to enable the patient to be more independent and/or to assist her when family or friends are not able. Meals may be provided in a congregate setting or through home delivery. Sponsored by the Title III nutrition program of the Older Americans Act, congregate meals are available for low-income elderly stroke survivors at centrally located senior centers, public agencies, schools, or churches. This program is especially helpful to patients who have difficulty shopping or preparing food because of impaired physical ability, for those with a low income, and those who may be socially isolated.

Another program also sponsored by Title III is Meals on Wheels. This program delivers a nutritionally balanced, hot, noon meal, and sometimes cold food for supper or breakfast the next day, to homebound elderly persons age 60 years and older. Typically, the meals are prepared at different institutional facilities and delivered by volunteers. This program can be helpful to stroke patients who are unable to prepare their own food and to get out into the community because they have decreased endurance or sensorimotor impairments. Information regarding available food services and eligibility requirements may be obtained by contacting the local Council on Aging.

Special accommodations for transportation may be provided by the local public transit system or by specific agencies. Some of the services provided by the local public transit system may include reduced fares for elderly travelers, wheelchair lifts in some of the vehicles (buses, trains, or vans), specialized modes of transportation by an appointment-only basis, and a driver who assists the patient in getting on and off the vehicle. Certain agencies may also provide specialized types of vehicles and escort service in which someone travels with the patient. This may be particularly helpful for stroke survivors who have decreased endurance, moderate or severe physical impairments, poor vision, or communication difficulties. Stroke survivors may need assistance with transportation to keep health care appointments, to go grocery shopping or to the pharmacy, or to participate in community activities. The nurse should discuss home-going needs for meals and/or transportation with the patient and family before discharge and provide them with the necessary information.

Equipment and Supplies

In many cases, equipment and supplies used by the stroke patient may be paid for by insurance. Medicare, Medicaid, and private insurers may pay partial or total costs, if there is a prescription from the physician; however, the amount of coverage varies, depending on the policy. To facilitate a smooth transition into the community, it is essential that the patient and family know what supplies are needed and how to get them. The nurse can assist the patient in getting prescriptions for supplies and equipment before discharge to maximize insurance coverage; she may also direct the stroke patient to specific suppliers who are competitively priced.

Stroke Clubs and Stroke Support Groups

Stroke clubs and stroke support groups help stroke survivors and families to get educational information, to share experiences, and to get support. Sponsored by the National Easter Seals Society, the American Heart Association, or local hospitals, stroke clubs provide social and educational opportunities in a positive supportive environment where members share experiences and resources. Though professionals may attend the meetings, the stroke club is a consumer group coordinated and run by stroke survivors and families (National Stroke Association, 1989).

In contrast, a stroke support group is a group counseling program for stroke survivors, families, and caregivers (National Stroke Association, 1989). Meetings are informal but structured and provide educational information, support for emotional needs, and assistance with resolving personal concerns. Meetings are coordinated and run by a professional, often a rehabilitation expert. The nurse can inform the patient and family about the purpose of these groups and provide information about meeting times and location. In some cases there may be an opportunity for the patient and/or family to attend a meeting before discharge.

Homemakers

Homemakers work under the supervision of a professional nurse or therapist who assesses the type of services needed. Services provided by a homemaker include meal preparation, housecleaning, and laundry and may be combined with providing personal assistance to the stroke survivor for ADL. The frequency of use may range from every day for a few hours to occasional help to go grocery shopping or shovel snow. Referrals for homemaker services can be obtained from home health agencies, Social Service departments, the local Council on Aging, and senior citizen centers. Sometimes these services can be provided by neighbors or church members on a volunteer basis or for a nominal fee. Services such as these can make a difference for the stroke survivor, enabling him to carry out his daily activities safely and with minimal support.

Adult Day Care

This service is targeted at semiambulatory or otherwise impaired patients to provide maintenance, custodial care, and social activities, usually in a group setting. Stroke survivors may benefit from this type of program if they need assistance or supervision with ADL and/or cognitive tasks. Depending on the program, adult day care may also provide limited medical assistance and rehabilitative services, such as physical, occupational and/or speech therapy, reality orientation, social stimulation, and family counseling (Huttman, 1985). Adult day care services are often affiliated with a formal health agency, such as a hospital or nursing home, that provides services for a few to several hours per day. The type of adult day care center determines whether or not Medicaid reimburses for services. Those centers providing medical care and therapy are more expensive but may be certified for reimbursement; more commonly, centers that provide social programs are not reimbursed by Medicaid and are a third to half the cost of day care centers that provide medical services. The nurse should evaluate home care issues with the patient and family and provide information about day care, as appropriate, before discharge.

Respite Care

The focus of respite care is to give intermittent relief to caregivers from their caregiving responsibilities by having a respite care worker assist the stroke survivor at home or in an adult day care program. Respite workers may be nurses or trained home health aides who provide companionship and/or any necessary emotional or physical care, including homemaking and health monitoring of the survivor and/or the caregiver (Lubkin, 1986). The duration of respite care can range from a few hours to 2 or 3 days, depending on the caregiver's needs. Some benefits to respite care include providing physical relief for the caregiver, preserving the relationship between patient and caregiver, and preventing caregiver burnout. When a stroke survivor needs a caregiver at home, the nurse should discuss respite care with the patient and designated caregivers, giving them information about local programs and encouraging them to take advantage of respite care when needed.

Organizations for Information and Referral

Many organizations offer information about stroke in the form of pamphlets for patients, families and professionals. The box on p. 294 lists some of the pamphlets about stroke available from different organizations. Additional books about stroke are listed in Appendix A. Audiovisual aids about various aspects of stroke have been produced by professionals and are available to the general public (see Appendix B). In addition to providing written information, organizations provide referrals and act as resources for stroke survivors, families, and health care professionals interested in stroke patients. By belonging to professional organizations, health care professionals have opportunities to access the most current information about stroke care, and for professional development. Membership fees and donations are an important source of funding and help organizations continue to provide community services to stroke survivors and families. A list of consumer and professional organizations for the nurse can be found in Appendix C.

In summary, several resources to support the stroke survivor exist in the community. Other services are available that provide alternative living arrangements for stroke survivors. Some of these include enriched housing, shared housing, or institutional care in a nursing home setting.

Enriched Housing

Enriched housing is a type of congregate housing where the individual has a studio or one bedroom apartment and shares a common kitchen and living room. In addition to some shared living space other services may be included, such as prepared meals, laundry, light housekeeping, and some assistance with ADL. Sponsored by community and local religious groups, the cost of enriched housing may be covered by Supplemental Security Income (SSI) (National Stroke Association, 1989). Stroke patients who are independent but would prefer not living alone can potentially benefit from this arrangement.

Shared Housing

Shared housing is when people with extra living space share their homes with others who need housing. The person needing housing pays rent and may participate in household chores in exchange for a room and some shared living space. Stroke patients who are homeowners may benefit from this arrangement by offering living space to someone who can assist with chores and with the financial burden of managing a household. Stroke patients who need a place to live can benefit from this arrangement also by not having to live alone and by not having the sole responsibility for meal preparation, shopping, and household chores. Arrangements between people in shared housing vary a great deal, depending on the needs and mutual agreement of the people involved. In addition to the practical aspects of sharing housing, it also can provide companionship and minimize social isolation. Shared housing is a creative but underutilized alternative to living in an institution.

Institutional Care

Several types of institutional care provide different types of living space and personal care. Boarding homes, also called adult homes and sheltered care, are inexpensive group living arrangements that provide a protective environment and minimal help with preparing meals and ADL (Huttman, 1985). Because no medical or nursing care is provided, these are not covered by Medicare or Medicaid.

A more supervised living environment is the intermediate-care facility (ICF). This type of institutional care provides 24-hour service and health supervision of ambulatory, medically stable individuals who need minimal help with ADL. Social and recreational activities may also be provided. A nurse is available at least 8 hours a day to evaluate health conditions and assist the patient with medications.

STROKE PAMPHLETS AVAILABLE

AMERICAN HEART ASSOCIATION

Aphasia and the family (50-002-A)
Body language (51-003-A)
Facts about strokes (51-1001)
1990 Heart and stroke facts (55-0376)
Heartline newsletter
Six hopeful facts about stroke (51-1014)
Risk factors in stroke (71-022-A)
Stroke: Why do they behave that way? (50-035-A)
Strokes—a guide for the family (50-025-B)
Up and around: A booklet to aid the stroke patient in activities of daily living (50-026-A) (availability limited)

EASTER SEALS SOCIETY

First aid for aphasics
Handy helpful hints for independent living after stroke
Organizing a stroke club
Understanding stroke

NATIONAL STROKE ASSOCIATION

Be stroke smart (newsletter)
Communication difficulties (3 pamphlets)
Emotional aspects (5 pamphlets)
Dental health care for the stroke survivor
Depression—a natural reaction to stroke
Home and work adaptations (5 pamphlets)
Home exercises for stroke patients
Living at home after a stroke
Prevention and warning signs (3 pamphlets)
Rehabilitation guidelines and resources (10 pamphlets)
Stroke: Questions and answers
Stroke: Reducing your risk
Stroke: What is it, what causes it?
Suggestions for communication with an aphasic person
The importance of a proper diet after stroke
Understanding speech and language problems after stroke
What every family should know about stroke

U.S. DEPARTMENT OF HEALTH AND HUMAN SERVICES

Stroke update (NIH Pub No 88-2989)
Stroke: Hope through research (NIH Pub No 83-2222)
Stroke (NIH Pub No 86-1618)
National survey of stroke (NIH Pub No 83-2069)
What you should know about stroke and stroke prevention (NIH Pub No 81-1909)

The most supervised nonacute institutional living environment is the skilled nursing facility (SNF), which provides 24-hour nursing care of ambulatory and nonambulatory individuals. Possibilities for care include providing whatever level of nursing care is required, physical and occupational therapy, more frequent visits from the physician, and social and recreational activities. This type of care may be necessary if the stroke patient is unable to manage self care and has no caregiver in the home. Because the services are more extensive, the SNF is the most costly alternative to home care. Usually the facility is Medicare-certified, which indicates that for a limited time, Medicare will cover a portion of the cost. The decision to place a stroke survivor in an institution may be a very delicate issue and requires care and sensitivity on the part of the nurse. Sometimes the family will not consider this option in spite of their difficulty in caring for the person at home. Having the family involved in the stroke patient's care early in the hospitalization often helps them in making the best and most realistic decision about placement after discharge.

ASSESSMENT

To facilitate reintegration to normal living, the nurse must accurately determine patient and family beliefs, skills, and resources by making a comprehensive nursing assessment. While the nurse discharging the patient from hospital or rehabilitation facility collects much of this data through an ongoing nursing assessment, the community health nurse continues assessing the stroke survivor and family after discharge. An ongoing nursing assessment provides valuable information to guide patient and/or family to seek appropriate resources as well as to alert the nurse to difficulties they may be having with current services. When patient and/or family needs are complex or when multiple agencies are involved, there are more opportunities for miscommunication, for patient and family caregivers to become overwhelmed, and for client needs to go unmet. Thus the nurse is a valuable liaison between the patient and family and available supportive resources. Guidelines for nursing assessment are listed in the box at right. Information about the patient's baseline physical, psychologic, and social functioning will also help the nurse to guide patient and family to appropriate community resources.

NURSING ASSESSMENT OF PATIENT AND FAMILY COMMUNITY NEEDS

What are the patient and family skills, resources?
In what areas does the patient and family need assistance?
Does stroke survivor have physical and/or functional deficits?
Effect of stroke survivor's physical deficits on family interaction, role functioning?
Does the stroke survivor have any residual cognitive and/or behavioral deficits?
Effect of stroke survivor's cognitive and/or behavioral deficits on family interaction, role functioning?
Does stroke survivor require a caregiver?
Who is patient comfortable with providing her or his care?
Are there single or multiple caregivers?
Are caregivers providing sufficient and appropriate care?
Does the caregiver have time away from caregiving?
Is the caregiving situation in the home compatible with needs of all family members?
Patient and family knowledge of community services (is it current and accurate)?
Types of community support currently being utilized?
Previous use of community services (types, frequency)?
Patient and family beliefs and values about asking for help?
Patient and family beliefs and values about accepting help?
Are the patient's or family's current use of community resources appropriate and sufficient?

INTERVENTIONS

Interventions must be customized to meet the needs of the patient and family; these are formulated jointly between the nurse, the patient, and the family. Interventions focus on stroke prevention, patient and family education, securing the necessary resources, and facilitating communication among the patient, the family and the community resources they will be utilizing.

The nurse must educate the patient and family about types and ways of accessing community resources. After obtaining a baseline assessment of the patient's and family's knowledge of resources, the nurse must identify relevant information to give the family, using the most effective teaching strategies. The type of teaching strategy will vary a lot with the client and will be influenced by individual learning styles, educational backgrounds, and interest.

Securing the necessary resources is crucial to preserving the integrity of the family support system and to maintaining or improving the stroke survivors's health status in the community. Once the nurse identifies patient and family needs for resources, the options should be discussed with the patient and assistance provided in the selection of what will best meet their needs. Often, social workers or discharge planners are excellent resources to facilitate this process. Once the patient and family determine the types of resources needed to facilitate reintegration, communication to agencies is the next step. Whenever possible, this should be done by the patient or family with the guidance of the nurse to promote independence in problem-solving and to help the patient develop a sense of mastery.

A broad-reaching goal that directs stroke rehabilitation in the hospital, rehabilitation center, extended care facility, and after discharge into the community, is helping the stroke patient to learn the skills necessary to enable him to function at an optimum level. To function at optimum level means being as independent as possible, without compromising overall state of health. Though there may be a lack of needed services to enable an elderly stroke victim to live in the home, more services are not necessarily better. The goal should be to identify the optimum amount of support needed that will enable the stroke survivor to be as independent as possible and provide the necessary support to the family.

Now, nursing diagnoses relevant to patient reintegration to normal living will be discussed. One pertinent nursing diagnosis for the stroke patient in the community is:

Social Isolation Related to Stroke-Related Deficits

The patient may feel socially isolated after a stroke for many reasons, including limited physical mobility; inability to drive; altered mood, cognition or communication; embarrassment about physical limitations and/or use of adaptive equipment; and/or role changes (i.e., imposed retirement, loss of job, temporary medical leave). Moreover, social isolation may be imposed on the stroke victim if significant others and/or friends are uncomfortable being around the stroke victim. The patient is not the only one at risk for feeling socially isolated. Significant others and family members may feel isolated because of caring for the stroke survivor. The goal of nursing interventions its to help the patient and family to identify causes for feelings of loneliness and to facilitate ways for them to participate in diversional activities and to interact with others.

Nursing interventions might include finding transportation for the stroke patient to participate in enjoyable activities, facilitating the stroke patient's return to work, facilitating a few hours of respite care to relieve family caregivers, connecting the stroke victim with other stroke survivors in the community, or identifying a stroke support or caregiver support group for patient and/or family. Other interventions include encouraging patient and family to talk about their feelings and thoughts about the stroke, promoting the optimum level of independence in self-care, and encouraging the patient to participate in normalizing social activities as much as they are able.

Altered Family Processes Related to Stroke

The experience of stroke can affect family functioning during hospitalization as well as after discharge from the rehabilitation unit. Family functioning may be disrupted by specific stroke-related factors, such as a patient who has significant physical and/or cognitive deficits, mood changes, or aphasia. On the other hand, the stroke may be one of many other stressors taxing the resources of family members. Alterations in family process brought on by a stroke can threaten the integrity of the family structure by exhausting the family resources and creating conflict between family members.

To a great extent, nursing interventions will depend upon the family resources and the extent to which the family is a functional unit. If communication and relationships within the family are healthy, the nurse can encourage realistic expectations between the patient and family, and facilitate open communication regarding feelings, concerns, and problems that arise. If the family resources are limited or the family is dysfunctional, nursing interventions might include educating the family about effective ways of coping, modeling open communication, and/or assisting the family to seek outside counseling and appropriate support services. It is critical that the nurse accurately assess family process in the community and any difficulties the family is having. This assessment provides the foundation for the nurse to intervene appropriately, enabling the family to learn how to adapt and use their own resources as much as possible.

Noncompliance Related to Lack of Necessary Resources

Though the patient and family may be noncompliant for many reasons, sometimes patients are unable to carry out necessary health behaviors (i.e., special diet, regular medications, visiting the physician for follow-up) because they lack the necessary resources to do so. For example, stroke survivors may be noncompliant because they lack the money to buy medications or pay for health care, they have no accessible transportation, they are unable to prepare their own meals, or they have not been educated about the reasons for specific health behaviors. Nursing interventions might include identifying potential community resources (i.e., financial assistance to purchase medications, accessible transportation, Meals on Wheels) for which the patient qualifies, educating the patient about rationales for certain health behaviors and options available to her or him, and assisting the patient and family to initiate contact with appropriate agencies.

Keeping in mind that noncompliance is rarely related to a single cause, the nurse must determine as carefully as possible reasons why a patient is noncompliant with the prescribed health regimen. Identifying the cause(s) of noncompliance is crucial to determining the most appropriate nursing interventions. The goal of nursing interventions is to accurately evaluate the reason for noncompliance; once this is determined, the nurse assists the patient and family to use the necessary resources that will aid them in following the prescribed health routine.

A care plan for patient and family community needs along with additional nursing diagnoses the nurse should consider when caring for the stroke patient and family are listed on p. 299.

PRIORITIES FOR STROKE CARE AND RESEARCH IN THE 1990S

A discussion of community reintegration could not be complete without identifying priorities for stroke care in the 1990s. When considering the needs of this population, it is essential to evaluate available resources and to identify strategies for change in policy-making and in the directions for future stroke nursing research.

In spite of a large and diverse body of research-based literature on stroke, few research studies have been nursing-focused. The great majority of research has been done by physicians and some by physical therapists, occupational therapists, and psychologists. Although stroke research in other disciplines has greatly contributed to the knowledge base in nursing, it is time for us to strengthen our understanding and to develop the scientific basis for interventions in the care of the stroke patient by conducting clinical nursing studies.

This is not to imply that research done in other disciplines and in other patient populations does not provide excellent data relevant to the nursing care of stroke patients. Nurses have researched relevant issues in different patient populations that can be applied to our understanding of stroke. A good example is that of coping research. Nursing studies have looked at coping with Alzheimer's disease (Quayhagen and Quayhagen, 1988), coping in hypertensive emergency room patients (Jalowiec and Powers, 1981), coping with hemodialysis (Gurklis and Menke, 1988), and coping with myocardial infarcts (Christman and others, 1988; Riffle, 1988). Though each group has its own unique set of circumstances, the clinical questions we ask from one population to another and the design and measurement issues are similar. The answers lie in doing research and sharing the results, in replicating studies in the stroke population, and in identifying aspects unique to the stroke experience that require further research.

A review of recent nursing literature reveals that nurses have investigated a variety of issues in the care of the stroke patient. Nurses have studied nurses' knowledge and attitudes toward sexuality of stroke patients (Mitchelson, 1988); stroke and the impact on families (Stroker, 1983); perceived loss in patients and spouses (Mumma, 1986); and perceived social support, coping focus, and coping (Mahoney, 1985). Other studies of coping after stroke have looked at coping strategies of stroke patients (Bronstein, 1986) and hope and coping in stroke patients (Popovich, 1990). Other outcome-oriented nursing research has evaluated the effects of stroke recovery groups (Pasquerello, 1987), the use of Bobath principles (Passarella and Lewis, 1987), the relationship of lesion location to emotional and functional outcomes (Williams, 1986; Whitney, 1987), the quality of life after cerebral bypass surgery (Stewart-Amidei and Penckofer, 1988), and the quality of survivorship following stroke (Kelly-Hayes, 1987). One ethnographic study explores the course of stroke recovery in depth over 12 months in a small group of patients (Doolittle, 1988).

Additionally, nurses are reviewing the stroke literature and recommending nursing interventions based on current clinical research. Examples of this review process include detection of vasospasm after subarachnoid hemorrhage (Flynn, 1989), the etiology and management of spasticity (Ferido and Habel, 1988), the relationship between aphasia and depression (Tanner and others, 1989), psychological responses in aphasia (Keller and others, 1989), sexuality concerns of the stroke patient (Burgener and Logan, 1989), and stroke family support and education programs (Kernich and Robb, 1988).

Recommendations for future nursing research in stroke care encompass a variety of settings and research designs. Nursing research in stroke care is needed in the acute and postacute care setting and in rehabilitation and the community. Research methods are equally diverse and should include ethnographic, descriptive, and quantitative studies that incorporate a longitudinal design whenever possible. Recommendations for stroke research are made according to the current status of nursing-focused studies and research priorities identified by the American Association of Neuroscience Nurses, the National Institute for Neurological Disorders and Stroke, and the National Center for Nursing Research. Recommendations for nursing research in stroke care include:

1. Investigate health-promoting behaviors and stroke prevention in at-risk populations and in stroke survivors
2. Investigate different aspects of stroke in minority populations
3. Validate nursing diagnoses that are relevant to stroke patients (i.e., incidence and severity of altered mental status, and changes in mobility, perception, sensation, pain, coping, sexual functioning, communication)
4. Evaluate effectiveness of nursing interventions on physiologic, psychologic and behavioral outcomes during all phases of stroke recovery
5. Identify more global measures of stroke outcomes (i.e., quality of life and community reintegration) and develop meaningful ways to measure the multidimensional domains of function
6. Evaluate effectiveness of educational content and methods with stroke patient and families
7. Evaluate long-term outcomes in recovery from stroke, including ability for achieving optimum independence in self-care, patient and caregiver coping, and long-term adaptation to stroke.
8. Evaluate outcomes of nursing care and recovery from stroke in specialized stroke rehabilitation units, especially in elderly stroke patients.
9. Describe the effect of stroke on families in relation to issues such as role change, and family functioning

Finally, nurse researchers should consider a collaborative, interdisciplinary approach and recognize the contributions of the staff nurse in clinical research studies. The staff nurse plays a crucial role in successful clinical research and can contribute in the following ways: researching the literature, recruiting and screening subjects, facilitating pilot studies on the unit, and collecting data. By pursuing a collaborative, interdisciplinary approach and involving the staff nurse, the nurse researcher minimizes obstacles in the clinical setting and uses all available resources to enhance the quality of the research.

NURSING CARE PLAN

Nursing Diagnosis	Interventions	Expected Outcomes
Social Isolation related to stroke-related deficits (i.e., altered mood, communication, physical mobility, perception/cognition) **Defining Characteristics** ■ Expresses feelings of loneliness, uselessness ■ Feels different from others ■ Feels inadequate, doubts own abilities	**Ongoing Assessment** ■ Assess feelings of isolation; patient's appraisal of source of and strategies for dealing with isolation ■ Assess aesthetic stroke-related changes that contribute to isolation (i.e., incontinence, facial paralysis, use of adaptive equipment) ■ Evaluate physical symptoms that may reflect feelings of isolation (anorexia, insomnia, fatigue, increased sensitivity) ■ Determine barriers to social contacts for the patient (i.e., physical immobility, altered mood, communication, perception/cognition) ■ Determine barriers to social contacts in the environment (i.e., architectural, transportation, lack of access to resources)	■ The patient will identify reasons for feeling isolated ■ The patient will plan appropriate diversional activities ■ The patient will participate in social activities and meaningful relationships

Continued

NURSING CARE PLAN — cont'd

Nursing Diagnosis	Interventions	Expected Outcomes
■ Little to no contact with community, peers ■ Supportive, significant others are absent ■ Inability to concentrate and make decisions ■ restlessness ■ irritability ■ apathy	■ Assess recent losses adding to the patient's sense of isolation (i.e., relocation, death of a significant other, divorce) **Therapeutic Interventions** ■ Encourage patient to express feelings; be a good listener ■ Identify causative or contributing factors for isolation ■ Promote social interaction ■ Decrease barriers to social contacts (i.e., suggest alternative for transportation, diversional activities, opportunities for socializing, stroke support groups, stroke club) ■ Assist the patient in managing aesthetic problems (i.e., incontinence, impaired physical mobility, use of adaptive equipment) ■ Make referral to community agencies as indicated	
Family processes, altered related to stroke **Defining Characteristics** ■ Difficulty adapting to change in role related to disability ■ Ineffective communication among	**Ongoing Assessment** ■ Assess the current relationships, roles, health practices, and resources of the family unit ■ Assess patient and family's knowledge about stroke and the recovery process ■ Determine family's ability to make appropriate and timely decisions ■ Determine whether family communication is clear, direct, and effective in most situations	■ The patient and family will receive and/or provide the physical, emotional, and spiritual care necessary ■ The patient and family will be knowledgeable about stroke, the

NURSING CARE PLAN — cont'd

Nursing Diagnosis	Interventions	Expected Outcomes
family members ■ Conflict among family members ■ Difficulty accepting help when needed ■ Family unable to meet physical, emotional, spiritual needs of its members ■ Rigidity in family functions, role ■ Lack of involvement in community activities ■ Difficulty making decisions	■ Identify sources of stress for the patient and family ■ Determine how conflicts are resolved among family members ■ Determine whether family roles are flexible and accommodating to the physical and emotional abilities of the stroke survivor ■ Assess the family's ability to meet its own physical, emotional, and spiritual needs within the scope of its resources ■ Determine the family's ability to ask for and accept help appropriately ■ Evaluate family's adaptation to changes brought on by the family member's stroke **Therapeutic Interventions** ■ Provide information about stroke, disability, resources as needed ■ Facilitate open communication among family members; model open communication for family ■ Encourage family to verbalize feelings ■ Refer to counseling, support groups, and community resources as appropriate ■ Facilitate accurate appraisal of the situation and realistic expectations ■ Encourage family members to support one another	health regimen, potential complications, and stroke prevention ■ The patient and family will communicate openly and constructively with one another ■ The patient and family will make appropriate and timely decisions ■ The patient and family will handle conflict constructively ■ The patient and family will seek and accept help appropriately ■ The patient and family will maintain flexibility in roles and promote independence of stroke survivor as appropriate

Continued.

NURSING CARE PLAN — cont'd

Nursing Diagnosis	Interventions	Expected Outcomes
Noncompliance related to lack of necessary resources **Defining Characteristics** ■ Failure to keep appointments ■ Develops complications or exacerbation of symptoms ■ Verbalizes noncompliance or nonparticipation ■ Does not participate in health regimen	**Ongoing Assessment** ■ Determine patient and family's appraisal of the situation ■ Assess patient and family's understanding of the necessary health behaviors ■ Assess patient and family beliefs about current state of health and the stroke ■ Determine what resources are necessary for the patient and family to comply with necessary health behaviors ■ Assess obstacles to patient obtaining resources to facilitate compliance (i.e., cognitive, motor, sensory deficits) **Therapeutic Interventions** ■ Facilitate open communication with patient and family; encourage them to express feelings, rationale for noncompliance ■ Actively involve patient and family in health routine ■ Promote patient control of situation when possible ■ Use visual aids (calendars, clocks, medication cards) as appropriate ■ Inform about community resources and facilitate access to resources as needed ■ Contract with patient and family for a commitment to be accountable for their own health behaviors	■ The patient and family will follow health regimen as closely as possible ■ The patient and family will understand the consequences of not complying with health routine ■ The patient and family will express feelings and/or thoughts about difficulties in complying with health routine ■ The patient and family will demonstrate adequate problem-solving to achieve compliance with health routine as much as possible

NURSING CARE PLAN — cont'd

Patient Education

- Educate patient and family about community resources and opportunities for social contact
- Educate patient and family about stroke and recovery process to facilitate patient's understanding and sense of control
- Educate patient and family about problem-solving to manage environmental barriers
- Educate patient and family about problem-solving to manage aesthetic physical problems
- Educate family in care of stroke survivor, if appropriate
- Provide health teaching for stroke prevention, necessity of following health regimen (i.e., medications, diet, follow-up visits)
- Educate family on potential complications (i.e., depression, medication, side effects)
- Educate family on communication skills, constructive decision-making, expressing feelings
- Educate patient and family about accessing resources that may facilitate compliance
- Educate patient and family about potential health consequences of not following health regimen

Other relevant nursing diagnoses

- Social interaction, impaired
- Role performance, altered
- Diversional activity deficit
- Home maintenance management, impaired
- Health maintenance, altered

REFERENCES

Anderson TP: Quality of life of individual with disability, Arch Phys Med Rehabil, 63:55, 1982.

Bronstein K: Coping strategies and adaptation post-stroke, unpublished doctoral dissertation, Chicago, 1986, University of Illinois.

Burgener S and Logan G: Sexuality concerns of the post-stroke patient, Rehabilitation Nursing 14:178, 1989.

Christman NJ, McConnell EA, Pfeiffer C, and others: Uncertainty, coping, and distress following myocardial infarction: transition from hospital to home, Res Nurs Health 11:71, 1988.

Dombovy ML, Bamford JF, Whisnant JP, and others: Disability and use of rehabilitation services following stroke in Rochester, Minnesota, 1975-1979. Stroke, 18:830, 1987.

Doolittle N: Stroke recovery: review of literature and suggestions for future research, J Neurosci Nurs 20:169, 1988.

Ferido T and Habel M: Spasticity in head trauma and CVA patients: etiology and management, J Neurosci Nurs 20:17, 1988.

Flanagan JC: Measurement of quality of life: current state of the art, Arch Phys Med Rehabil, 63:56, 1982.

Flynn EP: Cerebral vasospasm following intracranial aneurysm rupture: a protocol for detection, J Neurosci Nurs 21:348, 1989.

Freed, MM: Quality of life: the physician's dilemma, Arch Phys Med Rehabil 65:109, 1984.

Fugel-Meyer AR, Jaasko L, and Norlin V: The post-stroke hemiplegic patients, II: incidence, mortality, and vocational return in Goteborg, Sweden, Scand J Rehabil Med 7:13, 1975.

Granger CV, Hamilton BB and Gresham GE: The stroke rehabilitation outcome study—part I: general description, Arch Phys Med Rehabil 69:506, 1988.

Gresham GE, Fitzpatrick TE, Wolf PA, and others: Residual disability in survivors of stroke—the Framingham Study, N Engl J Med 293:954, 1975.

Gurklis JA and Menke EM: Identification of stressors and use of coping methods in chronic hemodialysis patients, Nurs Res 37:236, 1988.

Huttman ED: Adult day care centers. In Social services for the Elderly, New York, 1985, Free Press.

Jalowiec A and Powers MJ: Stress and coping in hypertensive emergency room patients, Nurs Res 30:10, 1981.

Keller C, Tanner D, Urbina CM, and others: Psychological responses in aphasia: theoretical considerations and nursing implications, J Neurosci Nurs 21:290, 1989.

Kelly-Hayes M: Quality of survivorship following stroke: cognitive, physical, and social factors, unpublished doctoral dissertation, Boston, 1987, Boston University.

Kelly-Hayes M, Wolf PA, Kannel WB, and others: Factors influencing survival and need for institutionalization following stroke: the Framingham Study, Arch Phys Med Rehabil 69:415, 1988.

Kernich CA and Robb G: Development of a stroke support and education program, J Neurosci Nurs 20:193, 1988.

Kottke FJ: Philosophic considerations of quality of life for disabled, Arch Phys Med Rehabil 63:60, 1982.

Lubkin, IM: Chronic illness: impact and interventions, Boston, 1986, Jones and Bartlett Publishers.

Mahoney E: The interaction of physical illness, coping focus, and perceived social support and their relationship to recovery from stroke, unpublished doctoral dissertation, San Francisco, 1985, University of California.

Mayo NE, Hendlisz J, Goldberg MS, and others: Destinations of stroke patients discharged from the Montreal area acute-care hospitals. Stroke, 20, 351-356, 1989.

Mitchelson JK: Rehabilitation nurses' knowledge and attitudes toward sexuality of stroke patients, unpublished master's thesis, Denton, Texas, 1988, Texas Woman's University.

Mumma C: Perceived losses following stroke, Rehabilitation Nursing 11:19, 1986.

National Stroke Association: The road ahead: a stroke recovery guide, Englewood, Colo., 1989, The Association.

Pasquarello MA: Developing, implementing, and evaluating a stroke recovery group, Rehabilitation Nursing 15:26, 1990.

Passarella PM and Lewis N: Nursing application of Bobath principles in stroke care, J Neurosci Nurs 19:106, 1987.

Popovich J: Hope, coping, and rehabilitation outcomes in stroke patients, unpublished doctoral dissertation, Rush University College of Nursing, Chicago.

Quayhagen MP and Quayhagen M: Alzheimer's stress: coping with the caregiving role, Gerontologist 28:391, 1988.

Riffle KL: The relationship between perception of supportive behaviors of others and wives' ability to cope with initial myocardial infarctions in their husbands, Rehabilitation Nursing 13:310, 1988.

Schmidt SM, Herman LM, Koenig P, and others: Status of stroke patients: a community assessment, Arch Phys Med Rehabil 67:99, 1986.

Scmidt, EV, Smirnov VE, and Ryabova VS: Results of the seven-year prospective study of stroke patients, Stroke 19:942, 1988.

Stewart-Amidei C and Penckofer S: Quality of life following cerebral bypass surgery, J Neurosci Nurs 20:50, 1988.

Stroker R: Impact of disability on families of stroke clients, J Neurosci Nurs 15:360, 1983.

Tanner DC, Gerstenberger DL, and Keller CS: Guidelines for treatment of chronic depression in the aphasic patient, Rehabilitation Nursing 14:77, 1989.

Whitney FW: Relationship of laterality of stroke to emotional and functional outcome, J Neurosci Nurs 19:158, 1987.

Williams AM: Relationship between right hemisphere stroke and a passive behavioral response (depression), unpublished doctoral dissertation, Phoenix, Arizona, 1986, University of Arizona.

Wood-Dauphines S, and Williams JI: Reintegration to normal living as a proxy to quality of life, Chronic Dis 40:491, 1987.

Appendix A

Books for Stroke Patients, Families, and Health Care Professionals

After a stroke: a journal
(Sarton M, 1988)
Norton & Co.
New York, NY

Aphasia: family's guide to the psychology of loss, grief, adjustment
(Tanner DC, 1987)
Pro-Ed Publishers
8700 Shoal Creek Blvd.
Austin, TX 78758

Aphasia: communication and the family
(Brady WM, Vulanich N, and Cera RM, 1989)
Pro-Ed Publishers
8700 Shoal Creek Blvd.
Austin, TX 78758

As I am: an autobiography
(Neal P, 1988)
Simon & Schuster
New York, NY

A stroke patient's own story
(Prazich MN, 1985)
Pro-Ed Publishers
8700 Shoal Creek Blvd.
Austin, TX 78758

A stroke family guide and resource
(Gray, Grady P, and Clark GS, 1984)
Charles C Thomas Publisher
Springfield, IL

A stroke in the family
(Griffith VE, 1959)
Delacorte Press
New York
(Available from Volunteer Stroke Rehabilitation Program, 96 Westwood Road, New Haven, CT 06515)

Blitzed by a stroke
(Krehbiel JL, 1987)
Standard Press
Hutchinson, KS

Can you hear the clapping of one hand? learning to live with a stroke
(Veith I, 1988)
University of California Press
Los Angeles, CA

Clinical evaluation of dysphagia
(Cherny LR, Cantieri CA, and Pannell J, 1986)
Aspen Publishers
Rockville, MD

Clinical management of right hemisphere dysfunction
(Burns MS, Halper AS, and Mogil SI, 1985)
Aspen Publishers
Rockville, MD

Adapted from the Suggested Reading List, National Stroke Association, Englewood, CO, 1990.

Disability and rehabilitation handbook
(Goldenson RM, editor, 1978)
McGraw-Hill Inc
1221 Avenue of the Americas
New York, NY 10020

Disability rights guide
(Goldman CD, 1987)
Media Publishing
Lincoln, NE

Family caregiver's guide
(Foyder JE, 1986)
Futuro Company
Cincinnati, OH

Family's guide to stroke, head trauma, and speech disorders
(Tanner DC, 1987)
Pre-Ed Publishers
8700 Shoal Creek Blvd.
Austin, TX 78758

How to prevent a stroke
(Donahue PJ, 1989)
Rodale Press
Emmaus, PA

Reprieve
(de Mille A, 1981)
New American Library
New York, NY

Sourcebook for the disabled, an illustrated guide to easier, more independent living for physically disabled people, their families and friends
(Hale G, editor, 1979)
Paddington Press Ltd
Grosset & Dunlap Inc.
51 Madison Avenue
New York, NY 10010

Sourcebook of patient education materials for physical medicine and rehabilitation
(Koch SJ, 1986)
Armstrong Publishing
Houston, TX
(Available from Sourcebook Orders, Center for Disability and Rehabilitation
Comanche County Memorial Hospital, P.O. Box 129, Lawton, OK 73502)

Speech/language treatment of the aphasias: an integrated clinical approach
(Burns MS and Halper AS, 1988)
Rehabilitation Institute of Chicago
345 East Superior Street
Chicago, IL 60611

Stroke . . . a family affair
(Hewson L, 1988)
Collins Dove
Melbourne, Australia

Stroke: a guide for patient and family
(Toole JF and Freye-Peirson J, 1987)
Raven Press
New York, NY

Stroke: from crisis to victory
(Lavin JH, 1985)
Franklin Watts
New York, NY

Stroke/head injury: a guide to functional outcomes in physical therapy management
(Charness A, 1986)
Rehabilitation Institute of Chicago
345 East Superior Street
Chicago, IL 60611

Stroke! Surrenders to love!
(Borsch RG, 1989)
Sandia Publishing Corporation
Albuquerque, NM

Ted's stroke—the caregiver's story
(Paullin E, 1988)
Seven Locks Press
Cabin John, MD

The road ahead: a stroke recovery guide
(National Stroke Association, 1986)
Denver, CO

The long way home: spiritual help when someone you love has a stroke
(Cole HA, 1989)
Westminister/John Knox Press
Louisville, KY

The 36-hour day
(Mace NL and Rabins PV, 1981)
John Hopkins University Press
Baltimore, MD

We are not alone, learning to live with chronic illness
(Pitzele SK, 1985)
Workman Publishing
New York, NY

Understanding stroke and aphasia
(Eisenson J, 1990)
Pro-Ed Publishers
8700 Shoal Creek Blvd.
Austin, TX 78758

Workbook for aphasia
Wayne State University Press
5959 Woodword Avenue
Detroit, MI 48202

Appendix B

Audiovisual Aids About Stroke*

A stroke survivor's workout
Courage Stroke Network
Courage Center
3915 Golden Valley Road
Golden Valley, MN 55422

Feeding techniques for adult dysphagic patients (1979)
Rehabilitation Institute of Chicago
345 East Superior Street
Chicago, IL 60611

High blood pressure (1990)
Milner-Fenwick
2125 Greenspring Drive
Timonium, MD 21093

High blood pressure compliance (1990)
Milner-Fenwick
2125 Greenspring Drive
Timonium, MD 21093

More alive
Adult Corporation
12345 East Cedar Circle
Aurora, CO 80012

Nursing management issues in right and left stroke (1979)
Rehabilitation Institute of Chicago
345 East Superior Street
Chicago, IL 60611

Senior fitnessize
Mike Cinquanto
P.O. Box 2567
Morgantown, NC 28655

Stroke-a-cize
Occu-Ther Inc.
3905 North College Avenue
Indianapolis, IN 46205

Stroke awareness and prevention (1978)
Milner-Fenwick
2125 Greenspring Drive
Timonium, MD 21093

Stroke: focus on family (1987)
Oracle Film & Video
1820 14th Street, Suite 202
Santa Monica, CA 90404

Stroke: focus on feelings (1986)
Oracle Film & Video
1820 14th Street, Suite 202
Santa Monica, CA 90404

Stroke: recovering together (1985)
Oracle Film & Video
1820 14th Street, Suite 202
Santa Monica, CA 90404

Materials are included in this list on the basis of content and availability and have not necessarily been previewed by the author.

Swing into shape
Lutheran Hospital
1910 South Avenue
LaCrosse, WI 51601-9980

Theracise
Theracise Inc
Jody Kaufman O.T.R./L.
P.O. Box 9100, Unit 107
Newton, MA 02159

Appendix C

Organizations and Professional Associations

American Association of Neuroscience Nurses
218 North Jefferson Street
Chicago, IL 60606
(312) 993-0043

American Congress of Rehabilitation Medicine
130 South Michigan Avenue, Suite 1310
Chicago, IL 60610
(312) 922-9368

American Heart Association
7320 Greenville Avenue
Dallas, TX 75231
(214) 750-5300

Association of Rehabilitation Nurses
5700 Old Orchard Road, 1st Floor
Skokie, IL 60077-1024
(708) 966-3433

Commission of Accreditation of Rehabilitation Facilities (CARF)
101 North Wilmot Road, Suite 500
Tucson, AZ 85711
(602) 748-1212

Joint Commission of Accreditation of Health Care Organizations
875 North Michigan Avenue
Chicago, IL 60611
(312) 642-6061

National Easter Seals Society
70 East Lake Street
Chicago, IL 60601
(312) 726-6200

National Heart, Lung, and Blood Institute Education Programs Information Center
4733 Bethesda Avenue, Suite 530
Bethesda, MD 20814
(301) 496-2563

NIH National Institute of Neurological Disorders and Stroke (NINDS)
Office of Scientific and Health Reports (pamphlets on stroke)
9000 Rockville Pike
Bethesda, MD 20892
(301) 496-5751

NIH National Institute of Neurological Disorders and Stroke (NINDS)
Division of Stroke and Trauma (grant applications)
Federal Building/Rm 8A13
7550 Wisconsin Avenue
Bethesda, MD 20892
(301) 496-4226

National Stroke Association
300 East Hampden Avenue, Suite 240
Englewood, CO 80110
(303) 762-9922

Stroke Clubs International
805 12th Street
Galveston, TX 77550
(409) 762-1022

Index

B

C

D

Q

R

S